DISEASE-PROO

4.WEEKS TO
Maximum Immunity

BY THE EDITORS OF **Prevention**®
with Kim Galeaz, RD, CD

RODALE®

© 2008 by Rodale Inc.

Direct edition was published as *Prevention's Maximum Immunity* in 2007. Trade edition published in 2008.

All rights reserved. No part of this publication may be reproduced or transmitted in any form or by any means, electronic or mechanical, including photocopying, recording, or any other information storage and retrieval system, without the written permission of the publisher.

Rodale books may be purchased for business or promotional use or for special sales. For information, please write to: Special Markets Department, Rodale Inc., 733 Third Avenue, New York, NY 10017

Prevention is a registered trademark of Rodale Inc.

Printed in the United States of America

Rodale Inc. makes every effort to use acid-free ♻, recycled paper ♻.

Interior design by Tara Long

Cover design by Susan Eugster

Front cover photo © Stockbyte/Getty Images

Contributing writers: Rick Ansorge, Elizabeth Shimer Bowers, Jennifer Bright Reich, Julia VanTine-Reichardt

Library of Congress Cataloging-in-Publication Data is on file with the publisher.

ISBN-13 978–1–59486–711–8   paperback
ISBN-10 1–59486–711–9   paperback

Distributed to the trade by Macmillan

2   4   6   8   10   9   7   5   3   1   paperback

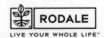

RODALE
LIVE YOUR WHOLE LIFE™

We inspire and enable people to improve their lives and the world around them

For more of our products visit rodalestore.com or call 800-848-4735

Contents

PART III   IMMUNE ESSENTIALS: THE 4-WEEK PLAN

PART IV   IMMUNE EXTRAS: SMART STRATEGIES TO BOOST IMMUNITY

PART V   IMMUNE ACCELERATORS: FIGHT BACK AGAINST ILLNESS

PART I

Meet Your Immune System

Your Best Ally against Illness

Compared to the deadly "hot zone" viruses such as Ebola and Lassa—now confined to continents half a world away—the influenza viruses that arrive here each winter seem tame. After all, there's a flu vaccine available, and most people have some immunity.

But seasonal flu *is* dangerous. Each year, about 36,000 Americans die from it or its complications. It's also possible that an entirely new influenza virus will emerge—one for which humans have no immunity—unleashing a worldwide outbreak, or pandemic. The world hasn't seen an influenza pandemic since 1968, and more than a few scientists believe that we're overdue. Its potential cause: a strain of flu that typically infects only birds.

This avian (bird) strain of influenza, named H5N1, first spread from bird to human in 1997. As of this writing, H5N1 has killed less than 200 people worldwide. But if the virus learns to spread from human to human, it could ignite the world's next plague.

Scientists have reason for concern. In 2005, a team of researchers re-created the 1918 Spanish influenza virus, which killed between 20 million and 50 million people around the globe. The team discovered that the Spanish flu strain had started out as an avian influenza virus that eventually learned to infect humans.

The Spanish flu—which killed more people in 6 months than AIDS has in 25 years—isn't the only threat. Biological weapons such as smallpox, botulism, and plague could be unleashed. Lethal viruses flare and disappear, only to flare again. Hantavirus, which broke out in the Southwest in 1993, recently re-erupted in Washington and Colorado. HIV (human immunodeficiency virus), which causes AIDS, continues to kill.

Currently, no vaccines exist for any of these threats. What, then, is our best defense?

A strong immune system.

Scientists often compare the immune system—the body's elegant and complex mechanism of defense—to an army. Its two trillion cells are organized into separate but integrated divisions of organs, tissues, and special cells that share a common mission: to defend their "country" (that's you). And like an army, the immune system

Bird Flu: Prepare, Don't Panic

TV movies about a global outbreak of bird flu portray doomsday scenarios—mandatory quarantines, emergency rooms overrun with panicked citizens, mass burials. But *pandemic* doesn't necessarily equal *plague*, and it's important to separate fact from fiction.

First, the facts: Avian influenza is caused by influenza viruses that typically strike birds and poultry. In 1997, one strain of the virus, H5N1, began to infect humans. In the current outbreaks, occurring in Asia and parts of Europe, the Near East, and Africa, more than half of those infected with H5N1—many previously healthy children and young adults—have died. Most cases resulted from contact with infected birds, mostly chickens, turkeys, and ducks raised for food.

Having never been exposed to the H5N1 virus, we have no immunity to it, explains bird-flu expert William Schaffner, MD, of Vanderbilt University School of Medicine in Nashville. So far, the virus virtually always spreads from birds to people. But some experts believe that H5N1 may acquire the ability to jump from human to human, igniting a pandemic. On the other hand, the changes required for the virus to spread among people could make it less dangerous than the current strain.

There's no way to know if a pandemic will strike, says Dr. Schaffner. But if it does, it will most likely begin in Asia, arriving in the United States within a few weeks. Local, state, and federal governments have begun to formulate plans for dealing with a pandemic. The federal Web site www.pandemicflu.gov offers guidelines on how families and communities can prepare. One suggestion: Stockpile a 2-week supply of food, water, and necessary prescription medications.

While even the strongest immune system can't protect against bird flu, good hygiene habits can help prevent its spread. Get into the practice of washing your hands frequently with soap and covering your coughs and sneezes with your inner arm rather than your hand. Teach your family to do the same.

Scientists haven't yet developed a vaccine that protects against H5N1, but clinical trials are under way. In the meantime, says Dr. Schaffner, don't panic—prepare. "The regular flu costs lives every year," he says. "Get your flu shots."

attacks foreign invaders that threaten its security, including illness-causing viruses and bacteria, icky fungi, and even cancer cells. But it lives in peace with the "good" bacteria that inhabit the gut and other organs.

The protection our immune systems afford us in part depends on genetics, but a lot rides on how well we care for ourselves. "There's no question that a healthy life-style benefits the immune system," says Michael Zasloff, MD, an immunologist and professor in the departments of surgery and pediatrics at Georgetown University Medical Center in Washington, DC. Terry Phillips, PhD, an immunochemist in the division of bioengineering and physical science at the National Institutes of Health, agrees. "If you have good health and your immune system is doing its job, the best way to keep it healthy is to do all the things that keep it naturally strong, like exercising, eating right, and coping with stress as best you can," he says.

That means that regardless of your genetics and current health, you can power up your immune system's ability to fight illness and speed healing. This book shows you how.

Our "Keys" Unlock Immune Power

We've interviewed a select group of physicians and researchers who specialize in immunology, preventive medicine, nutrition, alternative medicine, and environmental health. With their guidance and with groundbreaking research from leading medical journals, we've identified seven crucial lifestyle factors that unlock the immune system's healing potential. The 7 Keys to Maximum Immunity are:

Nutrition. As it destroys invaders, then repairs the damage, the immune system creates free radicals—molecules that damage cells and cause chronic inflammation, which sets the stage for disease. Research shows that certain substances in fruits, vegetables, and whole grains help protect the immune system from the destructive effects of free radicals. Some nutrients enhance specific aspects of immune function; for example, vitamin C raises levels of interferon, the chemical that coats cell surfaces and protects them from any virus that tries to hijack them. Other plant substances, called bioflavonoids, protect cell membranes against environmental pollutants.

Exercise. Physical activity does more than melt away pounds and tone muscles. It also boosts immune response. It's thought that working out may help flush disease-causing viruses and bacteria from the lungs; expel potentially cancerous cells through urine and sweat; and speed antibodies and white blood cells through the body so they identify and destroy marauding microbes more quickly than they might otherwise.

Chronic Inflammation: A Smoldering Volcano

The short-term inflammation that helps repair a cut or other wound is a protective response to infection or injury and an essential part of the healing process. It does its job, then stops. Chronic inflammation, on the other hand, never "turns off" and actually hastens the disease process. You might liken long-term inflammation to a volcano that smolders for years, ready to erupt at any time.

Research links chronic inflammation to heart disease, cancer, diabetes, and autoimmune disorders such as lupus and rheumatoid arthritis, among other serious illnesses. Fortunately, healthy living can help quiet that volcano within.

WHITTLE YOUR MIDDLE. Body fat fuels chronic inflammation. Research has found that overweight adults and children have higher levels of several inflammatory substances in their blood. When extra pounds are lost, levels return to normal.

FLOSS DAILY. When the bacteria behind advanced gum disease (periodontitis) enter the bloodstream, they can travel to major organs and cause chronic inflammation. Flossing gets rid of periodontal bacteria.

EAT FRESH. A diet heavy on processed foods and fatty red meats contributes to chronic low-grade inflammation. Load your plate with fresh fruits and vegetables instead. They're packed with antioxidants, which disarm cell-damaging free radicals, and flavonoids, which block the production of inflammation-promoting hormones.

FEAST ON GOOD FATS. Walnuts, canola oil, cold-water fish such as salmon and sardines, and pumpkin and flaxseed are rich in healthy omega-3 fatty acids, the raw materials of anti-inflammatory hormones called eicosanoids (eye-KAH-sa-noids). While some eicosanoids fan the fire, those made with omega-3s quench it.

Sleep. Logging 8 hours of shut-eye each night allows the immune system to fortify its defenses. For example, the sleep hormone melatonin inhibits the growth of tumors and raises the concentration of infection-fighting antibodies in saliva. By contrast, sleep deprivation appears to compromise the immune system by altering the blood levels of immune molecules called cytokines, raising the risk of chronic inflammation and infection. For example, studies have shown that six nights of partial sleep deprivation lower blood levels of antibodies produced in response to the flu vaccine, weakening protection.

Stress. Stress that lasts only a few minutes or hours temporarily mobilizes immune cells, says Monika Fleshner, PhD, associate professor in the department of integrative physiology and the Center for Neuroscience at the University of Colorado in Boulder. Temporary stressors trigger the release of corticosteroids and epinephrine, stress hormones that warn immune cells to prepare for imminent danger, such as an injury that needs protection from infection. But chronic stress—the kind caused by long-standing family, money, or relationship issues—has been found to suppress the ability of the immune system to battle viral, bacterial, and parasitic infections, according to a meta-analysis of almost 300 studies. Moreover, the immune systems of people who are older or whose immune systems are already suppressed due to illness are more prone to stress-related change.

Mood. Think positive and unroll the yoga mat. Research into the connection between the brain and immune system suggests that your outlook on life may affect your immune response. In a 1985 study, for example, people who used humor to cope with stress showed increases in levels of an immune system protein called salivary immunoglobulin A (sIgA), the body's first line of defense against respiratory illnesses. In another study, researcher Janice Kiecolt-Glaser, PhD, of Ohio State University in Columbus, taught a relaxation technique called progressive muscle relaxation to a group of elderly patients. Blood tests revealed that those who practiced the technique had more active natural killer cells, which help destroy viruses and tumors.

Sunlight. While slathering yourself with sunscreen helps protect against skin cancer, it may deprive your immune system of vitamin D, a nutrient that research now links to immune function, says Dr. Zasloff. A review of more than 100 studies of vitamin D and respiratory diseases found that low levels of the vitamin allow flu viruses to breach the immune system—one theory as to why seasonal flu strikes only in winter, he says. Sun exposure and vitamin D production tend to be at their lowest during the winter months.

Environment. Every day, we're exposed to chemicals and products that affect immune response. For example, antibacterial soaps and cleansers wipe out harmful bacteria—of benefit to hospitals or people with immune systems already weakened by illness—but these products also kill beneficial bacteria that live in the gut, colon, and bladder and on the skin, protecting us from infection. In fact, there's some evidence that using antibacterial products at home (as opposed to in hospitals) may help breed antibiotic-resistant strains of bacteria. (See "Beat Bugs without Drugs" on page 8.)

We've Got a Plan

In Part II of this book, you'll learn all about the 7 Keys to Maximum Immunity. Then in Part III, we'll show you how to use them. Our 4-week Immune Essentials

Beat Bugs without Drugs

Have you ever popped leftover antibiotics when you felt a urinary tract infection brewing? You're not alone. But misusing antibiotics this way—or demanding them when they're not medically necessary—allows bacteria to withstand the effects of antibiotics. This ability, called antibiotic resistance, is becoming a worldwide public-health problem.

Of the two million bacterial infections that Americans develop in hospitals each year, 70 percent are resistant to at least one antibiotic commonly used to cure them, according to the Centers for Disease Control and Prevention (CDC). That's cause for concern. If standard drugs don't work, doctors may need to use stronger but more toxic alternatives. In some cases, these last-resort antibiotics cause irreversible liver or kidney damage—and they may not wipe out the infection. Antibiotic resistance kills about 70,000 Americans each year—more than car accidents and murders combined.

The main problem: We're misusing antibiotics. US doctors write prescriptions for about 100 million courses of antibiotics each year. More than half are for colds, flu, and other viral infections that antibiotics don't treat.

No drug can match the power of the immune system at its peak. Enhancing its strength doesn't just help you and your family; it benefits the planet itself. When you commit to a healthy lifestyle, you tend to get sick less often, which means you'll use antibiotics less often, thus helping to thwart resistance. These tips can help you do your part.

■ Don't request antibiotics for a cold, flu, bronchitis, or middle-ear infection. These illnesses are caused by viruses, and antibiotics won't help.

■ If you are prescribed an antibiotic, finish it, even if you feel better before you get to the last dose. No saving a few pills for the next time you get sick.

■ Do not take an antibiotic prescribed for someone else.

■ If you must take an antibiotic, try to avoid the broad-spectrum kind, which kill good bacteria along with the bad. Broad-spectrum antibiotics include clindamycin (Cleocin) and the fluoroquinolones (Cipro, Floxin, and Levaquin).

Plan includes the practical information that you need to build an immune-friendly lifestyle. We've thought of everything—menu plans; week-by-week workouts; daily relaxation breaks; and tips for getting restful sleep, boosting your mood, and creating a healthier environment at work and at home.

Part IV of our "immune makeover" addresses the less-than-healthy lifestyle factors and habits shown to weaken the body's ability to protect against illness and infection. For example, carrying extra pounds can cause chronic, low-grade inflammation thought to play a role in many illnesses, including cancer, heart disease, stroke, diabetes, and autoimmune disorders such as lupus and rheumatoid arthritis. (For more information on autoimmune disease, which develops when the immune system mistakenly attacks the body, see "How the Immune System Works.") The specific supplement described on page 239 may help cool this harmful inflammation.

If you smoke, see page 252 to learn which foods and supplements can help reduce the effects of cellular damage caused by tobacco.

As mentioned earlier, chronic stress is a huge immune-buster. To soothe it, catch a catnap, walk around the block, or enjoy a cup of tea. The herbal tea on page 268 contains a substance shown to promote relaxation, which can help reduce the wear and tear on your immune system.

Fight Back against Illness

Perhaps you suffer from allergies or asthma. Maybe you'd like to prevent cancer, food poisoning, or seasonal colds or flu. Part V shows you how to prevent *and* treat a variety of maladies for which research has identified a potential immune component.

Take cancer. Studies have shown that when the immune system breaks down or is overwhelmed, tumors can develop and thrive. Fortunately, simple lifestyle strategies may reduce your risk of the disease. For example, one study found that drinking coffee every day—or close to it—cut the risk of a certain type of liver cancer in half. In another study, people who ate more than five servings of yellow, orange, and dark green leafy vegetables a day were half as likely to develop pancreatic cancer as those who ate fewer servings. Our experts offer even more simple ways to beef up your immune system, helping it fight back against common ailments.

■ Do you suffer from allergies? Turn to page 293 to find out which nutritional supplement caused allergy sufferers to produce 32 percent fewer immune proteins that trigger symptoms of airborne allergies. You'll also find out why you may not want to dry your sheets and clothes on the line and which houseplants may actually aggravate allergy symptoms.

■ If you or a member of your family has asthma, you'll be interested to know that asthma sufferers who took 20-minute hatha yoga classes three times a week for 6 weeks were able to breathe easier. Turn to page 306 to find out which common supplements may keep symptoms at bay and why you might want to switch your workout from your lunch hour to the end of the day.

■ If you cough, sniffle, and sneeze from October through March, page 317 offers some surprising strategies for beefing up your immune system. You'll also discover one inexpensive home improvement that kills off many of the viruses that cause the common cold.

■ Concerned about the recent outbreaks of food-borne bacteria? See page 331 to discover a powerful way to protect yourself when you dine out.

Flex That Immunity Muscle

We believe the information in this book can have a positive impact not just on how long you live but how *well* you live. Small steps—a daily walk, a much-needed nap, a few stress-busting laughs, and, yes, lots of hand-washing—add up to big benefits that go far beyond cold and flu protection. You stand to gain newfound energy; control allergies; and reduce your risk of chronic, age-related diseases like arthritis, heart disease, diabetes, and cancer. And should you come down with the flu, food poisoning, or shingles or develop an autoimmune disease, you'll be able to take steps to heighten your body's natural healing powers. As the immune system goes, so goes your health and vitality.

How the Immune System Works

Without an immune system, we'd wake each morning covered with mold. Die from colds or blisters. Be forced to live in sterile bubbles—never to touch a loved one, feel the sun on our hair, or savor a warm breeze tickling our skin.

Few systems in nature are as complex as the human immune system. Any attack on the body, from a mosquito bite to a cancerous cell, mobilizes a specific, coordinated defense. Some immune cells mark suspicious microbes or organisms with chemicals that identify them as threats. Others devour infectious invaders or blast them with toxic chemicals. A variety of chemicals coordinate the immune response, much as a conductor leads a symphony orchestra.

Despite its extraordinary powers, the immune system isn't infallible, and sometimes we fall sick. The viruses that waft up our noses and burrow into our lungs cause fevers, sore throats, and stuffed noses. Bacteria that sneak into the gut through contaminated food result in diarrhea and vomiting. Slice your finger with a paring knife, and the area swells as damaged cells release distress chemicals that trigger the cascade of chemical events known as the inflammatory response. While these responses cause discomfort or pain, they also signal that the body's defenses are working as they should.

At the heart of the immune system's ability to heal and protect is its ability to distinguish between "self" cells and organisms that belong in the body and "strangers" that pose a threat. Virtually every cell in the body carries specific molecules that identify it as self and prevent the immune system from attacking it. However, when immune defenses meet up with molecules it considers strangers, the troops move in for the kill.

Three Defense Systems in One

The immune system actually consists of several systems, each with its own set of functions.

The *innate* or *passive system* of immunity includes the defenses we came into the world with. Babies receive protective molecules called *antibodies* while in the womb and, after birth, through breast milk. (More on antibodies later on.) Innate immunity also includes our skin, specialized cells, and mechanisms such as inflammation, the cough reflex, and fever. The innate system provides a generic, generalized defense and can't "remember" specific invaders.

The *adaptive system* of immunity, however, has a long, long memory. It even remembers that bout of measles or chickenpox you had when you were 4. The adaptive system is also called acquired immunity because we acquire it by being exposed to *antigens*. An antigen is anything that the immune system doesn't recognize as self and triggers an immune response, including disease-causing viruses and bacteria (collectively known as *pathogens*), chemicals in the environment, pollen, pet hair,

Remembrance of Things Past

The immune system's ability to recall past encounters with millions of antigens and disease-causing microbes is called immunological memory. It's one of evolution's most impressive innovations, the basis of both natural immunity and artificial immunity from vaccinations.

"Immune systems remember the things they've seen beneath our skin because immune systems believe that someday those things will be back," says Gerald N. Callahan, PhD, professor of immunology at Colorado State University in Fort Collins. But how does the immune system "remember" its first run-in with every invader?

Like a pack rat hoards bits of string, old magazines, and scraps of aluminum foil, the immune system saves fragments of every antigen it encounters—childhood diseases like mumps and chickenpox; bouts of flu and food poisoning; tetanus. The fragments are "stored" in the lymph nodes.

These bits of antigens help the immune system remember the threat they posed once—and may pose again—"by maintaining a low-grade, barely perceptible immune response against the pieces of the invader inside of our lymph nodes," says Dr. Callahan. "The next time the same virus or bacterium shows up beneath the skin, that smoldering immune response quickly flares into a systemic immune response—one that is much faster and more specific than the first time the body was threatened. Because of that, a second exposure to many infectious diseases is much less likely to be life-threatening."

even cancer cells. (The word *antigen* is derived from the phrase *"anti*body *generating."*) The adaptive system remembers each of the millions of antigens it encounters and develops a specific response to each one.

The *lymphatic system* consists of the organs of the immune system, including the bone marrow, thymus, lymph nodes, and tonsils. Among other functions, the lymphatic system defends against foreign invaders and removes cellular waste, cancer cells, bacteria, and toxins from tissues.

Let's examine each of these systems in more detail.

Innate Immunity: Built-In Protection

As mentioned above, even a newborn has a system of immunity, which encompasses the protections that come with our standard human packaging.

■ The skin is the body's first defense against bacteria, viruses, and other undesirables. When it's intact, without cuts or breaks, it's the most effective barrier against foreign invaders. Skin even secretes chemicals that kill bacteria.

■ Saliva and tears contain enzymes that break down the cell walls of many types of bacteria and viruses.

■ Stomach acid kills most bugs. Our intestines shelter permanent colonies of helpful bacteria that protect against invading germs.

■ *Natural killer (NK) cells,* a specific type of white blood cell (or lymphocyte), destroy infected and cancerous cells before the adaptive immune system is alerted.

■ When tissues are infected or damaged—whether by bacteria; trauma such as a cut, bruise, or sprain; or something else—the pain, swelling, and redness of inflammation occur. The injured tissues release substances that cause blood vessels in the affected area to dilate, which increases bloodflow to that area. Fluid leaks from the vessels, diluting harmful substances that might be there. Immune cells called *macrophages* devour microorganisms and dead or damaged cells.

While short-term inflammation is a critical part of the body's healing process, research implicates chronic inflammation in several serious illnesses, including heart disease and Alzheimer's. For more on chronic inflammation, see page 6.

Adaptive Immunity: Learned Protection

While the innate system responds almost immediately to invaders, the adaptive immune system takes days or even weeks to respond because its attack is triggered by the presence of antigens. Once the adaptive system swings into action, however, it mobilizes an army of special fighter cells called B and T cells to search out and destroy invaders.

Both B cells and T cells begin their lives as stem cells in bone marrow, the soft tissue that fills most bones. However, B cells mature in the marrow, while T cells mature in the thymus, a small gland located under the breastbone. B cells and T cells also have different missions.

B cells. B cells work chiefly by making antibodies—molecules produced in response to antigens. Each antigen has a corresponding antibody, which attaches to its surface much like a key fits a lock, and marks it for destruction. B cells never forget an enemy. They can remain in the body for years, ready to wage war when antigens they've met before reappear. This is how vaccination works (see opposite page). The ability of B cells to produce antibodies is critical to a healthy immune response. However, they can destroy only those microbes that show themselves in the blood and lymph, such as those that cause the hepatitis virus and HIV (the precursor to AIDS). B cells are less effective against germs that hide in cells and make thousands of copies of themselves (such as the herpes virus).

T cells. T cells don't recognize antigens like B cells do. Rather, T cell surfaces contain receptors that recognize pieces of antigens on infected or cancerous cells. There are several types of T cells: helper, killer, and suppressor.

Helper T cells are the generals of the immune system. They activate and direct the troops, coordinating the immune response by signaling other cells. Some helper T cells stimulate nearby B cells to make antibodies. Others direct microbe-gobbling cells called phagocytes. Yet others activate other T cells. Without helper T cells, your body could not mount an effective immune response.

Killer T cells are the ninjas of the immune response. They directly attack body cells whose surfaces carry certain foreign or abnormal molecules. Killer T cells are especially good virus slayers. Viruses often hide from other parts of the immune system as they grow inside infected cells. Killer T cells recognize fragments of these viruses and launch an attack, killing infected cells by releasing substances that punch holes in their membranes and trigger a process called programmed cell death (or *apoptosis*). Although it sounds bad, this is the body's way of eliminating abnormal cells. When apoptosis doesn't occur, cancer can result.

Once an infection or disease is eliminated, *suppressor T cells* step in to slow or stop the action of B and T cells.

The Lymphatic System

A home filtering system strains bacteria and other impurities from tap water. Likewise, the lymphatic system is the body's filtering system, sifting out pathogens, abnormal cells, and other foreign bodies. This network of organs, nodes, ducts, and vessels makes and transports lymph from tissues to the bloodstream. In Greek, *lymph* means "a pure, clear stream." In our bodies, this clear fluid contains white blood

How Vaccines Work

In 1762, 13-year-old Edward Jenner, a doctor's apprentice, heard a milkmaid say that she'd never get smallpox because she'd had cowpox, a mild viral disease related to smallpox. Thus, she believed, she was naturally protected from the often lethal virus.

More than 3 decades later, Jenner put this folk wisdom to the test. He placed pus from a dairymaid's cowpox sore on a needle, then scratched the arm of an 8-year-old boy. The boy developed cowpox and quickly recovered. Two months later, Jenner repeated the process, this time using smallpox pus. The boy stayed healthy.

Jenner's experiment paved the way for the development of modern vaccines, which today protect against more than 20 infectious diseases. Before vaccines, the only way to acquire immunity to a disease was to get it—and survive. Vaccines, which confer immunity artificially, prevent disease in the first place.

Vaccines contain forms or derivatives of particular pathogens, which trick the body into thinking that it's under attack. The immune system then produces antibodies to destroy the invader—that is, the vaccine. If the immune system encounters that particular microbe again, the antibodies will attack and kill it. There are several types of vaccines.

■ *Live, attenuated vaccines,* such as those for measles, mumps, and chickenpox, use live viruses that are weakened (attenuated) in the laboratory. It's the closest thing to actual infection, triggering a strong immune response that can confer lifelong immunity with one or two doses.

■ *Inactivated vaccines,* such as the inactivated polio vaccine, use dead (inactivated) microbes. Made by killing pathogens with chemicals, heat, or radiation, inactivated vaccines are safer than live vaccines because dead microbes can't cause disease.

■ *Toxoid vaccines,* like those for diphtheria and tetanus, are made from killed bacterial toxins (toxoids). They cause the immune system to produce antibodies that attach to and block the toxin.

■ *Subunit vaccines,* which include the hepatitis vaccine, use only the parts of a pathogen that stimulate the immune system.

Children in the United States currently receive 11 vaccines to protect against 15 diseases. Years of immunization have pushed most of these formerly life-threatening diseases to their lowest levels in history.

cells and other immune cells that destroy foreign substances. Lymph vessels drain into lymph nodes found in clusters in the neck, armpits, and groin. These tiny, bean-shaped structures produce lymphocytes and other infection-fighting cells and filter foreign matter—including cancer cells—out of the body. When the lymph nodes

Vaccines for Cancer

For decades, surgery, chemotherapy, and radiation have been the standard treatments for cancer. Soon that may change, as scientists develop cancer vaccines that tap into the immune system's healing powers.

Prophylactic vaccines, for people without cancer, stimulate the immune system to attack cancer-causing viruses. The FDA has approved two prophylactic vaccines. The hepatitis B vaccine prevents infection with that virus, which causes liver cancer. (Thus, it's the first true "anticancer" vaccine.) The other vaccine, Gardasil, prevents infection with the two types of human papillomavirus (HPV) that together cause 70 percent of cervical cancer cases worldwide.

Therapeutic vaccines, for people with cancer, are designed to boost the immune system's ability to recognize and attack cancer cells without harming normal cells. These vaccines are still in the testing stage but someday may be used to stop the growth of existing tumors, prevent the return of a previously treated tumor, or kill cancer cells not destroyed by previous treatments. There are several different types of therapeutic vaccines.

■ *Tumor cell vaccines* are made of cancer cells removed during surgery. In the laboratory, the cells are treated with radiation to prevent them from forming more tumors. Chemicals or new genes may be added to make them more visible to the immune system. Then the cells are injected back into the patient. Recognizing their antigens, the immune system seeks out and attacks any other cells with these antigens. Tumor cell vaccines are being tested on various cancers, including those of the kidney, ovary, breast, and lung.

■ *Antigen vaccines* use whole or parts of proteins called peptides to coax the immune system to fight cancer cells. Antigens are combined with other chemicals to enhance the immune response. Several antigens can be combined in a single vaccine. Antigen vaccines are being studied for use against several different cancers, including those of the breast, prostate, ovary, and kidney.

■ *Dendritic cell vaccines* use specialized white blood cells taken from the blood of a person with cancer. These cells are taught to recognize cancer antigens by exposing them to the antigens in a dish or by modifying them to make their own antigens. The trained dendritic cells are then injected back into the patient, theoretically helping T cells better recognize and destroy cancer cells that show those antigens. Early studies are promising.

recognize foreign substances, they enlarge as they pump out additional white blood cells to fight the infection.

Other organs of the lymphatic system include the spleen, thymus, and tonsils. Located in the upper left abdomen, the *spleen* is the immune system's command central and contains special compartments where immune cells gather and work. The *thymus* transforms white blood cells into T cells. The *tonsils* trap and destroy bacteria, helping to protect against many of the germs we inhale or swallow. Sometimes the tonsils themselves become infected, a condition known as tonsillitis. Chronic tonsillitis may require surgical removal of the tonsils (tonsillectomy).

Some practitioners of alternative medicine use what's known as manual lymph drainage (MLD). In this light massage-therapy technique, the skin is manipulated in certain directions based on the structure of the lymphatic system. Practitioners believe that MLD stimulates lymph flow and enhances immune function. They also use MLD to treat lymphedema, a swelling of the lymph nodes caused by skin infections, injury, tumors, or radiation therapy.

When Immunity Attacks

Pathogens attack the body; immune cells target and wipe them out. At least, that's the way they're supposed to work. Sometimes immune cells mistake the body's own cells as the enemy, causing autoimmune disease. For instance, T cells that attack pancreas cells contribute to diabetes, while an autoantibody called rheumatoid factor is common in people with rheumatoid arthritis. (Produced by the immune system, an autoantibody attacks self tissues, often causing autoimmune disease.) People with systemic lupus erythematosus develop antibodies to many types of their own cells and cell components.

Experts have identified more than 80 autoimmune diseases. While they don't know for certain what causes them, they suspect that several factors, including viruses, certain drugs, and excessive sun exposure—all of which may damage or alter normal cells—may be involved.

Hormones may also play a role. About 75 percent of autoimmune diseases occur in women of childbearing age. Some women with autoimmune disorders improve during pregnancy, with flare-ups after delivery; for other moms-to-be, symptoms worsen. A few autoimmune diseases occur more often after menopause.

Autoimmune disease may also run in families, though it may strike as different illnesses. For example, one family member may have rheumatoid arthritis; another, lupus erythematosus; yet another, type 1 diabetes. One of the most difficult aspects of dealing with an autoimmune disease is getting a correct diagnosis. Symptoms

The Ebb and Flow of Hormones

Virtually every organ in a woman's body—the heart, the gut, the brain—is different from a man's. The immune system is no exception. "The female immune system is exquisitely sensitive to any aberration—smoking, shifts in hormone levels, changes in diet, environmental influences," says Robert G. Lahita, MD, professor of medicine at Mount Sinai Medical School in New York City. "The male immune system is less complex. It is designed to reject foreign invaders and combat bacteria and other pathogens, but it does not have the female immune system's degree of sensitivity."

For example, doctors have long observed that women tend to develop yeast infections just before their periods. Studies conducted at Cornell University in New York City confirmed it. It's also known that a woman's immune system peaks before ovulation and declines once the egg is released. Researchers from Sweden have theorized that a woman's preovulatory rise in immunity is designed to rid her body of germs in preparation for conception and pregnancy, while immune function is suppressed after ovulation or conception to prevent her body from rejecting the sperm or fertilized egg, which the immune system perceives as invaders.

Other research shows that women who experience morning sickness (which can occur at any time of day) are significantly less likely to miscarry. The theory: A pregnant woman's suppressed immune system makes her and her fetus more vulnerable to infectious microbes in food. Morning sickness may be an adaptation that predisposes pregnant women to avoid foods that tend to contain high levels of parasites and toxins, such as meat, fish, and eggs.

---

often come and go or disappear completely for a time, only to flare again. Doctors may even dismiss these elusive symptoms as "all in the head." In fact, a survey of people with autoimmune disease, conducted by the American Autoimmune Related Diseases Association, found that 45 percent had been labeled as hypochondriacs before they were diagnosed.

There's no cure for autoimmune disease, but following a healthy diet, getting regular sleep and gentle exercise such as yoga, and managing stress often help reduce symptoms. Treatment aims to control symptoms and protect affected organs; for example, people with lupus may need medication to control kidney inflammation.

Why Your Immune Function May Be at Risk

A healthy immune system is a fortress that protects you from the marauding hordes of microorganisms beyond your skin. When it's on its game, the immune system routs harmful bacteria, viruses, fungi, parasites, and cancerous tumors before you get sick. When it's not, it often finds a way to let you know. Symptoms of sluggish immune function include a cold or flu that lingers for weeks, frequent yeast infections or rashes, fatigue, and wounds that are slow to heal.

Factors beyond our control can weaken immunity—aging, chemicals in the environment, medications that suppress immunity (such as large doses of oral corticosteroids or the antirejection drugs prescribed after organ transplants), chemotherapy, and HIV infection. The typical crash-and-burn American lifestyle—too much stress, too little sleep, and a steady diet of takeout—also takes its toll on immune function.

Is your immune system in harm's way? This chapter lays out the five lifestyle factors that research suggests place the biggest strain on immune function.

Risk #1: You Smoke

Hooked on cigarettes? Then you probably know that smoking raises the risk of heart disease as well as cancers of the lung, esophagus, bladder, breast, and cervix. You also may know—from bitter experience—that smokers develop more upper respiratory infections (colds, bronchitis, pneumonia) than nonsmokers do and that a smoker's wounds heal more slowly.

Smoking wreaks its systemwide havoc in part by suppressing immune function. Studies show that smoking lowers blood levels of several kinds of antibodies, reduces the function of T cells and natural killer (NK) cells, and hinders the ability of macrophages in the lungs to gobble up and kill bacteria. Smoking also floods the body with free radicals, molecules formed naturally when the body uses oxygen. Free radicals damage cellular DNA, which raises the risk of cancer and causes immune-suppressing inflammation.

The latest research suggests a possible link between smoking and autoimmune disease. In a study of 22,000 Norwegians, for example, smokers were 1.8 times more likely to develop multiple sclerosis than nonsmokers were. The risk was highest for women. Similarly, an analysis of the records of more than 30,000 women enrolled in the Iowa Women's Health Study since 1986 found that, compared with nonsmokers, smokers had double the risk of developing rheumatoid arthritis.

Researchers aren't sure why smoking might increase the risk of autoimmune disease. Some are focusing on the fact that smoking damages the endothelial cells, which form the lining of blood vessels. It may be that when these cells sustain injury, the immune system becomes overactive and turns against the body's own cells.

The good news: Stop smoking, and immune function begins to improve within 30 days.

Risk #2: You're Constantly Stressed

Brief bouts of stress triggered by, say, giving a presentation at work or taking a test don't harm the immune system. But ongoing stress—a side effect of caring for a chronically ill child or parent or coping with financial worries or family crises—can take a toll.

Chronic stress trips an alarm in the brain—the so-called fight-or-flight response, the body's automatic physiological reaction to danger. Activated by the nervous system, the fight-or-flight response triggers the release of stress hormones that prepare the body to defend itself against a threat or to flee from it. Heart rate and blood pressure rise. Blood is directed away from the extremities and digestive system to the large muscles. The pupils dilate—the better to see the enemy—and hearing sharpens.

Studies suggest that short bursts of stress actually cause a temporary boost in immune response. But when stress never lets up, and the body remains in a constant state of fight or flight, the immune system's ability to repair and defend declines. Chronic stress has been shown to reduce levels of B and T cells, affect the responsiveness of NK cells, and lower levels of antibodies secreted in saliva.

What's more, long-standing stress appears to result in inflammation. This physiological process is regulated by *cytokines*—hormonelike proteins that deliver chemical "messages" to immune cells—and is linked to heart disease, diabetes, arthritis, and other chronic illnesses.

Can Your Pet Make You Sick?

When you share kisses or a pillow with your pets, you share what they get into—dead varmints, toilet water, their own leavings. Can our best friends infect us with anything more than passionate devotion?

It's possible but rare, says Bruno Chomel, DVM, professor of zoonoses (the diseases that pass from animals to humans) in the School of Veterinary Medicine at the University of California, Davis. "If your pet is regularly checked by a vet and gets its immunizations, the risks are low," says Dr. Chomel. "On the other hand, pets do carry dirty stuff."

The "dirty stuff" includes ringworm (a fungus), salmonella and campylobacter (bacteria that cause vomiting and diarrhea), and—rarely—more dangerous bugs. Recently, a 3-year-old pet cat in San Francisco was found to carry a strain of the superbug MRSA, short for methicillin-resistant *Staphylococcus aureus*. Often found in hospitals, MRSA is resistant to most antibiotics.

Infants and toddlers, whose immune systems are not fully developed, and the elderly, whose immune systems are fragile, are vulnerable to contracting illnesses from pets. So are people whose immune systems are weakened by chemotherapy, HIV, or an organ transplant. These tips can help reduce the risks.

WASH YOUR HANDS—OFTEN. Pets carry a variety of bugs on their fur and in their mouths and can shed them in their droppings. Wash your hands with soap and running water after you handle or clean up after a pet, especially if it has diarrhea.

NIX THE LICKS. Easier said than done, but if you're concerned about contracting a pet-borne bug, don't let Fido or Fluffy kiss or lick you, says Dr. Chomel.

DELEGATE LITTER-BOX DUTY IF YOU'RE PREGNANT. Cat droppings can carry toxoplasmosis, a parasite that can trigger a miscarriage or cause birth defects.

CHOOSE PET CHEWS WISELY. Dried pig ears, a popular chew for dogs, are often contaminated with salmonella, says Dr. Chomel. You can pick up the bug when you handle the chew or clean up after the dog with diarrhea caused by the virus. Get other treats instead.

RECONSIDER REPTILES. If your household contains a young child, an elderly person, or someone whose immune system has been compromised, pass on lizards, snakes, and other reptiles. They're notorious for shedding the salmonella virus.

Risk #3: You're Sleep-Deprived

Not logging enough pillow time? Join the club. The National Sleep Foundation's 2005 Sleep in America poll found that 71 percent of us get less than 8 hours of sleep a night on weekdays. That's not enough for the immune system.

Like stress, a sleep deficit—even a small one—is associated with chronic, low-grade, systemwide inflammation. A team of researchers led by Alexandros N. Vgontzas, MD, professor of psychiatry at the Pennsylvania State University College of Medicine in Hershey, found that the blood of sleep-deprived folks contains higher levels of inflammatory cytokines such as interleukin-6 and tumor necrosis factor. Sleep deprivation also affects NK cells. In a study from the University of California, San Diego, involving 23 men, one night of interrupted sleep reduced NK cell activity to 72 percent of normal levels.

The immune system returns to normal function once we get the sleep we need. The problem is that "damage might have been done during the time that your immune system left you undefended and susceptible to infection," says Stanley Coren, PhD, author of *Sleep Thieves* and a professor of psychology at the University of British Columbia in Vancouver.

Risk #4: You Move Too Little—Or Too Much

If you're among the 25 percent of Americans who are completely sedentary, you probably know that an inactive lifestyle raises the risk of chronic health problems like heart disease, diabetes, and cancer. But inactivity also may lower immunity. In one study, researchers compared people who were inactive with those who took brisk walks nearly every day. Over a 4-month period, the walkers took half as many sick days as the nonwalkers.

Research shows that moderate exercise, such as a brisk walk, has a positive effect on the activity and number of NK cells and neutrophils, immune cells that kill foreign invaders and trigger the immune response. Moderate exercise also helps regulate the immune system and hormones that influence the healing process.

Scientists at Ohio State University in Columbus delivered a small puncture wound to 28 inactive men and women ages 55 to 77. Half of the volunteers then exercised on a treadmill or stationary bike and trained with weights three times a week, while the other half remained inactive. The workout group's wounds healed an average of 10 days sooner than the sedentary group's did—29 days versus 39. While the researchers studied only healthy people, they theorized that exercise may also help people with diabetes, whose wounds tend to heal slowly.

You might think that when it comes to exercise, more is better. That isn't the case, at least as far as immune function is concerned. Working out too hard and for too long actually suppresses the immune system, which may explain why people who do marathons often get sick after the 26.2-mile run. (In fact, in one study, marathoners were six times more likely to catch colds after completing the event than those who dropped out during training.) Intense exercise lowers antibodies in saliva and reduces the activity of NK cells and neutrophils. Stress hormones, which tend to suppress immune function, may be the cause.

Risk #5: You're on the Drive-Thru Diet

"Poor diet is the biggest cause of a weakened immune system in healthy people," says William Boisvert, PhD, assistant professor of medicine at Harvard Medical School.

If you don't take in enough calories, you may not get enough nutrients that are critical to good health. Malnutrition reduces the immune system's ability to fight infection. Those at risk for malnutrition include the elderly, people with eating disorders or certain diseases such as celiac disease or cancer, and people who are addicted to drugs or alcohol. Fortunately, "when you restore the person to normal nutrition, the immune system improves," says Jeffrey Blumberg, PhD, chief of the antioxidants research laboratory at the USDA Human Nutrition Research Center on Aging at Tufts University in Boston.

However, even people who consume enough calories may be malnourished if their diets don't have enough nutrient-rich foods. A junk-food diet doesn't give the immune system what it needs to function at its peak. For example, refined sugar inhibits *phagocytosis,* the process by which viruses and bacteria are engulfed and then literally chewed up by white blood cells. A diet high in fat, especially polyunsaturated fat, also tends to suppress the immune system. (On the other hand, healthy omega-3 fatty acids—found in flaxseed, fish, and canola oil—support the manufacture of immune cells that help control the inflammatory response.)

A junk-food diet can lead to obesity, another factor in suppressed immunity. One animal study conducted at the University of North Carolina at Chapel Hill suggests that obesity may prevent the body from properly switching on the immune system, leaving it more vulnerable to flu virus. Researchers fed one group of 35 laboratory mice a high-fat diet and a second group a high-carbohydrate diet. The fat-fed mice had 31 percent body fat, compared with 21 percent for the carb-fed mice. After 5 months, the researchers infected both groups with a flu virus. Compared with the leaner mice, the obese mice were 10 times more likely to die when infected. The researchers found that the obese mice had significantly lower levels of two types of cytokines—antiviral cytokines,

Yo-Yo Dieting Starves Immunity

Constantly losing and regaining weight—also known as yo-yo dieting—won't just leave you weak with hunger. It also may weaken your immune system.

Researchers at the Fred Hutchinson Cancer Research Center and the University of Washington in Seattle measured the activity of NK cells in the blood of 114 healthy but overweight women. These immune cells help fight off the viruses that cause the common cold and herpes, as well as human papillomavirus (HPV), which can cause cervical cancer. Research links low activity in NK cells with higher rates of cancer and increased susceptibility to colds and infections.

The study found that the more frequently a woman reported intentionally losing weight, the more her long-term immune function declined. Women who maintained the same weight for 5 or more years had 40 percent greater NK cell activity, compared with those whose weight had remained stable for fewer than 2 years. "Those who reported losing weight more than five times had about a third lower natural-killer-cell function," says study leader Cornelia Ulrich, PhD, an assistant member of the division of public health services at the Hutchinson Center. The findings are intriguing, but more research is needed, says Dr. Ulrich. "Clearly, there's evidence that weight loss is beneficial for your health," she says. "What we're concerned about is this pattern of weight cycling, where women go up and down."

---

which help control the initial spread of a virus, and proinflammatory cytokines, which trigger the recruitment of immune cells. Moreover, the NK cells in the obese mice were 50 percent less able to kill the virus, compared with those of the slimmer mice.

Although the researchers studied animals, their findings "suggest that the growing obese population is at increased risk for immune dysfunction during influenza infection, which may lead in humans, as it did in the mice, to increased mortality," says study leader Melinda A. Beck, PhD, professor in the departments of pediatrics and nutrition at the University of North Carolina at Chapel Hill School of Medicine.

Make Over Your Immune System

While immune function can't be quantified without a blood test, it *can* be measured with a more general "test": how you feel. Do you bounce out of bed in the morning or drag yourself out of it? Do you dread cold and flu season or sail right through? Every healthy lifestyle choice you make is a key that can help unlock—and unleash—the power of your immune system.

The risk factors for poor immunity outlined in this chapter, plus many others, are well within your control. Change them and watch a healthier, more vibrant you emerge. Besides enhancing your immune function, you'll sleep better, shrug off stress more easily, and perhaps even lose weight. Best of all, you'll reap the satisfaction of knowing that you're taking an active role in your health.

It won't take long for you to notice immediate, positive changes in how you feel once you begin making the sorts of lifestyle adjustments outlined in Part II and in the Immune Essentials Plan in Part III. But first, take the Immunity IQ quiz starting on page 26 to get a sense of your current immune status.

What's Your Immunity IQ?

By now you know that lifestyle has a significant effect on the immune system's ability to serve and protect. The question is, how about *your* lifestyle? Do your health habits support immune vitality or hinder it?

This quiz (actually, a series of miniquizzes) measures your "immunity IQ"—how well your health habits bolster your immune defenses. You'll score yourself on each miniquiz, as well as overall. If you "flunk," no worries. Brush up on healthy-lifestyle basics, make a few simple changes, and you're sure to raise your score.

Miniquiz 1: Healthy Eats

Give yourself zero points for each A, two for each B, and one for each C. *If you score three or more points in this section, see Key #1, page 33.*

1. Describe your eating style.
    a. Health nut. I crave fruits and veggies, shun white flour and sugar, and consume moderate amounts of lean protein (chicken, fish).
    b. Junk-food junkie. I crave fatty, salty, or sugary food served in a bag, box, or can.
    c. Health-conscious. I eat well most of the time but occasionally indulge in a slice of cake or an order of fries.

2. How many servings of fruits and vegetables do you eat each day?
    a. Nine or more. I have several with every meal.

b. Do fruit roll-ups count?

c. Five to eight. I add them in when I can.

3. Describe the source of fats in your diet.

   a. Most come from healthy sources, like fish, nuts, and olive oil. I limit my intake of trans fats and saturated fats.

   b. My diet is heavy on red meat, full-fat cheeses, doughnuts, and fast food.

   c. I eat mostly healthy fats but occasionally splurge on a doughnut or drive-thru meal.

4. How much water do you drink each day?

   a. Eight or more glasses. I sip constantly at the office, the gym, even in my car.

   b. None, usually. I guzzle soda or coffee but can go days without a drop of water.

   c. One or two glasses, whether or not I'm thirsty.

Miniquiz 2: Rest and Motion

Give yourself zero points for each A, two for each B, and one for each C. *If you score four or more points in this section, see Keys #2 and #3, pages 63 and 81.*

1. How often do you work out?

   a. Four or more times a week, either at home or at the gym.

   b. Every day, if you count Internet- or channel-surfing.

   c. At least three times a week.

2. How would you describe your workout's intensity?

   a. Moderate. My heart pumps a little faster, and I break a sweat.

   b. I don't exercise.

   c. Intense. I sweat buckets and can't hold a conversation.

3. When you wake up in the morning, how do you typically feel?

   a. Well rested. I'm ready to face the day.

   b. Exhausted. I either toss and turn all night or wake up and stay up.

   c. A bit sleepy. After a few minutes, though, I'm good to go.

4. How often do you take naps?

   a. Rarely. I sleep well at night, so no need for a catnap.

b. Often. I fall asleep on the couch after work or take 2-hour naps on the weekend.

c. Once in a while. An occasional 15- or 20-minute catnap recharges my batteries.

Miniquiz 3: Outlook on Life

Give yourself zero points for each A, two for each B, and one for each C. *If you score three or more points in this section, see Keys #4 and #5, pages 92 and 108.*

1. If life is like a box of chocolates, describe your box.

   a. Half full with my favorites. I tend to take an optimistic view of life.

   b. Half empty, no favorites. I tend to be a pessimist.

   c. Neither half full nor half empty. I'm a realist who takes and savors chocolate when it's offered.

2. How often do you laugh each day?

   a. Often. I love to send and receive e-mail jokes, and it's easy to tickle my funny bone.

   b. Rarely. Life's a serious matter; not much to laugh about, is there?

   c. A few times. Laughter is like money; you can always use more.

3. Describe your social circle.

   a. I'm always around family or a wide circle of close friends.

   b. I don't really have one. I'm a bit of a loner.

   c. I'm close with a few people but would like to expand my circle.

4. How do you handle stress?

   a. I find healthy ways to release tension. I might sweat it out at the gym, vent to a friend, or curl up with my knitting needles or a good book.

   b. I tend to fall apart. I complain, rage, or neglect my health.

   c. I may have a few sleepless nights or mini meltdowns, but I treat myself with TLC to get through the worst of it.

Miniquiz 4: Colds, Flu, and Bugs

Give yourself zero points for each A, two for each B, and one for each C. *If you score three or more points in this section, you'll want to pay close attention to all of the chapters in Part II.*

1. During cold and flu season, how often do you get sick?

   a. Never. The sniffle season doesn't faze me, even when those around me fall ill.

   b. Often. Viruses seem to love me.

   c. Rarely—once or twice, tops.

2. If you do fall ill, how severe are your symptoms?

   a. Minor. Maybe I have a stuffy nose or a sore throat for a day.

   b. Severe. I cough and honk until April.

   c. Moderate. My colds rarely last more than a week.

3. How often do you experience skin rashes, swollen glands, or postnasal drip?

   a. Rarely or never.

   b. Quite often.

   c. Once in a while.

Miniquiz 5: Clean Living

Give yourself zero points for each A and two points for each B. *If you score two or more points in this section, see Key #7, page 133.*

1. During the day, how often do you wash your hands?

   a. Often, especially after using the bathroom, during cold and flu season, and before and after preparing food.

   b. Rarely. There's just no time—or no soap.

2. How would you describe your kitchen hygiene?

   a. I'm a germaphobe, compelled to scour counters, sponges, and cooking utensils.

   b. I'm not as vigilant as I could be when washing fruits and vegetables, handling raw meat or poultry, and storing leftovers.

3. Do you use antibacterial soaps and cleansers?

   a. No. I find that plain old soap and standard household cleansers like bleach or pine cleaner work just as well.

   b. Yes. I won't use anything else. They kill everything, right?

Your Immunity IQ

While your score in each category helps you zero in on your personal strengths and weaknesses, your overall score reflects the general health of your lifestyle. Here's your immunity IQ.

0 to 6 points: genius. Your lifestyle supports a strong, healthy immune system, but it can't hurt to do even better. Turn to Part II, 7 Keys to Maximum Immunity, for simple, natural ways to enhance immunity.

7 to 12 points: superior. By and large, you live an immune-friendly lifestyle. If one bad habit affected your score—perhaps you stress too much, sleep too little, or smoke—see Part IV, Immune Extras: Smart Strategies to Boost Immunity.

13 to 18 points: average. Healthier choices could enhance your immune system and protect your health. If your score is high because you have a health condition, such as asthma, diabetes, or cancer, turn to Part V, Immune Accelerators: Fight Back against Illness.

19 or more points: back to school. A lifestyle makeover can help raise your immunity IQ. Part III, Immune Essentials: The 4-Week Plan, makes adapting healthy habits a no-brainer.

PART II
7 Keys to Maximum Immunity

Key #1—Nutrition: An Apple a Day Can Keep the Doctor Away

Immune Rx: Eat a Well-Balanced Diet Rich in Immune-Boosting Foods

A sound, balanced diet is essential to achieving maximum immunity, protecting yourself from illness, and improving your overall health.

But just what is a sound, balanced diet?

The US Department of Agriculture defines it as one with a proper mix of grains, vegetables, fruits, low-fat or fat-free dairy products (specifically, milk, yogurt, and cheese), and proteins (such as lean meats and poultry, fish, beans, nuts, and seeds). Collectively, these foods deliver the necessary nutrients to keep your body—and your immune system—performing at their best.

The conventional wisdom has been that fruits and vegetables are the most important food groups for immune function, primarily because they're so rich in antioxidants. But emphasizing one or two groups at the expense of the others isn't to your advantage, according to Kim Galeaz, RD, CD, an Indianapolis-based nutrition and culinary consultant who created the menus that appear in the 4-week Immune Essentials Plan beginning on page 157. "You need to have a certain amount of every food group to be healthy, stay healthy, and feel good," she explains.

In this chapter, you'll learn how each of the major food groups influences your immunity and overall health and how to incorporate them into your diet. You also will discover how proper hydration and dietary "extras" such as tea, coffee, red wine, and dark chocolate can complement the immune-boosting effects of a balanced diet.

Poor Nutrition Leads to Poor Immune Function

If you think hard enough, you probably can remember your initial introduction to the principles of proper nutrition in junior-high health class. Though the rules have changed over the years, the underlying message remains the same: Your body needs certain nutrients in certain amounts just to perform its basic functions. Without that solid foundation, it falters.

Even in this land of plenty, nutritional deficiencies are common—especially among older adults. Surveys conducted in the United States, as well as in Canada, Europe, and India, suggest that as many as 35 percent of apparently healthy adults over age 50 aren't getting enough of at least one essential vitamin or mineral that enhances immune function. The result: a higher incidence of respiratory, urinary, and other common infections.

"Infections and malnutrition aggravate each other," observes Ranjit K. Chandra, MD, PhD, director of the World Health Organization Center for Nutritional Immunology, in a 2002 review article published in the *European Journal of Clinical Nutrition*. "However, nutrition does not influence all infections equally. For some infections—such as pneumonia, bacterial and viral diarrhea, measles, and tuberculosis—there is overwhelming evidence that the clinical course and final outcome are affected adversely by nutritional deficiency."

Some essential vitamins and minerals are antioxidants, which protect your cells—including immune cells—from free radical damage. *Free radicals* are unstable oxygen molecules that attack cells and their DNA. As we get older, our antioxidant levels tend to decline, while our free radical levels rise.

A growing body of evidence supports the so-called free radical theory as the most plausible cause of aging and age-related decline, a process known as senescence. Free radical damage is thought to be responsible for immunosenescence—age-related decline in immune function, resulting in increased susceptibility to infection and to cancer.

Immunosenescence isn't inevitable. "Aged [adults] who maintain their immune function at an exceptionally high level have a long life span and may even become centenarians," notes M. De La Fuente, MD, of the Universidad Complutense de Madrid in Spain, in a 2002 article published in the *European Journal of Clinical Nutrition*. "Several laboratories, including our own, have shown that antioxidants preserve . . . adequate function of immune cells. The protection of this system afforded by dietary antioxidant supplementation may play an important role in order to achieve . . . healthy aging."

In 1992, Dr. Chandra and his colleagues conducted a landmark randomized, double-blind, placebo-controlled study of 96 healthy men and women over age 65. For 1 year, half of the volunteers took multivitamin-mineral supplements that supplied the essential nutrients at Recommended Daily Allowance (RDA) levels, except for beta-carotene (a precursor to vitamin A) and vitamin E, which were at four times their RDAs. The remaining volunteers took a placebo.

The study's results were dramatic and conclusive. The supplement takers showed significant rises in their levels of vitamins A, B$_6$, and C and the minerals iron and zinc, as well as increased production of infection-fighting T cells and natural killer (NK) cells. They also showed an enhanced immune response to flu vaccines. None of these improvements occurred among the placebo takers.

Although adequate nutrition is essential for optimal immune function, overeating that leads to obesity can impair immunity, opening the door to infection, cancer, and possibly premature death. This finding has prompted researchers to explore whether calorie restriction and reduced body mass can improve immune function and extend life span. According to animal studies, at least, they do.

The most tantalizing clue that calorie restriction might benefit humans emerged from a 2006 study that appeared in the *Proceedings of the National Academy of Sciences*. For the study, researchers from the Vaccine and Gene Therapy Institute of Oregon Health and Science University in Portland observed one of our closest relatives: the rhesus monkey. They placed 13 monkeys on a diet supplying 30 percent fewer calories than usual and 28 monkeys on a regular diet. All of the monkeys were between ages 18 and 23—which is 60 and 70 in human years.

By the end of the 42-month study, the calorie-restricted monkeys showed significant improvements in their T-cell function, along with reductions in inflammatory compounds, compared with the control monkeys. The results suggest that calorie restriction in primates—including humans—may delay immunological aging, improve disease resistance, and extend life span.

Even a modest reduction in calories may produce similar benefits. In a 2005 study of slightly overweight people, researchers at Tufts University in Boston found that cutting just 100 to 200 calories a day led to weight loss, improved cholesterol levels, and a significant boost in immune response to disease-causing microorganisms. If a couple hundred calories seems like a lot, think of it this way: The next time you eat out, skip the baked potato with sour cream and order steamed vegetables instead. You'll save 200 calories with this simple switch.

The Essential Vitamins and Minerals for Maximum Immunity

Each of the menus in the 4-week Immune Essentials Plan supplies roughly 1,800 calories per day, the recommended intake for someone who's getting about 30 minutes of exercise most days of the week, beyond the normal activities of daily living. In addition, many of the menus supply more than the established Daily Values (DVs) of key immune-boosting vitamins and minerals. Among these nutritional superstars:

Selenium. A potent antioxidant, selenium plays an essential role in immune function by protecting immune cells against free radical damage. It also helps regulate T cells' production of proteins called cytokines, a process that's essential for launching a quick and vigorous immune response to an acute infection. Studies have shown that selenium deficiency contributes to impaired immune function, and supplementation improves the immune system's production of antibodies in response to foreign invaders.

DV: 70 micrograms; *top food sources:* whole grains, nuts, seeds, broccoli, and fish

Vitamin A. Sometimes it's called the anti-infective vitamin, because a deficiency of vitamin A has a strong correlation with an increased risk of infection. Researchers long have known that vitamin A is necessary to maintain healthy levels of circulating T cells. Even a modest deficiency can weaken the immune defenses of a child's respiratory tract by damaging mucous membranes that form a naturally protective barrier against viruses and bacteria. Vitamin A also enhances the activity of white blood cells, which attack, engulf, destroy, and clean up infected cells.

DV: 5,000 IU; *top food sources:* dark-green leafy vegetables, bell peppers, butternut squash, cabbage, cantaloupe, carrots, and sweet potatoes. All of these contain large amounts of beta-carotene, which the body converts to vitamin A on an as-needed basis.

Vitamin B$_6$. This B vitamin supports the activity of white blood cells. When researchers from Tufts School of Nutrition temporarily removed vitamin B$_6$ from the diets of healthy older adults, immune function plummeted. Interestingly, it took as much as 50 milligrams of vitamin B$_6$ per day to restore immune function to a level equal to or better than before the study.

DV: 2 milligrams; *top food sources:* fish, poultry, lean meats, whole grains, leafy greens, bananas, prunes, peanuts, walnuts, and chickpeas

Vitamin C. A potent antioxidant that protects immune cells from free radical damage, it's also vital to the production of white blood cells. Although large amounts of vitamin C do not significantly lower your risk of catching a cold, supplemental doses may reduce the duration and severity of symptoms by inhibiting the release of histamine, an inflammatory chemical that causes a runny nose and respiratory congestion.

DV: 60 milligrams; *top food sources:* oranges and grapefruit (either whole or as juice), bell peppers, broccoli, cantaloupe, kiwifruit, rutabagas, strawberries, sweet potatoes, and tomatoes

Are Supplements a Substitute for a Healthy Diet?

Between balancing family, work, and the myriad other distractions of 21st-century life, you may be wondering if there are any shortcuts to achieving maximum immunity—like nutritional supplements, for example. It would be so much easier to just pop a pill and forgo the hassle of shopping for and preparing fresh, nutrient-packed foods!

Alas, such a supersupplement doesn't exist—not yet, anyway. Although nutritional supplements can help correct some deficiencies, they don't come close to matching the immune-enhancing benefits of a balanced diet. Whole grains, fruits, vegetables, low-fat dairy products, and lean proteins—which together form the foundation of the Immune Essentials Plan—contain so many thousands of beneficial substances that no pill could possibly duplicate all of them. Besides, megadoses of certain nutrients, such as vitamin A and selenium, can be toxic.

That said, some experts believe that a little nutritional insurance may help. For example, Andrew Weil, MD, clinical professor of medicine at the University of Arizona in Tucson and director of its Program in Integrative Medicine, recommends this daily immune-enhancing regimen:

- B-complex vitamin: Choose a supplement that supplies 400 micrograms of folic acid.
- Selenium: 200 micrograms
- Vitamin C: 200 to 250 milligrams
- Vitamin E: 400 IU (80 milligrams) as mixed tocopherols and tocotrienols

---

Vitamin D. Long known as essential for maintaining strong bones and preventing osteoporosis, it also helps the thymus gland generate a sufficient number of immune cells. Vitamin D is present in most multivitamins and calcium supplements. A few minutes of sunlight per day also can help restore your supply (see page 122).

DV: 400 IU; *top food sources:* eggs, butter, and fortified milk

Vitamin E. This potent antioxidant sacrifices its own electrons to cell-damaging free radicals, effectively neutralizing them. Vitamin E also raises levels of interferon and interleukin, chemicals produced by the immune system to fight infection.

DV: 30 IU; *top food sources:* wheat germ, molasses, whole grains, nuts, and seeds

Zinc. A mineral known for its ability to lessen the severity and duration of colds, zinc plays a critical role in maintaining a strong immune system. Specifically, it helps stabilize and protect your primary barriers against infectious organisms—your skin and mucous membranes—and promotes the normal development of immune cells.

Most Americans run low on zinc, which raises the risk of many different kinds of infection. Zinc also has antioxidant properties.

DV: 15 milligrams; *top food sources:* fish, shellfish, skinless poultry, and lean cuts of pork and beef. (The leanest cuts of pork are labeled "loin"; the leanest cuts of beef, "loin" or "round.") Whole grains also contain some zinc.

A Closer Look at the Five Food Groups

As mentioned earlier, by eating a variety of foods across all five food groups, you are virtually guaranteed to meet your body's—and your immune system's—daily nutritional requirements. Though our Immune Essentials Plan does recommend a multivitamin as nutritional insurance, most experts agree that it's best to get nutrients from foods whenever possible. This is because foods offer a variety of vitamins, minerals, and compounds called phytonutrients that may work synergistically inside your body. With this in mind, let's explore the health- and immune-enhancing benefits of each food group in turn.

Whole Grains: The Staff of Life

Grains—especially whole grains—are essential to an immunity-friendly diet. They're good sources of the immune-enhancing vitamins B_6 and E, as well as the minerals selenium and zinc. They also contain generous amounts of other B vitamins such as thiamine, riboflavin, niacin, and folate, plus minerals such as iron and magnesium. The fiber in whole grains may help reduce blood cholesterol (and heart disease risk), enhance bowel function, and prevent constipation and diverticulosis.

"In the Immune Essentials Plan, you'll be aiming for 6 ounces of grains a day, but not much more," Galeaz says. How much is an ounce—or an ounce equivalent—of grains? Here are several examples.

- Bread: one regular whole wheat slice

- Corn bread: one 3-inch-square piece made from refined grain

- English muffin: half a muffin made from whole wheat or refined grain

- Oatmeal: ½ cup cooked, one packet instant, or 1 ounce dry (regular or quick)

- Pancakes: one pancake (4½ inches in diameter) made from whole wheat or buckwheat; two pancakes (3 inches in diameter) made from refined grain, buttermilk, or plain wheat

- Popcorn: 3 cups, popped, from whole corn

Oatmeal's Secret Immune-Booster

In addition to their many other healthy nutrients and fiber, oats and (to a lesser extent) barley contain large amounts of beta-glucan. A polysaccharide component of fiber, beta-glucan appears to have potent antitumor and immune-stimulating activity. It also speeds wound healing, enhances the therapeutic effects of antibiotics, and strengthens immune resistance to viral, bacterial, protozoan, and fungal diseases.

Interestingly, the reishi mushroom contains beta-glucan—which just goes to show that you really can fight fungus with fungus! Other fungi, yeast, and algae also have high concentrations of beta-glucan.

According to a Norwegian study, beta-glucan is more potent than echinacea as an antimicrobial and antioxidant agent. When animals consume this compound, they're more resistant to diseases such as the flu, herpes, and anthrax.

Beta-glucan is immune stimulating because it activates macrophages, the immune cells produced deep in the bone marrow that roam the bloodstream and engulf and ingest invading viruses and bacteria. Animal studies suggest that beta-glucan may boost immunity and increase disease resistance in athletes during immunity-suppressing periods of intense training. Studies are under way to determine if these benefits translate to humans.

Our recommendation: Make oatmeal one of your three daily servings of whole grains. A good choice is steel-cut oats, like McCann's Irish Oatmeal, with twice as much beta-glucan as the rolled, quick-cooking variety.

■ Rice: ½ cup cooked whole grain, brown, or wild; 1 ounce dry enriched, white, or polished

The menus in the Immune Essentials Plan emphasize whole grains. Refined grains—which have been milled to remove the bran and germ—supply smaller amounts of many vitamins and minerals, plus virtually no fiber. The most common refined grain is white flour, which you'll find in many commercially available breads, baked goods, pastas, and cereals.

To increase the proportion of whole grains in your diet:

■ Substitute whole wheat or oat flour for up to half of the white flour called for in pancakes, waffles, muffins, and other flour-based recipes.

■ Stuff brown rice into baked green peppers or tomatoes.

■ Use whole wheat pasta in macaroni and cheese.

■ Add whole grain barley to vegetable soups and stews.

■ Use crushed, unsweetened whole grain cereal or rolled oats to coat baked chicken, fish, veal cutlets, or eggplant Parmesan.

Vegetables: Vital to a Healthy Diet

Pick a veggie, any veggie. No matter which is your favorite, you can't go wrong, nutrition-wise. As a group, vegetables are top-notch sources of an array of immune-boosting nutrients—including vitamins A, B_6, C, and E and the mineral selenium. They also are packed with fiber and *phytonutrients*, compounds that protect immune cells by neutralizing free radicals. Among the best-known phytonutrients is lycopene, a potential cancer fighter that gives tomatoes their bright red color. (We'll talk more about lycopene in a bit.)

A vegetable-rich diet can help protect against infection and illness. Specifically, it may lower the risk of heart disease, type 2 diabetes, osteoporosis, and certain cancers, including those of the mouth, stomach, and colon.

As one of the five major food groups, vegetables consist of four subgroups.

■ Dark-green vegetables—such as bok choy, broccoli, collard greens, kale, leaf lettuce, mesclun, mustard greens, romaine lettuce, spinach, turnip greens, and watercress

■ Orange vegetables—including acorn squash, butternut squash, carrots, hubbard squash, and sweet potatoes

■ Starchy vegetables—including corn, green lima beans, green peas, and white beans

■ Other vegetables—such as artichokes, asparagus, bean sprouts, beets, Brussels sprouts, cabbage, cauliflower, celery, cucumbers, eggplant, green beans, green and red bell peppers, iceberg lettuce, mushrooms, okra, onions, parsnips, tomatoes, tomato juice, vegetable juice, turnips, wax beans, and zucchini

If you follow the Immune Essentials Plan, you'll be eating at least 2½ cups of vegetables per day. For most veggies, a serving is 1 cup raw or cooked (exceptions: spinach and iceberg lettuce, for which a serving is 2 cups raw). "More is better," Galeaz says. "You can't overdose on vegetables."

The best cooking methods for vegetables are steaming and microwaving, Galeaz says. Boiling leaches out some (though not all) of the immune-enhancing nutrients. So does overcooking. "Vegetables are best eaten when they're tender or crisp," she says. "Avoid cooking them for so long that they lose their natural beautiful colors and turn mushy." Still, she adds, "if the only way you'll eat your veggies is to cook the heck out of them, it's better to do that than to eat no veggies at all."

Looking for more ways to make the most of vegetables? These tips can help.

■ Buy fresh vegetables in season when they contain the largest amounts of immune-enhancing nutrients and are at their peak flavor.

■ Choose canned vegetables labeled "no salt added." Even if you sprinkle on a little salt at mealtime, you probably will get less sodium than you would from the regular canned product.

■ Do you like to grill? Try making vegetable kebabs with tomatoes, mushrooms, green bell peppers, and onions.

■ Cut up vegetables and refrigerate them so they're ready to eat when you're in the mood for a snack. Instead of the usual carrot and celery sticks, consider broccoli florets, cucumber slices, and red and green bell pepper strips.

Perhaps like some people, you just aren't a big fan of vegetables. Galeaz recommends finding at least one or two that appeal to you and sticking with them. Although dark-green and orange vegetables are among the best sources of immune-enhancing nutrients, even starchy vegetables such as corn supply some vitamins, minerals, and fiber. Another alternative to eating vegetables is to "drink" them in the form of tomato or other juices, she says.

TERRORIZE GERMS WITH TOMATOES

Multiple studies have found a correlation between regular consumption of tomatoes and tomato products and reduced risk of certain cancers, as well as cardiovascular disease. This is because tomatoes contain many immune-boosting nutrients, the most potent of which may be the carotenoid lycopene. Tomatoes also are good sources of vitamin C, vitamin A, potassium, coumaric acid, and cholorgenic acid.

According to a 2005 study, published in the *American Journal of Clinical Nutrition,* lycopene acts as an antioxidant, helping white blood cells resist the harmful effects of free radicals. For this study, researchers tracked 10 volunteers who ate a tomato-rich diet for 3 weeks, followed by a tomato-free diet for another 3 weeks. The volunteers' white blood cells showed 38 percent less free radical damage during the tomato phase, compared with the tomato-free phase.

This finding came on the heels of a 2004 study involving a group of men with low blood levels of lycopene and beta-carotene (also a carotenoid). In the men who drank a serving of tomato or carrot juice a day, production and activity of immune cells—including NK cells—improved by as much as 25 percent.

Not all studies show that tomatoes have a stimulating effect on immune cells. In a 2006 study, for example, researchers from the University of Milan in Italy asked half of a group of 26 volunteers to drink a tomato beverage containing lycopene, phytoene, phytofluene, and alpha-tocopherol. The remaining volunteers drank a placebo that looked and tasted just like the real thing. The researchers concluded that the tomato drink didn't boost immunity. It did, however, significantly reduce the production of tumor necrosis factor–alpha by T cells and macrophages. Although the compound may play a role in destroying cancer cells, it also contributes to systemic inflammation. Elevated levels are associated with rheumatoid arthritis and other autoimmune diseases.

Among the best sources of lycopene are cooked tomato products such as ketchup, jarred and canned tomato sauce, and salsa. Raw tomatoes supply a generous amount, too, but not as much as cooked. This is because the heating process makes lycopene more bioavailable.

To get the full nutritional benefit of tomatoes and tomato products, you may want to pair them with a healthy fat such as olive or canola oil. Carotenoids need a small amount so the small intestine can efficiently absorb them. When researchers from Iowa State University in Ames drew blood samples from volunteers who had eaten a salad with either fat-containing or fat-free dressing, those with the fat-free dressing failed to absorb the carotenoids from the salad.

TOMATO AND BROCCOLI: A KILLER COMBINATION

Like tomatoes, broccoli appears to help protect against certain cancers. Just as tomatoes are packed with carotenoids (among other nutrients), broccoli contains two well-known cancer fighters: inole-3-carbinol and sulforaphane.

It's not surprising, then, that tomatoes and broccoli may deliver an even stronger anticancer punch when eaten together. "We think it's because different bioactive compounds in each food work on different anti-cancer pathways," says John Erdman, PhD, professor of food science and human nutrition at the University of Illinois at Urbana-Champaign. He and his colleagues conducted an animal study—published in the journal *Cancer Research* in 2007—in which the combination was more effective at shrinking prostate tumors than Proscar (finasteride), a commonly prescribed drug for men with enlarged prostates. The researchers implanted six groups of laboratory rats with prostate cancer cells. Then one group was fed a diet containing 10 percent tomato powder and 10 percent broccoli powder, with the powders made from whole foods. Another group received only tomato powder; the third, broccoli powder; the fourth, a supplemental dose of lycopene; and the fifth, finasteride. The sixth—and unluckiest—group was castrated.

After 22 weeks, the researchers examined the rats' prostate tumors. The tomato-broccoli combination had outperformed all of the other interventions, not only shrinking the tumors but also slowing the growth of cancer cells. The only other intervention that came close to achieving this effect was castration. "It was very exciting to compare this drastic surgery to diet and see that tumor reduction was similar," says doctoral candidate Kirstie Canene-Adams, who participated in the study. "Older men with slow-growing prostate cancer who have chosen watchful waiting over chemotherapy and radiation should seriously consider altering their diets to include more tomatoes and broccoli."

How much would the average guy need? Canene-Adams and Dr. Erdman did the math. A 55-year-old man who's concerned about his prostate health could achieve the same effect as in the study by eating 2.5 cups of fresh tomato, 1 cup of tomato sauce, or half a cup of tomato paste plus 1.4 cups of raw broccoli every day.

One of the study's take-home messages is that whole foods are more effective immune boosters than individual food components. "It's better to eat tomatoes than to take a lycopene supplement," Dr. Erdman says.

SWEET POTATOES: A SMART CHOICE

One vegetable with almost universal appeal is the sweet potato. It's a major source of beta-carotene, the carotenoid your body converts into vitamin A. One of your most important germ barriers—your 16 square feet of skin—depends on vitamin A to maintain its integrity and fend off attacks. "Vitamin A plays a major role in the production of connective tissue, a key component of skin," adds David Katz, MD, director of the Yale-Griffin Prevention Research Center in Derby, Connecticut.

A ½-cup serving of sweet potatoes supplies 2,000 IU of beta-carotene, which equals about 40 percent of the Daily Value of vitamin A (5,000 IU). Just don't smother that nutritious goodness under a thick layer of butter! Other foods rich in beta-carotene include carrots, squash, canned pumpkin, and cantaloupe.

GARLIC AND ONIONS: BODACIOUS GERM-FIGHTING BULBS

James A. Duke, PhD, former chief of the USDA Medicinal Plant Resources Laboratory and author of *The Green Pharmacy*, takes garlic almost daily—both as a supplement and as a food. "There's a clove in my soup, another in my New England boiled cabbage (vegetarian style), and . . . one in my broccoli/carrot/celery juice combo," he writes in the *Wild Foods Forum*.

According to Dr. Duke, raw garlic contains at least 13 different compounds that boost immunity. Its active ingredient is allicin, which fights viruses and bacteria. When British researchers randomly assigned 146 people to take either a garlic extract or placebo for 12 weeks, those in the garlic group caught two-thirds fewer colds. Other studies show that consumption of six or more garlic cloves a week may help reduce the risk of colorectal cancer by 30 percent and the risk of stomach cancer by 50 percent.

In addition to allicin, garlic contains S-allylcysteine, diallyl trisulfide, and diallyl disulfide. All of these compounds help to lower cholesterol and also thin the blood, which may reduce high blood pressure.

You can take advantage of the therapeutic power of garlic, and you probably don't need to eat as much of it as Dr. Duke does. Research suggests that the optimal dose consists of eating two raw cloves a day, plus adding crushed garlic to your food several times a week. "Toss it into your cooking at the very last minute to preserve allicin's beneficial effects," Dr. Weil suggests.

All of the members of the allium family—which includes onions and leeks, as well as garlic—contain large amounts of quercetin, a flavonoid that may enhance immunity. To get the most benefit from onions, try varying Bermudas with flavonoid-rich red and yellow onions, as well as shallots. During cold and flu season, add them to soups, stir-fries, casseroles, and chili for a potent immune boost.

SHOOT DOWN INFECTIONS WITH MUSHROOMS

"Though the science is still developing, some mushrooms appear to prime the immune system," says Susan Percival, PhD, professor of nutritional science at the University of Florida in Gainesville. Mushrooms contain active compounds that boost the production of NK cells. They also are a good source of niacin, a B vitamin that fosters the formation of the enzymes necessary to metabolize fats, convert sugars into energy, and maintain healthy tissues.

Studies show that mushrooms increase the production and activity of white blood cells, making them more aggressive. "This is a good thing when you have an infection," says Douglas Schar, DipPhyt, MCPP, a clinically trained herbalist based in Washington, DC.

Dr. Weil recommends this trio of Asian mushrooms to strengthen immunity and help ward off illness.

- Cordyceps (*Cordyceps sinensis*)—increases the number of T-helper cells and the activity of NK cells; supports the production of lymphocytes

- Zhu ling (*Polyporus umbellatus*)—stimulates lymph and T cells; may help the immune system rebound after chemotherapy and radiation treatment

- Lingzhi (*Ganoderma lucidum*)—also known as reishi; contains compounds such as beta-glucan, a polysaccharide with potent antitumor and immune-stimulating activity, and acidic protein-bound polysaccharide, which has antiherpes activity

Dr. Percival considers shiitake and reishi mushrooms to be the most beneficial; she suggests eating ½ ounce, cooked or raw, at the first sign of cold symptoms and every day until you feel better. Schar identifies the shiitake and maitake varieties as among the most potent. They also are virtually indestructible. "Basically, you can burn them, and they still will powerfully stimulate the immune system," Schar says.

There is no universal recommendation regarding the number of servings of mushrooms per day, so try adding them to meals whenever you can. They're versatile enough to go with just about any dish. One suggestion: "You can cook them with peas, snap peas, green beans, and other vegetables," Galeaz notes.

Fruits: Take Your Pick!

Like vegetables, fruits offer an abundance of immune-boosting nutrients, such as vitamins A, B$_6$, and especially C. They also are good sources of potassium and folate, a B vitamin that helps the body form red blood cells. Because they're plant foods, they contain thousands of different phytonutrients, which means that they can protect immune cells by neutralizing harmful free radicals.

Fruits can be eaten fresh, frozen, canned, or dried. Juice is fine, too, as long as it's 100 percent fruit. As for which fruits are best, well, you have so many options that something is bound to please your palate. Here's just a sampling.

■ Apples	■ Nectarines
■ Apricots	■ Oranges
■ Bananas	■ Papaya
■ Blueberries	■ Peaches
■ Cantaloupe	■ Pears
■ Cherries	■ Pineapple
■ Grapefruit	■ Plums
■ Grapes	■ Prunes
■ Honeydew	■ Raisins
■ Kiwifruit	■ Raspberries
■ Lemons	■ Strawberries
■ Limes	■ Tangerines
■ Mangoes	■ Watermelon

The Immune Essentials Plan calls for at least 1½ cups of fruits per day. In general, people seem more partial to fruits than to vegetables, so eating enough isn't too much of a challenge. Still, if you're looking for ways to pump up your daily fruit consumption, or if you want to make sure you're getting maximum nutrition from your fruit servings, these tips can help.

■ Buy fresh fruits in season. This is when they taste best and their immune-enhancing nutrients are most abundant. They tend to be less expensive, too.

■ Choose products canned in either water or 100 percent fruit juice instead of syrup.

■ Top breakfast cereal with bananas or peaches, and pancakes with blueberries.

■ Check out recipes for meat dishes that include fruit, such as chicken with apricots or mango chutney.

■ Ditch high-calorie desserts in favor of baked apples, pears, and other fruits.

■ Toss a piece or two of whole fruit into your bag before going to work or out on the town. You'll have a healthy snack at your fingertips when hunger strikes.

APPLES: ONE A DAY REALLY COULD KEEP THE DOCTOR AWAY

Apples contain a variety of phytonutrients known as *polyphenols*. The most potent of these is quercetin, a flavonoid that fights oxidative stress and inflammation. Quercetin even might reduce immune suppression in elite athletes with intense training schedules.

To assess the effects of apples and other polyphenol-rich fruits on immune function, German researchers concocted two different super-juices. The first contained apple, mango, and orange juices, as well as anthocyanin-rich chokeberries, blueberries, and boysenberries. The second contained apple, mango, and orange juices, plus flavonoid-rich green tea, apricot, and lime. For 10 weeks, the researchers tracked the juices' immune effects on 27 healthy, nonsmoking men in their midthirties who had low-polyphenol diets. By the end of the study, both juices had produced dramatic increases in the men's antioxidant levels, reduced DNA damage to immune cells, and improved the activity of NK cells. The men also showed increases in interleukin-2, an immune hormone that is essential for fighting infection.

According to the researchers, who reported their findings in the November 2006 issue of the *Journal of Nutrition,* "No clear differences were observed between the two types of juices, suggesting that the observed effects of the fruit compounds are

Best Together: The Synergistic Effects of Vegetables and Fruits

Although vegetables and fruits boost immunity on their own, together they actually may intensify each other's effects.

Studies involving older adults with deteriorating immune systems have shown that eating more fruits and vegetables can dramatically boost immunity. Amazingly, this strategy also works in strapping college students whose immune systems are seemingly as strong as they ever will be.

In 2004, researchers from the University of Florida recruited 59 law students—36 women and 23 men, all healthy nonsmokers who didn't drink to excess and (for the women) weren't pregnant. The researchers randomly assigned the students to take either active capsules containing a fruit and vegetable juice powder made from concentrates of acerola cherry, apple, beet, broccoli, cabbage, carrot, cranberry, kale, orange, peach, papaya, parsley, pineapple, spinach, and tomato—or a placebo.

During the study, 17 members of each group developed one or two illnesses, but symptoms were much less severe for those taking the active capsules. After 11 weeks, blood tests showed that the active-capsule group had 30 percent more circulating B and T cells and 40 percent less DNA damage to immune cells than the placebo group. The researchers attributed the enhanced immune function to significantly higher blood levels of important nutrients such as vitamin C and the carotenoids beta-carotene, lycopene, and lutein.

---

rather unspecific or are caused by compounds [that] were provided by both fruit juices (apple, orange, and mango). Although it is difficult to deduce the biological significance of these physiological changes, one may speculate that these changes contribute over a long period of time to a reduction in the risk of developing common diseases such as cancer and cardiovascular disease."

You'll get the biggest nutritional benefit from apples if you eat the whole fruit, including the peel. Drinking apple juice or cider can be helpful, too. Just beware: Clear apple juice is a relatively poor source of polyphenols. In 2007, researchers from the Agricultural University of Wrocław in Poland published the results of their study comparing clear and cloudy apple juices. The cloudy variety had four times the concentration of polyphenols. Clear apple juice is far more popular with consumers, however—largely because of the mistaken belief that it's "purer" and, therefore, better. It also is favored by retailers because it has a longer shelf life than cloudy juice.

Dairy Products: They Do a Body Good

Mention dairy products, and most people think calcium. It's true that calcium is important for strong bones and teeth. But milk, yogurt, cheese, and other dairy foods have much more to offer nutritionally.

First and foremost, these foods supply protein, which is essential sustenance for every one of your body's cells—including your immune cells. They also are among the best dietary sources of vitamin D, which helps maintain a healthy immune system. (We discuss vitamin D at length beginning on page 122.) Fermented dairy products such as yogurt and kefir (a drinkable form of yogurt) contain large amounts of beneficial bacteria. As you'll see a bit later, these bacteria play a vital role in optimal immune function.

Not all dairy products are healthy choices, however. For example, if you regularly consume whole milk and full-fat yogurt and cheese, you may be taking in large amounts of saturated fat and cholesterol. These raise LDL cholesterol (the "bad" kind) and help set the stage for heart disease. You also may be taking in more calories than you should, which can cause you to gain weight rather than lose or maintain.

By opting for low-fat or fat-free dairy products, you'll get all of the immune-enhancing benefits without elevating your heart disease risk. So be sure to read product labels before buying, and remember what the various terms regarding fat content mean.

- *Reduced-fat* products contain 2 percent fat.

- *Low-fat* products contain 1 percent fat.

- *Fat-free* products contain no fat.

To further help you navigate the dairy terrain, consider this advice.

- Be wary of sweetened dairy products. They contain lots of sugar—and unnecessary calories.

- Steer clear of fruit-flavored yogurt, which also can be loaded with sugar. Instead, mix plain yogurt with fresh blueberries, strawberries, or raspberries, or use your blender to whip up a delicious yogurt-and-fruit smoothie.

- When ordering a cappuccino or latte, ask your server to use fat-free milk instead of whole milk or cream.

- If you're lactose-intolerant, you still can get the immune-enhancing benefits of dairy products by choosing lactase-treated milk or low-lactose products such as yogurt and cheese. Another option is to take supplemental lactase, an enzyme that helps digest lactose, before consuming dairy products.

On the Immune Essentials Plan, you'll be getting about 3 cups of low-fat or fat-free dairy products per day. For cheeses, 1 cup equals 1½ ounces of hard cheese (such as Cheddar, mozzarella, Swiss, or Parmesan) or 2 ounces processed.

PROBIOTICS: PUMMEL BAD BUGS WITH GOOD BUGS

Twenty-four hours a day, there's a struggle going on in your gut that's every bit as fierce as the battle scenes in *Lord of the Rings*—albeit on a microscopic level. It pits millions of bacteria against each other in a classic confrontation of good and evil. At stake is your very health.

You and the good bacteria have a symbiotic relationship. You give them a nice warm place to stay; in return, they help you digest food. They almost never cause any mischief. Just as important, they create a hostile environment for the bad bacteria, which are patiently waiting for the opportunity to cause a nasty gastrointestinal infection—or, possibly, escape into your bloodstream and infect your entire body.

The good bacteria keep the bad ones in check in part simply by overcrowding them. The good bugs also form a physical barrier on your intestinal walls, which prevents the bad bugs from venturing into your bloodstream. Without this barrier, your intestines would not be strong enough to keep the bad bacteria at bay.

Usually, the good guys win. But aging, illness, antibiotics, chronic stress, and poor diet can upset the delicate balance in your gut and allow the bad bugs to take over. When this happens, your gut becomes infected and inflamed—and you're likely to get sick.

Probiotics—the beneficial bacteria in cultured dairy products such as yogurt, acidophilus milk, and kefir (a fermented milk drink)—can restore the delicate balance in your gut, putting the good guys back in charge. This helps prime your immune system to fend off gastrointestinal infections. (It also may help lower cholesterol and inhibit certain cancers.)

The characteristic tart taste of cultured dairy products occurs as bacteria ferment the milk and convert milk sugar into lactic acid. The primary live active culture in yogurt is *Lactobacillus bulgaricus*. Other beneficial strains include *Streptococcus thermophilus* (not to be confused with the bacteria that cause strep throat), *Lactobacillus casei*, *Lactobacillus acidophilus*, and *Bifidobacterium lactis*. Stonyfield Farm yogurt contains six active cultures. Another concentrated culture source is DanActive, a dairy drink made by Dannon.

One recent study by researchers at the University of Vienna in Austria showed that a daily 7-ounce serving of yogurt boosts immunity just as effectively as probiotic supplements. For another study, this one from Sweden, researchers randomly assigned 181 factory workers to drink either a placebo beverage or one containing *Lactobacillus reuteri*—a strain of bacteria that stimulates white blood cells—every day. Over the course of 80 days, the workers in the probiotic group took 33 percent fewer sick days than those in the placebo group.

Still another study, conducted at several daycare centers in Israel, showed that children who received *L. reuteri* had fewer doctor visits and antibiotic prescriptions, shorter bouts of illness, and fewer daycare absences than kids who received *B. lactis*. The only brand of cultured dairy product on the US market that contains *L. reuteri* is Stonyfield Farm.

Regular consumption of probiotics may become even more important with age. Over time, the number of immune cells diminishes and the immune system becomes less responsive to infectious organisms and rogue cancer cells. This decline can start long before you experience a major health crisis.

At Massey University in New Zealand, researchers conducted a study of probiotic therapy involving 30 people between ages 63 and 84—18 women and 12 men, all healthy and living independently. For the first 3 weeks, all of the volunteers drank plain milk twice a day. During the next 2 weeks, they drank milk supplemented with *B. lactis*. For the final 2 weeks, they switched back to plain milk. The researchers found that fortifying milk with *B. lactis* dramatically increased the proportions of total, helper, and activated T cells and stimulated the anticancer activity of NK cells. The most significant improvement in immune function—between 9 and 82 percent— occurred in volunteers who had low immune function before the study began. This suggests that probiotics can help reverse some of the most serious effects of immunosenescence (age-related immune decline).

To maintain a battle-ready immune system, it's best to consume probiotics regularly. The optimal "dosage" is two 7-ounce servings of yogurt daily. Hint: When you open a container of yogurt, don't pour off the clear liquid that forms on top. This is pure whey protein, a rich source of an amino acid called cysteine that converts to glutathione, a potent antioxidant that fortifies cells against viral and bacterial infection.

If you ever happen to get sick enough to require a hospital stay, don't hang up your spoon. As an inpatient, you're at risk for hospital-borne infections such as *Clostridium difficile*—a bug that's difficult to beat with antibiotics but can be tamed with probiotics.

It's worth noting that ounce for ounce, kefir is a more concentrated source of probiotics than yogurt. This fermented milk product has the consistency of drinkable yogurt but contains twice as many good bacteria as plain yogurt. It's also a great source of nutrients. One 8-ounce serving provides more than 30 percent of the calcium and 25 percent of the protein that you need each day. Despite its rich consistency, kefir is a relatively modest 160 calories per serving. If you're taking antibiotics, a daily serving can help replenish the good bacteria that the medication has wiped out. Galeaz recommends low-fat or fat-free Lifeway Kefir, which contains 10 different live and active probiotic bacterial cultures. It comes in 12 flavors, including vanilla, strawberry, peach, and cappuccino.

Lean Proteins: Consider the Sources

Though proteins—which include meats, fish, and poultry as well as dry beans and peas, eggs, nuts, and seeds—get little attention as immune-boosting foods, they nevertheless are essential for a healthy immune system. As mentioned earlier, protein helps nourish all of the body's cells, including the immune cells. Protein foods provide generous amounts of the immune-boosting vitamins B_6 and E, as well as the mineral zinc. These foods also supply other B vitamins such as thiamine, riboflavin, and niacin, which together support the formation of red blood cells and tissues and help maintain a healthy nervous system, and are among the top dietary sources of iron and magnesium.

As with dairy products, you need to be selective about proteins, particularly those from animal sources. Many are high in saturated fat and cholesterol, which raise LDL cholesterol and can help set the stage for heart disease. Whenever possible, choose the leanest cuts available. Here's a sampling of what to look for.

■ Beef—round steaks and roasts (such as eye of round, top round, bottom round, and round tip), top loin, top sirloin, chuck shoulder, and arm roasts

■ Ground beef—should be at least 90 percent lean

■ Pork—pork loin, tenderloin, center loin, and ham

■ Poultry—boneless, skinless chicken breasts; turkey cutlets

To further reduce the fat content of meat and poultry, trim away visible fat before cooking. Also, opt for broiling, grilling, roasting, poaching, or boiling instead of frying. If you do fry, don't use breading. It adds unnecessary calories and soaks up extra fat. Sauces and gravies add fat and calories, too.

The Immune Essentials Plan allows for 5 ounces of lean protein every day. For your reference, all of the following equal 1 ounce.

■ 1 egg

■ 1 tablespoon peanut or almond butter

■ ¼ cup cooked dry beans (such as black, kidney, pinto, or white)

■ ¼ cup tofu

■ ¼ cup cooked dry peas (such as chickpeas, cowpeas, lentils, or split peas)

Can Turkey Tame an Overactive Immune System?

In a classic episode of the TV show *Seinfeld*, Jerry plies a female acquaintance with tryptophan-rich turkey, hoping to knock her out. His not-so-sinister motive: to play with her classic toy collection while she's fast asleep. This could work only in a scripted comedy, not reality TV: Scientists have debunked the notion that turkey causes excessive sleepiness. Tryptophan works on the brain only after it's ingested on an empty stomach. But research does suggest that the amino acid may help treat autoimmune diseases, in which the immune system attacks the body's healthy tissues.

In an animal model of multiple sclerosis (MS), researchers from Stanford University Medical Center found that certain tryptophan metabolites—molecules formed as the body breaks down tryptophan—suppress what is the hallmark of MS: an assault by the immune system on the myelin sheath, the layer of fatty cells that protect nerve cells. This natural intervention appears to work as well as some MS medications. The results of the study—published in a 2005 issue of the journal *Science*—suggest that tryptophan triggers the production of regulatory T cells that inhibit inflammation.

Further research is necessary to determine whether tryptophan can be beneficial for humans with MS. For now, the researchers say, it's uncertain how much turkey you'd need to eat to achieve a similar therapeutic effect.

THE BIG O: OMEGA-3 FATTY ACIDS

Fish and shellfish have become a staple of popular diet plans, and with good reason: They're the best dietary sources of the omega-3 fatty acids eicosapentaenoic acid (EPA) and docosahexaenoic acid (DHA). In studies, omega-3s have helped prevent or treat a remarkable array of health concerns, including heart disease, asthma, Crohn's disease, depression, and rheumatoid arthritis. These beneficial fats also support a healthy immune system.

In 2005, a team of British researchers studied the relationship between fat consumption and immune function in 150 people. Those who consumed the most omega-3 fatty acids had the highest levels of flu-fighting T cells and gamma-interferon. Other research suggests that omega-3s can help ward off colds and flu by reducing lung inflammation and increasing airflow.

Unfortunately, most Americans aren't getting enough omega-3 fatty acids in their diets to reap all of the health benefits. In 2003, per capita fish consumption was just 16.3 pounds in the United States, significantly less than in many other countries. Complicating matters is the fact that we're getting too few omega-3s and too many omega-6s, the fatty acids found in meats, dairy products, eggs, and seed oils. Although both fatty acids are vital to human health (which is why they're known as essential fatty acids), our overreliance on omega-6s may contribute to inflammation, immune dysfunction, and a greater risk of infection and cancer.

In late 2006, researchers from the Harvard School of Public Health reported new findings from the Physicians' Health Study, which tracked the health status and habits of more than 20,000 male physicians. After evaluating data from the study, the researchers concluded that the men who ate fish at least five times a week were 40 percent less likely to develop colorectal cancer than the men who ate fish less than once a week.

Other research has shown that women who consume lots of fish may reduce their risk of renal cell carcinoma—the most common form of kidney cancer—by 44 percent. "We already know that eating fish can reduce the risk of sudden cardiac death," says study author Megan Phillips, of Harvard. "This might provide another reason to add fish to your diet."

Although fish and shellfish are excellent sources of omega-3 fatty acids, certain

What about Mercury in Fish?

In 2004, the FDA and the Environmental Protection Agency (EPA) issued an advisory for pregnant and nursing women, prospective moms, and young children to avoid shark, swordfish, king mackerel, and tilefish. The reason: These species may contain unsafe levels of mercury. The FDA also suggested that pregnant women restrict themselves to 12 ounces of fish a week.

The advisory didn't address any other segments of the population. In fact, it commented on the wide-ranging health benefits of eating fish: "Fish and shellfish contain high-quality protein and other essential nutrients, are low in saturated fat, and contain omega-3 fatty acids. A well-balanced diet that includes a variety of fish and shellfish can contribute to heart health and children's proper growth and development."

But these positive statements were lost in the ensuing media frenzy over mercury, which prompted many Americans to cut back on fish—and, in some cases, eliminate it from their diets. In 2005, researchers from the prestigious Harvard Center for Risk Analysis tried to put the issue into scientific perspective with a five-part series of review articles in the *American Journal of Preventive Medicine.* Their key finding: Reducing fish consumption nationwide would lead to more heart attacks and strokes, while increasing fish consumption would have the opposite effect. The modest health risk associated with mercury was far outweighed by the potential health benefits of omega-3s.

"Although some mercury is present in most fish, the levels tend to be so low that most people don't need to worry about it," says Floyd Chilton, PhD, professor of physiology and pharmacology at Wake Forest University School of Medicine, in his book *Inflammation Nation.* "If you're pregnant or nursing, if you're trying to conceive, or if you have young children, follow the FDA and EPA guidelines to reduce but not eliminate fish consumption."

species also are high in arachidonic acid, an inflammatory fatty acid. So choosing the right fish and shellfish is critical, according to Floyd Chilton, PhD, professor in the department of physiology and pharmacology at Wake Forest University School of Medicine in Winston-Salem, North Carolina, and author of *Inflammation Nation*. Dr. Chilton's research shows that many popular varieties of fish—including some commonly thought to be healthy, such as halibut and farm-raised Atlantic salmon—actually contain so much arachidonic acid that eating them may have more health risks than benefits.

In his book, Dr. Chilton recommends about three servings a week of what he identifies as "Category 1: Best Fish," meaning they contain an extremely high ratio of omega-3 fatty acids to arachidonic acid. This category includes European anchovies, Atlantic or Pacific herring, Atlantic or Pacific mackerel, wild Chinook salmon, and wild sockeye salmon. "Category 2: Good Fish" refers to a lower but still acceptable ratio of omega-3s to arachidonic acid. For fish in this group—which include wild pink salmon, Greenland halibut, wild coho salmon, Alaskan king crab, blue crab, shrimp, wild and farmed oysters, mussels, sea bass, and white tuna—Dr. Chilton recommends four servings a week. (One serving equals 4 ounces.)

SAY SOY-O-NARA TO GERMS AND CANCER

Soybeans and other legumes are rich in isoflavones, a subclass of flavonoids that includes daidzein, genistein, and glycitein. Isoflavones may be best known as phytoestrogens because they have mild estrogen-like effects (though they're far weaker than natural estrogen). These phytonutrients also are potent antioxidants with the potential to fortify resistance to infectious disease. Laboratory animals that were fed a genistein-rich diet showed improvement in their immune response, while in humans, a high-soy diet appeared to increase the activity of NK cells.

In 2006, researchers from Washington State University in Pullman published a study in the *American Journal of Clinical Nutrition*, showing that soy boosts immunity in postmenopausal women. The 16-week, double-blind, placebo-controlled trial tracked 52 healthy, mostly white women between ages 50 and 65, who were randomly assigned to one of three groups. The first group drank 706 milliliters of soy milk containing 71.6 milligrams of isoflavones every day, the second drank the same amount of cow's milk with 70 milligrams of isoflavones, and the third drank cow's milk and took a placebo supplement. The researchers instructed all of the women to not eat any soy products during the study.

The women who drank soy milk and the women who drank cow's milk with isoflavones had significantly higher urine levels of isoflavones—a marker of high concentrations of these compounds in the body—than the women who served as controls. In fact, their levels were similar to those found in Asians and other ethnic groups who eat large amounts of soy.

But the most dramatic finding was that soy—either in milk or in supplement form—significantly increased the proportion of B cells in the immune arsenal. B cells produce antibodies that are released into the bloodstream for the sole purpose of attacking and destroying a specific target, such as a flu virus. A high proportion of B cells indicates that the immune system is alert and ready for action.

In the women who drank cow's milk with a placebo, the percentage of B cells held steady, starting at 8.5 percent and ending at 8.6 percent. In the women who drank soy milk, the percentage jumped from 8.1 percent to 11.3 percent. The B-cell population grew even more in the women who drank cow's milk with supplemental isoflavones, rising from 8.5 percent to 12.2 percent. In addition, both of the isoflavone groups showed much lower levels of 8-hydroxy-2-deoxyguanosine, an important indicator of DNA damage. "These findings suggest a protective effect of soy isoflavones regarding oxidative stress in postmenopausal women," the study's authors conclude.

Interestingly, the effects of soy appear to vary with age. In postmenopausal women, the antioxidant activity may be more important than the estrogen-like activity. In premenopausal women, however, the estrogen-like activity may profoundly influence breast cancer risk.

In late 2006, Larissa Korde, MD, of the National Cancer Institute, presented the findings of a soy study at the annual meeting of the American Association for Cancer Research. Dr. Korde and her colleagues had intensively examined the diets and lifestyles of 1,563 Asian American women, 597 of whom had breast cancer and 966 of whom did not. The results were startling. The women who had eaten the most soy as children (a little more than two servings of tofu, miso, or natto a week) were 58 percent less likely to develop breast cancer than the women who had eaten the least soy (about one-quarter of a serving a week). Similarly, those who ate the most soy as adolescents and adults had a 25 percent lower risk than those who ate the least.

"This is the first study to look at childhood soy exposure and the later risk of breast cancer," Dr. Korde says. "It suggests that there really is a biologic effect for soy, and we're excited about that. The hypothesis is that exposure to estrogen-like substances early in life can cause changes in developing breast tissue that decreases its sensitivity to carcinogenesis later in life."

Although soy remains a relative rarity on menus in Western countries, it's a dietary staple in Asian countries, where the breast cancer rate is about four to seven times lower than in the United States. When Asians immigrate to the United States and their families gradually adopt Western diets, their breast cancer rates usually match those of whites within several generations.

Still, Dr. Korde cautions, it's too soon to advise American women and girls to make a wholesale switch to soy as a staple for the sole purpose of reducing breast cancer risk. In the meantime, a serving or two per day could be beneficial for immune function. If you'd like to incorporate more soy into your diet, consider using precooked soy crumbles as a meat substitute in chili, spaghetti sauce, and tacos.

Beyond the Basics

By focusing your meals on the five food groups, you'll cover your body's nutritional bases and provide your immune system with the necessary raw materials to fend off illness. The Immune Essentials Plan will get you on your way, with immune-enhancing menus that provide for three hearty meals plus one satisfying snack each day.

But there's more in the immune arsenal than the five food groups. In fact, a few of the following ancillary immune-boosters may surprise you. If you're looking to give your immune system an extra kick, you might want to keep these in mind.

Be Fluent in Fluids

Although plain water contains no antioxidants or other immune-enhancing compounds, it nevertheless is essential for optimal immune function. Proper hydration keeps your mucous membranes supple and swimming with disease-fighting antibodies such as immunoglobulin A. It also keeps you alert, makes your skin glow, and helps protect you against diseases from kidney stones to cancer. It even helps you lose weight.

If you're not taking in enough fluids, however, your mucous membranes could dry out and become more susceptible to bacteria and viruses. What's more, dehydration forces cells to suck fluids from your bloodstream, leaving your blood thick and sludgy. As your heart works harder to pump the thicker blood through your arteries and veins, it can set the stage for fatigue. Even if you aren't thirsty, you may not be properly hydrated. The average woman drinks just 4.7 cups of water-based beverages—including juice, soda, and coffee—each day.

For many years, the standard recommendation for fluid intake was eight to ten 8-ounce glasses per day. This changed in 2004, when the Institute of Medicine of the National Academy of Sciences issued new hydration guidelines. For women ages 19 to 70-plus, the institute recommends a total of $11\frac{1}{2}$ cups of water a day, with beverages accounting for at least 9 cups and the rest coming from foods. For men in the same age range, the suggested intake is 16 cups of water, with beverages accounting for at least 13 cups.

The institute defines "beverage" as any nonalcoholic drink—even tea and coffee. Recent evidence shows that caffeine's diuretic effect is transitory and does not cause dehydration. (We'll talk more about the immune-enhancing effects of tea and coffee in the next section.) To make sure that you're getting the fluids your body, and your immune system, needs:

- Drink a beverage with every meal and snack.
- Eat those fruits and veggies. Besides being chock-full of nutrients, most produce is made up of 80 to 90 percent water.
- Don't wait until you're thirsty to drink; you could be mildly dehydrated by then. Keep water bottles with you—in your car, at your desk, in your bag—and take frequent sips throughout the day.
- Check the temperature. In studies, people tend to drink more when fluids are lukewarm rather than very cold or very hot.
- If the taste of plain water doesn't appeal to you, try flavoring it with a slice of lemon or lime.

How can you tell if you're getting enough water? When you wake up in the morning and use the bathroom, check the color of your urine. If it's dark yellow, then you need to increase your fluid intake.

Proper hydration is especially important when you engage in exercise, whether it's moderate or vigorous in intensity. In fact, the combination of dehydration and vigorous activity can increase your susceptibility to colds and flu, one of the main reasons that marathoners often get sick after a race. Elite competitive athletes should consider getting their liquid refreshment from a sports drink instead of plain water. In a 2005 study of 15 triathletes, published in the *International Journal of Sport Nutrition and Exercise Metabolism,* those who drank 1 cup of sports drink every 15 minutes during vigorous exercise showed a stronger immune response than those who drank a placebo beverage.

Coffee, Tea . . . Immunity?

It's a good thing both tea and coffee count toward your daily fluid quota, since both beverages contribute to healthy immune function.

For its part, tea of all kinds is packed with enzymes that help flush toxins from your body, plus polyphenols that protect cells against free radical damage. Over the years, many studies have linked drinking tea to a reduced risk of certain cancers. In the December 2005 issue of the *Archives of Internal Medicine,* for example, researchers published a study showing that women who regularly drank 2 or more cups of any kind of tea per day were 46 percent less likely to develop ovarian cancer than women who drank little or none. Each additional cup of tea a day correlated to an 18 percent drop in ovarian cancer risk.

Because tea significantly raises blood levels of antioxidants, it may help protect against colds and flu. In a study that appeared in the May 2003 issue of the *Proceedings of the National Academy of Sciences,* people who drank 3 cups of black tea a day had five times the number of certain immune cells as people who drank coffee.

Meanwhile, Harvard University researchers found that people who drank 5 cups of black tea every day for 2 weeks had 10 times as much virus-fighting interferon in their blood as people who drank a placebo beverage. The researchers attributed this effect to L-theanine, an amino acid in both black and green teas.

Black and green teas aren't the only varieties that enhance immune function. In 2005, researchers from Imperial College in London published a study in which people who drank 5 cups of chamomile tea every day for 2 weeks had much higher blood levels of polyphenols associated with antibacterial activity. The researchers also noted a rise in blood levels of glycine, a mild nerve relaxant and sedative—confirming chamomile's reputation as a sleep-inducing herb.

Even gargling with tea seems to offer some benefit. Japanese researchers found that people who gargled twice a day with black tea extract were less likely to catch the flu.

But the disease-fighting potential may be diminished—or even eliminated—with the addition of milk, according to a study that appeared in the January 2007 issue of the *European Heart Journal.* Using ultrasound, German researchers measured blood vessel function in 16 healthy postmenopausal women who drank either ½ liter of plain black tea, black tea with 10 percent fat-free milk, or plain boiled water. Compared with plain water, plain black tea significantly improved endothelial function—that is, the ability of the arteries to relax and expand. But the tea with milk had no such effect. The researchers determined that casein, a protein component in milk, reduced the concentration of catechins, the flavonoids in tea that help protect against cardiovascular disease.

"Our results thus provide a possible explanation for the lack of beneficial effects of tea on the risk of heart disease in the UK, a country where milk is usually added [to tea]," according to Verena Stangl, MD, the study's lead researcher. "Since milk appears to modify the biological activities of tea ingredients, it is likely that the antitumor effects of tea could be affected as well. I think it is essential that we reexamine the association between tea consumption and cancer protection to see if [this] is the case."

Keep in mind that tea without milk or sugar is a zero-calorie beverage, so you can drink as much as you want. "There's no reason you shouldn't drink at least 1 cup of tea per day—and many good reasons that you should," Galeaz says. Actually, you may want to aim for several cups a day during cold and flu season. Just be careful not to drink caffeinated tea too close to bedtime, as it could keep you from falling asleep.

Here's another hint: By bobbing the tea bag up and down in your cup, you'll dissolve far more of the tea and get up to five times as many antioxidants. Leaving the bag in the cup may be a breech of etiquette in some quarters, but it will net you a much bigger nutrient boost.

Though tea seems to be getting the lion's share of research attention, coffee can claim its own immune-enhancing properties—as long as it's without cream or sugar. "Green" coffee contains about 1,000 different antioxidants; roasting the beans adds another 300. According to some studies, coffee contains four times as many antioxidants as green tea. (Robusta varieties have twice as many antioxidants as arabica.)

The most fascinating research about coffee involves its protective effects against type 2 diabetes. Though the causes of this disease are complex, researchers believe that immune-mediated inflammation could be a major culprit. In one recent study, Finnish researchers concluded that men and women who drink 3 to 4 cups of coffee per day are 27 to 29 percent less likely to develop type 2 diabetes than those who drink none. But it has nothing to do with caffeine. The researchers believe that the effect may be due to coffee's high antioxidant content, which could help protect insulin-producing beta cells in the pancreas from free radical damage. The researchers also singled out another compound: chlorogenic acid, found in coffee as well as red wine and chocolate. In animal studies, chlorogenic acid appears to lower blood sugar levels.

Another study, published in a 2006 issue of the *Annals of Internal Medicine*, analyzed lifestyle data collected from 29,000 older women over the course of 11 years. After adjusting for other factors, the researchers concluded that women who drank at least 6 cups of any type of coffee per day were 22 percent less likely to develop diabetes than women who drank no coffee. Diabetes risk was 33 percent lower for women who drank the same amount of decaf.

The one major caveat with coffee is that its caffeine can disrupt your sleep, which in turn suppresses your immune system. To avoid trouble, stick with caffeine-free foods and beverages after 2:00 p.m. According to the National Institutes of Health, a moderate intake of caffeine—the equivalent of three 8-ounce cups a day, supplying a total of 250 milligrams of caffeine—does not appear to have any health risks.

Red Wine: A Toast to Better Health

If you drink red wine within the guidelines established by the FDA—no more than one 5-ounce glass a day for women, no more than two glasses a day for men—you may reduce your risk of certain infectious diseases and cancers. You also may be less vulnerable to health problems such as diabetes and Alzheimer's disease. If the findings of animal studies hold true, a specific compound in red wine could improve your endurance and extend your life span.

The compound is resveratrol, a polyphenol found beneath grape skins. (Red wine contains more resveratrol than white because the skin stays on longer during the fermentation process.) In 2006, researchers from the Institute of Genetics and Molecular and Cellular Biology in Illkirch, France, published the findings of a study in which they had fed large amounts of resveratrol to obese mice with an animal model of type 2 diabetes. The researchers found that resveratrol activated the enzyme SIRT1, which in turn stimulated mitochondria, the "energy factories" inside cells.

Because increased mitochondrial activity contributes to improved muscle performance, the mice were able to run twice as long on their treadmills as they previously could. These findings suggest that resveratrol could protect against fat accumulation and type 2 diabetes in humans. They also suggest that the compound might play a role in treating neurological diseases that would benefit from increased mitochondrial activity, such as Parkinson's and Huntington's.

There's a catch, however: The amount of resveratrol used in the study far exceeds the amount available in red wine or even supplements. To get the same benefits, you would need to drink hundreds of glasses of wine or take hundreds of pills each day, researchers say.

Still, red wine contains other compounds that offer a variety of immune-boosting, disease-fighting benefits. For example, researchers from Oregon State University in Corvallis found that wine—especially red wine—inhibits three common food-borne pathogens: *Escherichia coli*, *Listeria*, and *Salmonella*. Its combination of immune-enhancing compounds, alcohol, and low pH appears to scramble the genetic material of these bugs, which are common causes of food poisoning.

Another research team, this one from Université Laval in Quebec, conducted a test-tube study in which the polyphenols in red wine appeared to inhibit the bacterial inflammation associated with gingivitis and periodontitis. This is significant because chronic gum infections not only weaken gums and teeth, they also contribute to heart disease. According to the American Association for Dental Research, periodontitis—the most severe form of gum disease—affects 15 percent of Americans between ages 21 and 50 and 65 percent of adults over age 50.

Meanwhile, researchers from the State University of New York at Stony Brook found a correlation between red wine consumption and colorectal cancer risk. Their study involved a total of 1,741 people—245 red-wine drinkers, 115 white-wine drinkers, and 1,381 abstainers. The incidence of colorectal neoplasia—which includes cancers and polyps that can become cancerous—was 68 percent lower in those who drank at least three glasses of red wine a week.

Not all red wines contain equal amounts of immune-enhancing compounds. A 2006 study published in the journal *Nature* by researchers from Queen Mary's School of Medicine and Dentistry in London showed that red wine from France and

Sardinia—countries where traditional winemaking still is practiced—have procyanidin levels that are five to 10 times higher than those of red wines from other countries. The researchers suggest that French and Sardinian wines may have an especially protective effect on blood vessels.

Of course, while a moderate amount of red wine may be beneficial, too much of any form of alcohol could do more harm than good. In excess, alcohol suppresses immune function, including the production of B cells that make antibodies. This could increase your susceptibility to infections such as bacterial pneumonia, tuberculosis, and hepatitis C. Some studies suggest that even moderate alcohol consumption may increase breast cancer risk in women.

The bottom line is this: If you don't already consume alcohol, then don't start. A healthy diet and moderate exercise will do far more to enhance your immunity than a glass of Cabernet Sauvignon. Besides, a single glass of vino supplies 120 calories, at minimum. You don't want to give up other immune-boosting foods to make room for alcohol in your diet.

"It's your personal choice if you want to have a glass of red wine a day," Galeaz says, "but you certainly should not exceed that." Likewise, you shouldn't drink any alcohol if you have a health condition such as liver disease, depression, high blood pressure, or congestive heart failure—all of which can become worse with alcohol consumption. Needless to say, it's extremely risky for those who are in recovery to have even a small amount of alcohol.

The Bright Side of Dark Chocolate

Red wine isn't the only dietary indulgence with an immunity connection. Dark chocolate containing at least 70 percent cocoa is a concentrated source of flavonoids and procyanidins, phytonutrients that help safeguard immune cells and reduce inflammation. Dark chocolate also contains impressive amounts of magnesium and fiber.

Much of the research to date has focused on the relationship between dark chocolate and heart disease. In 2006, for example, researchers from the National Institute for Public Health and the Environment in Bilthoven, the Netherlands, published the results of a 15-year study involving 470 men between ages 65 and 84. The men who regularly ate or drank cocoa had significantly lower blood pressure than those who didn't. They also were half as likely to die from heart disease and significantly less likely to die from any cause during the course of the study. The reduction in risk remained significant even after the researchers adjusted for other lifestyle factors such as smoking, weight, calorie intake, physical activity, and alcohol consumption.

According to the researchers, the lower blood pressure was not responsible for the lower death rate. Instead, this benefit most likely had something to do with the

Feed a Cold, Starve a Fever

This traditional maxim, uttered by millions of mothers over the millennia, may be true. Preliminary research suggests that short-term fluctuations in diet really could modulate your immune status.

In a small study, researchers from the Academic Medical Center in Amsterdam, the Netherlands, tested the blood levels of chemical messengers called cytokines in six volunteers who ate a meal after fasting. Eating caused levels of the cytokine gamma interferon to spike by 450 percent. This particular cytokine is responsible for prompting the immune system to produce white blood cells that destroy infected cells.

Fasting, on the other hand, reduced levels of gamma interferon while increasing levels of another cytokine called interleukin-4. This cytokine stimulates the immune system to brandish its most lethal weapon: infection-fighting antibodies that target specific viruses and bacteria.

So feeding a cold and starving a fever may make sense, the researchers say, because colds tend to be less serious, longer-lasting infections, while fevers are signs of severe, swift-acting infection. But more research is necessary before this bit of folk wisdom wins acceptance as medical fact.

---

large amount of antioxidants in chocolate, which helped protect the men's blood vessels from oxidative stress.

Other recent research has shown that chocolate improves vascular function by relaxing blood vessels, which prevents cholesterol from forming plaque and reduces the risk of blood clots that lead to heart attack and stroke. In 2006, researchers from Johns Hopkins University School of Medicine in Baltimore announced the findings of their study involving 139 chocolate lovers who had been excluded from another trial because they kept sneaking treats. The chocolate eaters' blood platelets took significantly longer to clump together—130 seconds, on average, versus 123 seconds for a control group.

Because even dark chocolate delivers a hefty load of calories, sugar, and fat, most nutrition experts caution against eating more than 1 ounce per day. You can get many of the same immune-boosting nutrients from less energy-dense food sources, including green tea, black tea, and coffee.

The Immune Essentials Plan makes room for 1 ounce of dark chocolate as an occasional snack. Steer clear of milk chocolate, which contains fewer flavonoids but more saturated fat than dark chocolate. In human studies, only dark chocolate has consistently shown health benefits.

Key #2—Exercise: Keep It Moderate and Consistent

Immune Rx: Aim for 30 to 60 Minutes of Moderate Aerobic Activity Most Days—Preferably Every Day—Plus at Least 10 Minutes of Strength Training Most Days

As a health-conscious person, you likely are aware of the multitude of physical and psychological benefits that accrue with regular exercise. Now you can add "enhanced immune function" to the list.

"Your immune cells are like cops," explains David Nieman, PhD, professor of health and exercise science at Appalachian State University in Boone, North Carolina. "When you're sedentary, they sit in their station, which in this case is lymph tissue. Within minutes after you start exercising and for a few hours afterward, they leave the station and patrol throughout your body."

Moderate exercise—such as 30 to 60 minutes of walking at about 3½ miles per hour—triggers many hormonal and immunological reactions. For example, it increases blood levels of the stress hormone epinephrine, which in turn recruits natural killer (NK) cells—a type of white blood cell that springs into action before the rest of the immune system—into the bloodstream. Epinephrine also calls upon T cells and B cells, though they aren't quite as active.

This changes with vigorous exercise, as the blood levels of stress hormones climb even higher—the result of microscopic damage to muscle and other tissue. In response to the elevated stress hormones, the number and activity of circulating NK, T, and B cells escalate as well. But too much of a good thing, well, isn't such a good thing. If a vigorous workout lasts longer than 90 minutes, it floods the body with so many stress hormones that they actually suppress immune function, increasing the likelihood of infection. (We'll talk more about the adverse effects of too-vigorous exercise a bit later.)

After any workout, immune cell levels return to normal within several hours. But overall, the immune system is just a little bit stronger. The longer and more consistently you exercise, the greater the benefits you'll experience. If you continue exercising into your fifties, sixties, seventies, or beyond, you'll be significantly less likely to develop infections or chronic illnesses such as heart disease, diabetes, and certain cancers. You also will be less likely to become disabled.

Of course, we've just barely scratched the surface in discussing all the good that regular exercise can do. It helps maintain healthy bones, joints, and muscles. It improves endurance, flexibility, and energy level. It enhances mood and cognitive function. In short, exercise is an immunity elixir that preserves your muscle as well as your marbles.

In this chapter, we'll explore how regular exercise fortifies you against infectious and chronic illness, improves your overall health, and sets the stage for a long and vital life. We also will cover the basics of an immune-boosting fitness regimen, the details of which we'll present in the 4-week Immune Essentials Plan that begins on page 149.

Exercise Fights Fat

Along with proper diet, regular exercise can help melt away unwanted extra pounds. Why are we talking about weight loss when our goal is optimal immune function? Because studies have linked overweight and obesity to suppressed immunity. In other words, carrying even a few too many pounds can leave you more susceptible to infections. It also raises your risk of chronic illnesses such as heart disease and diabetes, in part because fat stores secrete inflammatory substances that injure internal organs as well as the linings of coronary arteries.

Most experts agree that a minimum of 30 to 60 minutes of moderate exercise most days of the week—preferably every day—is necessary to lose weight and enhance immunity. More than half of American adults aren't active enough to meet even the minimum standard for physical activity set by government health agencies: 30 minutes of moderate-intensity exercise most days of the week. Studies show that only about 25 percent of American adults get enough exercise to realize any true health benefits and that 20 percent of the population don't exercise at all.

The remaining 55 percent of the population follow an on-again, off-again exercise pattern, which has a strong connection to yo-yo dieting and frequent weight fluctuations. The more often you lose and then regain weight, the more it could affect your immunity, according to researchers at the Fred Hutchinson Cancer Research Center in Seattle. Their research identified a correlation between frequent gains and losses of 10 or more pounds and diminished activity of NK cells, one of the primary defenders against viruses.

Not surprisingly, people who are sedentary are more likely to be overweight or obese. In 2006, the *Journal of the American Medical Association* published some alarming statistics from the Centers for Disease Control and Prevention (CDC) about the looming weight crisis in the United States. CDC researchers had found that 66.3 percent of American adults are overweight, and of these, 32 percent are obese. Perhaps even more disconcerting, 5 percent of American adults are morbidly obese, meaning they're at least 100 pounds beyond their ideal weight.

If you weigh more than you should, even modest weight loss can help improve your immune status. A 2006 study, also published in the *Journal of the American Medical Association,* examined the effects of exercise and calorie restriction in 48 overweight men and women (average age 38). The researchers determined that exercise—in conjunction with a diet that reduced daily calorie intake by 12.5 percent—led to an average weight loss of at least 10 percent over 6 months. The exercise-and-diet regimen also inhibited DNA fragmentation, a sign of free radical damage. The researchers concluded that such a regimen may protect against acute and chronic disease and possibly increase longevity.

Have you ever noticed that you're more likely to get sick when you're trying to slim down? Weight loss suppresses the activity of NK cells, which is why many dieters come down with a cold or the flu. But, according to a study from Temple University in Philadelphia, light to moderate aerobic exercise and resistance training appears to preserve immune function while you're cutting calories.

Exercise Thwarts Infectious Disease

Multiple studies have shown that regular exercisers are more likely to stay healthy even during cold and flu season. When Dr. Nieman and his colleagues placed 150 people on a 12-week walking program, the walkers caught 50 percent fewer colds and sore throats than a less-active control group. Another study found that people who walked briskly for 12 to 15 weeks took only half as many sick days as those who were sedentary. And in a 2006 study conducted by researchers from the University of South Carolina, men who got 3 hours of moderate physical activity per week—the equivalent of walking briskly, climbing stairs, or playing tennis—were 35 percent less likely to catch a cold.

If you weigh more than you should, moderate exercise can help counter the immune-suppressing effects of those extra pounds, according to a 2006 study published in the *American Journal of Medicine.* For this study, Hutchinson Center researchers recruited 115 exercise-averse women in their early sixties, all of whom were overweight and postmenopausal. The researchers assigned 53 women to engage in moderate exercise such as brisk walking for 30 minutes a day, 5 days a week. The remaining 62 women attended a 45-minute stretching class once a week.

The researchers tracked the women for a year. At first, the exercisers caught only half as many colds as the stretchers, who served as the control group. The protective effect increased over time. During the final 3 months of the study, the exercise group caught only one-third as many colds as the control group. Although both groups developed the flu with about the same frequency, the researchers attributed this to a lower rate of flu vaccination among the exercisers than among the stretchers (23 percent versus 42 percent).

Even short-term moderate exercise may help prevent colds, if the findings of an animal study bear out for humans. For the study, which appeared in a 2003 issue of the *American Journal of Physiology—Regulatory, Integrative and Comparative Physiology,* researchers from the University of South Carolina tracked four groups of mice. The first group spent 20 minutes on a treadmill every day and received plain water. The second group also exercised on a treadmill, plus they received a liquid supplement of beta-glucan, a soluble fiber from oats that may help enhance immune function. The other two groups were the mouse equivalent of couch potatoes, remaining sedentary for the duration of the study; one group received water, while the other received beta-glucan. (In case you're wondering, all of the mice also received their regular chow!)

After 6 days, the researchers sprayed a respiratory virus—herpes simplex virus type 1—into the mice's nostrils to simulate how colds spread in humans. Only 13 percent of the active mice developed infections, compared with 58 percent of the couch-potato mice. To the researchers' surprise, the beta-glucan didn't appear to provide any extra protection against the virus.

Only about 8 percent of the active mice died during the course of the study; for them, the beta-glucan didn't have any effect on mortality. On the other hand, the supplement did seem to help the sedentary mice defy death. Only 33 percent of those given beta-glucan died, compared with 46 percent of those given plain water.

When the researchers looked more closely under the microscope to see what was going on, they found that the active mice had significantly stronger immune systems. Although these mice showed only slight increases in NK cell activity, compared with the control mice, they had dramatically higher viral resistance. All of this suggests that more complex creatures—such as us humans—could expect to see a quick immune boost from starting a moderate exercise program.

But don't stop eating your oatmeal! Although beta-glucan offered no additional protective effects in this particular study, the researchers believe that the compound deserves further study. In previous research, beta-glucan has stimulated important infection-fighting immune cells such as NK cells, neutrophils, and macrophages.

Exercise Reduces Cancer Risk

Perhaps one of the most compelling benefits of moderate exercise is its ability to protect against certain cancers. Though much of the supporting research is epidemiological in nature—in other words, it tracks certain populations to find correlations between behaviors and outcomes—the findings are worth mentioning here.

For example, when one research team tracked 1,806 women for 11 years, they found that moderately active women were 50 percent less likely to develop breast cancer than those who were inactive. Some women fulfilled their weekly exercise quota through everyday tasks such as gardening and yard work. More vigorous activity had an even greater effect: Women who ran, swam, or played tennis at least once a week were 80 percent less likely to develop breast cancer.

Exercise can be such a potent immune stimulant that it may help protect against lung cancer in women smokers. When researchers from the University of Pennsylvania's Center for Clinical Epidemiology and Biostatistics (CCEB) in Philadelphia analyzed data collected from 36,410 older women, they concluded that the smokers who were physically active were 35 percent less likely to develop lung cancer than sedentary smokers. Of course, quitting smoking reduces lung cancer risk most of all. The good news for those trying to kick the habit: Exercise increases the chances of succeeding.

Even for those already diagnosed with cancer, exercise can be beneficial both during and after treatment. In November 2006, the American Cancer Society released its newly updated guidelines regarding diet and exercise for cancer patients. Among its key recommendations: As little as 1 to 3 hours of exercise per week can significantly reduce the chances of a recurrence.

Exercise and the Aging Immune System

Immune function usually peaks in early adulthood, then steadily declines. But exercise can help reverse this trend. Even if you're 65 or older, moderate exercise can boost your immunity by improving the function of infection-fighting T cells and increasing production of immunoglobulin A (IgA), the antibody that protects mucous membranes. It also can improve the immune system's response to influenza vaccinations, which means that you're less likely to catch the flu, a common viral infection that claims thousands of lives each year.

The longer you engage in regular exercise, the greater its benefits. Numerous studies confirm that exercise can extend a person's healthy years deep into old age. In both men and women, long-term exercise is associated with a reduced risk of death from any cause at any age.

Yet only two-thirds of people age 65 and older—and fewer than half of those older than 75—engage in any leisure-time physical activity, according to a report published in July 2006 by the nonprofit Center for the Advancement of Health. The report advises older adults to work up to 30 minutes of exercise 5 days a week, with a focus on activities such as walking, swimming, and bicycling, which improve balance, strength, and flexibility. The report also recommends two strength-training sessions per week. The American Academy of Family Physicians seconds this opinion, recommending at least 30 minutes of aerobic activity almost every day, plus 20 minutes of strength training 2 days a week.

As older adults ease into their fitness routines, it restores balance to their immune systems, which in turn are better able to fend off viruses and bacteria. For a 2005 study published in the *Journal of Strength and Conditioning Research,* Japanese researchers compared the effects of a single 30-minute bout of exercise on a treadmill in two groups of women in their early sixties. The first group had participated in a recreational walking program for 4 years, logging 3 to 5 kilometers (about 2 to 3 miles) every day and 10 kilometers (about 6 miles) every Saturday. The second group of women had been sedentary. For the treadmill test, both groups exercised at 70 to 75 percent of VO_2 max, which is the maximum amount of oxygen (in milliliters) that the body can use in 1 minute per kilogram of body weight.

After the treadmill test, the women who had been sedentary showed higher NK cell counts but lower cell activity than the women who had been active. The net effect: diminished immunity. This finding confirms that for boosting immunity, consistency of exercise is important. "The results of our study indicate that daily exercise may enhance the natural immunity of elderly people, even if they initiated their exercise [programs] only a few years earlier," the authors conclude.

No matter how old you are, it's never too late to start a fitness routine. For a 2006 study published in the *Journal of Gerontology: Medical Sciences,* researchers from the University of Florida in Gainesville recruited 424 adults between ages 80 and 89. All of the participants had been sedentary, which the authors defined as exercising less than 20 minutes per week. Although the participants needed to be fit enough to walk about one-quarter mile in 15 minutes without sitting or using an assistive device such as a cane, all of them had low scores on three physical-performance assessments: walking speed, balance, and ability to get out of a chair.

For the study, half of the men and women enrolled in a supervised exercise program with an emphasis on endurance, strengthening, flexibility, and balance. The remainder, who composed the control group, attended a "successful aging" education program that addressed general health issues and included instructor-led flexibility exercises.

After 6 and 12 months, the exercisers performed significantly better on all three physical-performance assessments and had steadier speeds during the quarter-mile walking test. The researchers concluded that in most cases, it's safe for older adults to start a moderate exercise regimen. "As US life expectancy rises, functional decline and disability among older people are growing public health and clinical concerns," observes Richard J. Hodes, MD, director of the National Institute on Aging, which funded the study. "This pilot study helps us to understand better the relationship between exercise training and mobility, which is a key to maintaining older adults' independence and quality of life and provides a basis for designing more definitive large-scale clinical trials."

The Magic of Moderate Exercise

Throughout this chapter, we've been discussing how moderate exercise can enhance immune function and overall health. But just how moderate is "moderate"? Because of the way the media filter research findings as well as government recommendations, many people believe that even 30 minutes of light housework divided into three 10-minute chunks is enough to satisfy their exercise quotas for the day. That might be true for those who are prone to engaging in particularly frenetic bouts of housecleaning. Generally, however, the tasks of daily living—such as hand washing the dishes or walking at a casual pace while grocery shopping—don't elevate the heart rate enough to provide benefits for the immune system or otherwise. To get the full immune-enhancing effect of a moderate exercise program, you'll need to work at it, maybe even break a sweat. (Think of it as an immunity bonus: Perspiration contains substances that protect the skin from harmful bacteria.)

How can you tell if what you're doing is moderate? For starters, see how much time you need to walk a mile. If you're moving at a moderate pace, you should be able to cover that distance in 20 minutes. (If you can do it in 15 minutes, then you're in vigorous exercise territory.) Take note of how much effort it takes to walk that mile. Now apply the same amount of effort to all of the activities that are part of your daily exercise regimen.

To put it in more scientific terms: During moderate-intensity physical activity, your target heart rate should be between 50 and 70 percent of your maximum heart rate. You can calculate this by subtracting your age from 220. For example, the maximum heart rate for a 50-year-old man or woman is 170. Fifty to 70 percent of

170 equals a target heart rate zone of 85 to 119. (*Note:* This formula may not apply if you have high blood pressure, according to the American Heart Association. Some blood pressure medications can lower your maximum heart rate, which in turn lowers your target heart rate zone; ask your doctor whether you should be using a different target zone.)

The best way to monitor your heart rate during exercise is to wear a heart-rate monitor that straps around your chest and gives you a continuous digital readout. As a low-tech alternative, you can check your pulse by gently placing your index finger on either your carotid artery (located in your neck between the middle of your collarbone and your jawline) or your radial artery (on the underside of your wrist, near the thumb). Simply count the number of heartbeats in 10 seconds, then multiple by 6.

If you can't find time in your daily schedule for a single 60-minute session of moderate physical activity, two shorter sessions may provide the same immune-boosting effect, according to researchers at Texas Christian University in Fort Worth. For a small pilot study, 10 volunteers rode a stationary bike for 60 minutes twice a day, while another group of volunteers remained sedentary. A week later, the groups switched places. Though a single exercise session improved immune function, the effect became even more pronounced with the second session.

Bear in mind that this "divide and conquer" approach works only if you're getting at least 30 minutes of exercise at a time. Ten to 15 minutes is barely long enough to warm up your muscles, let alone reach your target heart rate zone. Although any physical activity is better than none, strive for at least 30 minutes of continuous moderate activity most days (and preferably every day).

When Exercise Does More Harm Than Good

You can get even more immune-enhancing benefits by exercising more intensely but for the same amount of time (30 to 60 minutes). If you push beyond that limit, though, you could do your immune system more harm than good. Vigorous workouts lasting 90 minutes or longer actually suppress your immune system.

When Dr. Nieman taught a running class at a small California college 25 years ago, he noticed that he often developed sore throats after long runs. Likewise, his students often came down with colds and flus after their final exam—running a marathon. These illnesses were especially likely to strike in winter and spring.

According to Dr. Nieman, running or cross-training for 30 to 90 minutes several days a week increases the circulation of immune cells. Yet surveys of hundreds of finishers in the Los Angeles Marathon and the Western States 100 Mile show that an unusually high percentage of them became ill within 2 weeks of their events—one in seven runners after Los Angeles, one in four after Western States. What's behind the seemingly paradoxical finding? More than 90 minutes of intense exercise increases production of the stress hormones cortisol and epinephrine, which not only suppresses the function of T cells and NK cells but also triggers the release of inflammatory cytokines, neutrophils, and monocytes.

To measure the effect of different exercise intensities on immune function, Turkish researchers enlisted the assistance of three groups of men between ages 40 and 54. The first group consisted of 10 elite athletes who ran competitively at distances of 3,000 to 10,000 meters. These men had been in intensive training for at least 10 years and at the time of the study were training for at least 7 hours a week. The second group were the regular Joes—11 recreational athletes who engaged in aerobic activities such as jogging, gymnastics, basketball, and football for at least 3 hours a week. The 11 men in the third group were sedentary and served as controls.

The elite athletes had an extremely high VO_2 max, which is considered the best indicator of cardiorespiratory endurance. However, as their VO_2 maxes rose, their T-helper cells declined. T-helper cells activate macrophages to ingest invading germs and stimulate production of B cells, which produce antibodies and killer T cells.

Among the recreational athletes, on the other hand, researchers found a correlation between increasing VO_2 max and higher levels of immunoglobulin G (IgG), the body's most abundant antibody and a potent weapon against viruses, bacteria, and fungi. IgG accounts for about 75 percent of the body's total antibody supply. These results suggest that moderate exercise could boost what's known as humoral immunity, the part of the immune system that produces antibodies. In other words, the regular Joes got a twofold benefit—a higher VO_2 max, which in itself may enhance immunity by ensuring a steady supply of oxygen to immune cells, and an actual increase in the number of circulating immune cells.

What Type of Exercise Should You Do?

Practically any physical activity that raises your heart rate into your target heart rate zone and keeps it there for 30 to 60 minutes is beneficial for your immune system. Which activity you choose depends on your personal preference. If you like to exercise in groups, you might consider joining a walking club, a recreational sport league, or a gym. If you're more of a solitary soul, you could set up an inexpensive home gym or take walks around your neighborhood.

Whenever you engage in an aerobic activity such as brisk walking, running, bicycling, or swimming—or use a machine such as a treadmill, a stationary cycle, or an elliptical trainer—you speed up your heart rate and bloodflow, which helps circulate infection-fighting white blood cells. This is just one of the many ways in which aerobic exercise helps prevent disease.

To study the effects of a single bout of aerobic activity, Japanese researchers recruited 24 healthy men ages 22 to 29 who hadn't been exercising regularly. The men were divided into three groups, each of which ran 5,000 steps but at different intensities. One group ran at a rate of 180 steps per minute, considered a vigorous workout; another at a rate of 130 steps per minute; and the third, 80 steps per minute. After collecting blood samples before and after the workout, the researchers determined that circulating levels of infection-fighting neutrophils had increased by 20 percent in the high-intensity group and by 15.5 percent in the middle-intensity group.

Next, the researchers exposed the blood samples to *Micrococcus luteus*, a non-pathogenic bacterium used in laboratories to assess immune response. Exercise increased antibacterial activity by 31.2 percent in the high-intensity group and 25.4 percent in the middle-intensity group. These findings suggest that even if you've been sedentary, you're likely to accumulate immune-enhancing benefits from your very first aerobic workout.

What about resistance training? It, too, appears to stimulate immune function by recruiting NK, T, and B cells into the bloodstream. Though it may not deliver as robust an immune boost as aerobic activity, it has other benefits that indirectly impact your immune system.

For a study that appeared in a 2003 issue of the *Sao Paulo Medical Journal,* researchers compared the immune effects of 5 minutes of vigorous exercise on a stationary bicycle, 90 minutes of moderate exercise on the bike, and a standard circuit of five resistance-training exercises performed on weight machines. The study involved eight moderately fit men, who engaged in multiple workout sessions over the course of 9 weeks. Although all three types of exercise raised blood levels of the immune cells, the counts were higher after aerobic activity—particularly the extended moderate-intensity workout—than after resistance training.

Another study, published in a 2004 issue of the *Journal of Strength and Conditioning Research,* assessed the immune effects of a single bout of resistance exercise in eight men—average age 30—who were moderately active but new to resistance training. The men performed a standard workout consisting of abdominal crunches, chest presses, leg curls, leg extensions, leg presses, seated rows, shoulder presses, and lat pull-downs (which work the latissimus dorsi, the large triangular muscles on both sides of the back). After one session, all eight men showed increases in NK, T, and B cells. But levels of all three immune cells returned to normal within 30 minutes. Because the increases were small and the recovery was rapid, the researchers

Tai Chi: A Mostly Sweat-Free Alternative

Qigong (pronounced "chee-gung") is the ancient Chinese practice of mind-body fitness. Actually, the term *qigong* applies to thousands of individual disciplines, from tai chi (which combines meditative breathing with slow, graceful movements) to kung fu.

Across hundreds of studies, qigong has proven helpful for treating conditions as diverse as arthritis, asthma, cancer, chronic pain, diabetes, heart disease, hepatitis, high blood pressure, osteoporosis, stroke, and ulcers. It also may increase the immune cells known as T-helper cells by as much as 50 percent.

According to UCLA researchers, tai chi in particular has dramatic effects on the immune system—including an ability to reduce production of catecholamine, a neurotransmitter that inhibits immune function. In a study involving adults with shingles, three tai chi sessions every week for 4 months improved immune cell function by 45 percent.

Tai chi also may help tame the overactive immune system that is characteristic of autoimmune disease. When researchers tracked the effects of an 8-week tai chi class in 19 people with multiple sclerosis—in which the immune system attacks the myelin sheaths that surround nerve fibers—the study participants experienced a 21 percent increase in their walking speed and a 28 percent increase in the flexibility of their hamstring muscles, which improved their mobility. They also reported better mental functioning.

A specific form of tai chi, called tai chi chih, consists of 20 slow movements that practitioners believe help balance the flow of vital energy, or chi. For a 2004 study published in *Psychosomatic Medicine,* lead author Michael Irwin, MD, a professor at UCLA's Neuropsychiatric Institute, and his colleagues evaluated whether tai chi chih could help healthy older adults avoid shingles. (In older adults, shingles—when the varicella zoster virus that causes childhood chickenpox emerges from its dormant state—usually is considered a sign of declining immune function.) The researchers monitored 18 people age 60 or older who'd had chickenpox as children. All of them took tai chi chih classes 3 days a week for 15 weeks. Another 18 people served as controls.

Blood tests confirmed that resistance to the varicella zoster virus increased by 50 percent in the tai chi chih group, compared with the control group, and these participants also reported more energy, improved mobility, and generally better health and well-being.

Dr. Irwin suggests that tai chi chih may enhance immunity to many different kinds of infections, especially if resistance is depleted because of depression or stress. You can find accredited tai chi chih instructors at www.feeltheqi.com (click on the tab for "Find an IIQTC Teacher"). As of this writing, an 8-week course costs between $45 and $100.

concluded that a single bout of resistance training was neither immune-enhancing nor immune-suppressing.

Of course, resistance exercise can help whittle a too-wide waistline—and, as we discussed earlier, maintaining a healthy weight is important for maximum immunity. Just two resistance-training sessions a week may help prevent middle-age weight gain and reduce abdominal fat.

At the American Heart Association's (AHA's) 2006 Conference on Cardiovascular Disease Epidemiology and Prevention, CCEB researchers presented the findings of a 2-year study involving 164 women between ages 24 and 44, all overweight or obese. One group participated in a 16-week program of supervised resistance-training classes, then continued working out independently. The women returned for four follow-up sessions each year. Another group received a brochure advising them to get 30 to 60 minutes of exercise most days of the week.

Not surprisingly, the women who received the brochure didn't lose weight. Such benign interventions seldom have any effect. The women who engaged in resistance training, on the other hand, lost 3.7 percent of their total body fat, on average—with much of it melting away from their midsections.

Another interesting effect of resistance training is that it stimulates production of growth hormone in women, according to a 2006 study published in the *American Journal of Physiology—Endocrinology and Metabolism*. Instead of testosterone, women's bodies rely largely on growth hormone for bone and muscle development. As a bonus, growth hormone enhances metabolic function and immune function. "We found that growth hormone was responsive to moderate and heavy exercise regimens [involving] three to 12 repetitions with varying weight loading," reports William J. Kraemer, PhD, the study's principal author. "Women need to have heavy loading cycles or workouts in their resistance-training routines, as it helps to build muscle and bone."

Ideally, your exercise program includes both aerobic activity and resistance training, along with stretching to help improve flexibility and reduce risk of injury. The 4-week Immune Essentials Plan (beginning on page 149) incorporates all three elements with weekly workout suggestions, plus daily checkpoints to ensure that you're getting enough exercise to support your immune system and overall health.

Tips for New Exercisers: Getting Started

If you've been spending so much time on the sofa that you've come to think of it as your conjoined twin, you know that you need to get up and get moving. But where do you begin?

Delicious Solutions for Exercise-Related Aches and Pains

You need a sufficient amount of protein to help maintain immune function during exercise. One of the reasons is that all of your immune cells rely on glutamine as an important source of fuel. "Glutamine comes from protein foods," explains Jose Antonio, PhD, CEO of the International Society of Sports Nutrition. "If you're not eating enough of those foods, your body will borrow from skeletal muscle, especially if you're working out."

But even with adequate protein intake, you may experience exercise-related muscle strain. What's a good way to prevent it? Cherry juice, according to a study published in the June 2006 issue of the *British Journal of Sports Medicine.* Cherries are rich in polyphenols, which protect cells from the oxidative damage caused by free radicals. Researchers from the University of Vermont in Burlington compared the effects of cherry juice, a cherry juice/apple juice combination, and a cherry-free juice on 14 healthy volunteers who drank one of the three beverages for 3 days before working out and 4 days afterward.

The results? The cherry juice, which contained about 50 to 60 cherries' worth of juice, virtually eliminated any adverse effects on muscle strength after exercise. Those who drank cherry juice lost just 4 percent of their muscle strength, compared with 22 percent of those who drank the other two juices. Pain scores in the cherry-juice group were significantly lower, too: just 2.4 percent, compared with 3.2 percent in the other two groups. Four days after working out, the cherry-juice drinkers actually had gained some muscle strength.

Not fond of cherry juice? Another study, this one published in the *International Journal of Sports Nutrition and Exercise Metabolism,* suggests what may be a more palatable alternative: chocolate milk. The study found that people who drank 17 ounces of chocolate milk after finishing a workout recovered as quickly as those who drank Endurox, a popular recovery drink.

As a rule, it's a good idea to check with your doctor before launching an exercise program if you meet any of the following criteria.

■ You're a woman over age 50 or a man over 40.

■ You have a chronic health problem such as heart disease, high blood pressure, diabetes, osteoporosis, or asthma.

■ You have significant risk factors for heart disease, such as a family history; smoking; a diet rich in saturated fat, trans fat, or cholesterol; or a sedentary lifestyle.

To make the first steps of a new exercise program as comfortable and safe as possible, the AHA offers these tips.

■ Buy comfortable, properly fitting shoes.

■ Wear clothing that's appropriate for your activity.

■ Select an exercise time (or times) that fits into your daily schedule, and stick with it.

■ Start slowly and increase gradually.

■ Drink water before and after exercise, and possibly during it. (Ask your doctor for specific recommendations.)

■ Enlist friends or family members as exercise buddies. This makes workouts more enjoyable and helps you stay motivated.

■ If you get bored easily, try varying your fitness routine by switching between different activities that you enjoy.

When Exercising Outdoors, Don't Get Burned

If you exercise outdoors—especially between 11:00 a.m. and 3:00 p.m., when the sun's ultraviolet rays are strongest—you may be at increased risk for skin cancer, according to research published in a 2006 issue of the *Archives of Dermatology.*

When researchers from the University of Graz in Austria compared 210 marathoners with 210 controls, they found that the marathoners had significantly more dysplastic nevi. These are atypical moles that can become precursors to malignant melanoma, the most serious form of skin cancer. The marathoners also had more age spots. The longer and more intensive their training, the greater their skin damage.

Admittedly, this is an extreme example; many of the marathoners had trained for years sans T-shirts and sunscreen. But too much sun can raise the risk of skin cancer in anyone who spends a lot of time outdoors. The researchers offered these tips for outdoor exercisers.

■ Avoid exercising at midday.

■ Before exercising, apply a sunscreen with an SPF of at least 15.

■ During workouts, wear a wide-brimmed hat and a long-sleeved shirt or at least a T-shirt.

If you haven't been a dedicated exerciser, it will take about a month for workouts to become second nature. Your body and brain need time to adjust to your new schedule. Experiencing changes in your body composition, strength, and energy level will provide the inspiration to stick with it.

Though part of the immune "prescription" for this chapter is to engage in moderate aerobic activity for 30 to 60 minutes a pop, you definitely shouldn't jump in at this level if you haven't been exercising regularly or you're out of shape. Instead, start by taking a 10- to 15-minute walk 4 days per week, then gradually work up to longer and more intense workouts.

Likewise, if going from zero to seven workouts per week seems daunting, try committing to just four workouts per week at first. Reserve Wednesdays as "hump days" in which you take a break from exercise. As you feel ready and able, add a workout a week until you're at five, then six, and finally seven.

It's not uncommon for beginning exercisers to experience shortness of breath. Still, it's frustrating, and it can quickly put a damper on motivation. The American Lung Association offers these tips for regulating your breathing during workouts.

■ Cough several times to clear your lungs of mucus.

■ Before you start exercising, relax and take three deep breaths. Continue to breathe deeply during your workout.

■ Make each exhalation twice as long as each inhalation. To maintain this ratio, count to two as you breathe in, then count to four as you breathe out.

■ If you do experience shortness of breath, either rest or slow your pace for several minutes before continuing with your workout.

Also, be sure to warm up before each workout with 5 minutes of stretching. Afterward, cool down with another 5 minutes of stretching. And take care not to exercise when you're sick. While it's noble to attempt to tough out a workout, it's better for your body if you don't. Your immune system needs to tap all of its available resources to bring about a quick and full recovery. (For more information, see "Under the Weather? Skip the Workout" on page 78.)

Staying Motivated

For many people, the hardest part of an exercise program is not starting it but sticking with it. Any number of factors can interfere, from family and work responsibilities to simple loss of interest. How can you stay on track?

Under the Weather? Skip the Workout

When you're sick, recuperative rest—not exercise—is the order of the day. Exercise places additional stress on your immune system, so a workout can leave you feeling worse instead of better. In general, you should skip exercise if you have symptoms of an infection, such as fever, headache, or nagging muscle pain. The same rule of thumb applies if you have an upset stomach or a hacking cough or you're spitting up a lot of phlegm.

Actually, it's a good idea to pay attention to how you're feeling before any exercise session. According to a study published in the *Journal of Applied Physiology,* exercise may leave you more susceptible to illness if you're:

■ Exhausted most of the time but have trouble sleeping at night

■ Feeling weak

■ Achy all over

■ Frequently injuring yourself (with sprains, pulled muscles, and so on)

If any or all apply to you, the researchers recommend reducing the frequency and duration of your workouts. Also, if you ever feel light-headed or experience chest pain during exercise, stop and call your physician right away.

Take a whiff of peppermint. In a study involving 15 male and 14 female NCAA Division II basketball players, researchers from Wheeling Jesuit University in West Virginia found that the athletes who took regular whiffs from peppermint inhalers during games reported higher levels of motivation, confidence, energy, speed, strength, and alertness. Although peppermint didn't actually improve the athletes' ability to sink free throws, it did give them a psychological edge. Inexpensive peppermint inhalers are available from retailers such as GNC. As an alternative, you can sprinkle a few drops of peppermint extract onto a handkerchief and inhale.

Sign an exercise "contract." Create a contract specifying when, where, and how often you intend to engage in physical activity. If you and a witness (a family member or friend) sign it, you may be as likely to follow through on your commitment as when you sign to purchase a car or a home.

Find an exercise buddy. As suggested earlier, you have a better chance of sticking with an exercise program if you pair off with a friend whose fitness level is similar to your own.

Visualize the results. Instead of dreading sweat, think of each drop of perspiration as an extra calorie draining from your body.

Cultivate an active frame of mind. Open your garage door manually. Get up to change TV channels instead of using the remote. Wash your dishes—and your car—by hand. Hang out your laundry instead of throwing it in the dryer. By finding ways to sneak "active minutes" into your day, you foster an active mind-set that can provide a much-needed mental edge for following through on a workout.

Be creative with your exercise time. Exercise needn't be limited to formal, regimented workouts. Almost any activity that gets you moving at a moderate pace—such as playing badminton, tilling the garden, or mowing the lawn—will help enhance your immune function.

Eat a big breakfast. If you consume most of your calories early in the day, you'll have more energy for daytime workouts. Just be sure to follow your big breakfast with a light lunch and dinner. Also avoid late-night snacking, which is likely to lead to weight gain.

Snack if you need to. If your energy is flagging, try eating a protein- and carbohydrate-rich snack—such as a hard-cooked egg and a slice of whole wheat toast—2 hours before your workout.

Give yourself a reward. When you reach a milestone—even if it's a modest one,

The Exercise Benefits of Dog Ownership

If you need extra motivation to start an exercise program and you like furry critters, consider getting a dog. The right pooch can be not only your best friend but also your best exercise buddy, according to a 2006 study published in the *American Journal of Preventive Medicine.*

When Canadian researchers examined the exercise habits of dog owners versus nonowners, they found that the owners walked almost twice as many minutes per week—300 minutes, on average, compared with 168 minutes for the nonowners. "There's an extra obligation that helps people get up and out for their exercise," says study coauthor Shane Brown, PhD, of the University of Victoria in British Columbia.

Interestingly, the dog owners actually got less total exercise than the nonowners, suggesting that they were walking their dogs more for fun and companionship than for health reasons. But the researchers theorize that some of the owners wouldn't have gotten any exercise at all if Sparky hadn't sparked them to head outdoors. "We're definitely not saying, 'Everyone go out and get a dog,'" Dr. Brown says. "We are saying that for those of us who have dogs or are thinking of getting a dog, this is an added benefit."

such as resolving to exercise 4 days a week and then doing it—treat yourself to something special, such as a subscription to a glossy magazine or a trip to a day spa. After all, you've earned it!

Get Fit, Fight Disease

Once you begin to experience the many benefits of exercise—including enhanced immune function and fewer illnesses, better sleep, and reduced stress—you may wonder how you got along without it. You may feel better and more energetic than you've felt in years—or perhaps better than you've ever felt, period!

As part of the 4-week Immune Essentials Plan that begins on page 149, you'll be able to mix and match aerobic activity, resistance training, and stretching to build a fitness routine that's just right for you. By exercising smart and gradually increasing the frequency, intensity, and duration of your workouts, you'll notice dramatic improvement in your fitness level—for maximum immunity and for optimal health.

Key #3—Sleep: Quality Matters as Much as Quantity

Immune Rx: Get 7 to 8 Hours of Restorative Sleep Every Night

You know how you feel after a short night's sleep. You're so drained that you can't think clearly; you have trouble paying attention; you simply can't perform as well as you usually do. It's as though your body and brain are mired in molasses.

Sleep deprivation takes a toll on virtually all of your body's systems, especially your immune system. It impairs the production of natural killer cells, leaving you more vulnerable to infection and chronic disease. It triggers the release of stress hormones such as adrenaline and cortisol, which further suppress immune function. It reduces the production of growth hormone, which not only is essential for proper immune function but also helps restore and maintain cells, tissues, organs, and metabolic pathways.

A growing body of research suggests that sleep deprivation prompts the immune system to release inflammatory proteins such as C-reactive protein, a risk factor for atherosclerosis. It also steps up production of tumor-necrosis factor, which may contribute to autoimmune conditions such as rheumatoid arthritis. The effects become even more pronounced with age. In postmenopausal women, for example, there is a strong correlation between age-related sleep impairment and elevated tumor-necrosis factor.

If you don't get the recommended 7 to 8 hours of sleep per night, it eventually catches up with you. Here's a sampling of how even short-term sleep impairment disrupts immune function.

■ Sleep deficit of 5 hours in one night: Levels of infection-fighting killer T cells decline by 30 percent. Levels of cancer-fighting interleukin-2 also drop. Normal sleep the next night may restore killer T-cell activity but not interleukin-2.

■ Sleep deficit of 4 hours a night over six nights: Hormone production falters, as does starch and sugar metabolism—which in turn prompts a rise in blood sugar.

■ Five nights with no sleep: Infection-fighting immunoglobulin-M (IgM) antibodies decline by 35 percent, and white blood cells decline by 30 to 50 percent. Meanwhile, stress hormones rise.

During normal sleep, your body is able to rest, refuel, and regroup. Your heart rate, blood pressure, and metabolism slow, allowing your brain and internal organs to steel themselves against the stresses of the coming day. In addition, your immune system is able to perform its tasks without the distraction of the immune-suppressing stress hormones that you normally produce as you go about your daily routine.

How important is a good night's sleep? Back in the 1950s, the American Cancer Society asked one million Americans about their lifestyle habits, including the amount of sleep they got. After 7 years, the researchers checked back to see how many of the survey participants were alive and how many had died. They came away with a startling finding: The lifestyle factor most strongly associated with an increased risk of death wasn't poor diet, lack of exercise, or even smoking. It was sleep loss. The death rate was highest among those men and women who averaged 4 hours or less of sleep a night. The death rate was lowest among people who slept about 8 hours a night.

The Science of Sleep

In September 2006, the *Archives of Internal Medicine* devoted an entire issue to sleep and its effects on overall health, including the immune system. One study, from the University of Lübeck in Germany, clearly showed restful sleep is essential for balancing immune function. The researchers looked at 11 healthy men, average age 25. All were nonsmokers who didn't take medications and had normal sleep patterns. The men participated in two sleep sessions: a normal sleep-awake cycle, in which they slept from 11:00 p.m. until 7:00 a.m.; and a sleep-deprived cycle, during which they remained awake for 24 hours. The researchers drew blood samples and analyzed them for levels of proinflammatory type 1 cytokines such as interleukin-2, interferon-y, and interleukin-12, as well as anti-inflammatory type 2 cytokines such as interleukin-4 and interleukin-10.

For optimal immune function, you need a proper balance of type 1 and type 2 cytokines. An overabundance of either one can cause a range of adverse effects—inflammation and tissue damage on the one hand, increased susceptibility to infection and allergy on the other. Several bodily processes help to maintain the proper balance between type 1 and type 2 cytokines. For example, the production of chemicals such as growth hormone and prolactin tends to increase during sleep, while levels of stress hormones such as norepinephrine and cortisol tend to fall.

The researchers identified a link between normal, restful sleep and higher levels of type 1 activity, which helped establish a rhythm in which type 1 cytokines dominated at night and type 2 dominated during the day. Because sleep supported a balanced, finely tuned immune system that was neither overactive nor underactive, the researchers concluded that shut-eye is essential for maintaining optimal immunity.

The study's sleep-deprivation segment completely disrupted this delicate balance, suppressing production of type 1 cytokines by 40 percent, while increasing type 2 production by 170 percent. This sort of severe cytokine imbalance is common in autoimmune diseases such as rheumatoid arthritis, which occur because of an overactive immune system. These results suggest that sleep deprivation can suppress some immune processes, increasing infection and poor response to vaccines, while overstimulating others, which could aggravate conditions such as allergies, eczema, and rheumatoid arthritis.

According to the study's lead author, Tanja Lange, MD, and her colleagues, "The most striking and novel result of our experiment is the clear dependence of the cytokines' rhythm on sleep and its complete absence during continuous wakefulness. Improving sleep could represent a therapeutic option to enhance the success of vaccinations and success in the treatment of diseases that are characterized by type 2 cytokine overactivity."

Researchers long have known that sleep deprivation blunts the immune system's response to the flu vaccine. In a 2006 study, a team from the University of Chicago found that men who slept only 4 hours a night for 1 week produced half as many flu-specific antibodies in response to the flu vaccine as men who were sleeping between $7\frac{1}{2}$ and $8\frac{1}{2}$ hours a night.

According to animal studies, sleep is as essential for survival as food. Rats that are completely deprived of sleep survive for just 2 to 3 weeks, an effect similar to that of starvation. Basically, sleep deprivation causes their immune systems to break down.

How long does it take to recover from a chronic sleep deficit? Longer than you might think. Researchers studying sleep-deprived animals found it took a full 15 nights of regular sleep for immune function to return to normal.

The Health Effects of Sleep Deprivation

Insomnia, whether occasional or chronic, affects about half of the adult population. Among its most common symptoms are decreased immunity, increased drowsiness, lack of motivation to exercise, reduced work productivity, mood shifts, depression and anxiety, impaired memory, and poor physical coordination.

In addition to its direct impact on immune function, sleep deprivation contributes to a host of health problems, including cardiovascular disease. During normal, restful sleep, your heart rate and blood pressure drop by about 10 percent. This gives your heart and vascular system a badly needed breather, which is essential for maintaining cardiovascular health. If you don't get enough sleep, this slowdown may not occur, raising your risk of heart attack, angina, irregular heartbeat, and stroke. Sleep deprivation also prevents the dip in stress hormones that usually occurs during sleep, further magnifying the risk of heart disease.

During sleep, your blood sugar rises and falls in a distinct pattern. If sleep deprivation interrupts this pattern, it can increase your risk of diabetes. In one study of healthy young men, those who got only 4 hours of sleep every night for six nights had insulin and blood sugar levels similar to those of people with prediabetes. Another study showed that women who slept less than 7 hours a night were more likely to develop diabetes than those who logged between 7 and 8 hours a night.

Sleep deprivation also may accelerate aging, according to a study involving younger men who were limited to 4 to 6 hours of sleep every night for several weeks. The resulting changes in hormonal levels and carbohydrate metabolism were typical of much older men.

Of course, sleep deprivation can seriously undermine your ability to perform complicated tasks that require complete focus and attention, such as operating a vehicle. When 39 people stayed awake for 17 to 20 hours before a driving test, their test cores were awful. They didn't perform any better behind the wheel than someone who is legally drunk. In fact, sleep deprivation is responsible for at least 100,000 traffic accidents and more than 1,500 accident-related fatalities every year. Notorious examples of human error resulting from sleep deprivation include the *Exxon Valdez* oil spill in Alaska, the meltdown at Chernobyl nuclear power plant in the Ukraine, and the near meltdown at Three Mile Island in central Pennsylvania.

For a 2006 study published in the *Public Library of Science—Medicine*, researchers from Brigham and Women's Hospital and Harvard Medical School recruited one of the most sleep-deprived groups in America: first-year medical residents, who often work hospital shifts lasting 24 hours or more. To measure the effects of this grueling schedule, the researchers conducted monthly surveys of 2,737 medical residents through their first year of residency.

The results were alarming. The participants who worked at least one shift of 24-plus hours in a month were three times as likely to report a significant fatigue-related medical error as they were during months when they worked no extended shifts. When they put in five or more shifts of 24-plus hours in a month, they were seven times as likely to report a significant medical error. The wiped-out residents often dozed off during lectures and ward rounds and sometimes during clinical activities such as surgery.

It isn't only working adults who are sacrificing shut-eye. For a 2007 study published in the *Journal of Clinical Sleep Medicine,* researchers from the University of Colorado School of Medicine in Pueblo pored over questionnaires filled out by middle-school and high-school students from 238 school districts. The researchers identified a high rate of sleep disturbances, which translated into poor academic performance. Students with lower grade point averages were significantly more likely to have restless legs syndrome and report nighttime snoring and difficulty waking up in the morning. During the day, they were more likely to lose concentration and even fall asleep during class.

Barriers to a Good Night's Sleep

A hundred years ago, when the pace of life was less frantic, most people slept about 9 hours a night. Since the 1950s, there has been a steady decline in the amount of time that most of us devote to sleep. Today, less than one-third of American adults get 8 hours of sleep a night—despite mounting evidence that adequate sleep is essential for immune function and overall health. Most of us are getting less than 7 hours a night, on average.

To make matters worse, it isn't necessarily good-quality sleep. The stresses of modern life—longer work hours and commutes, family and household responsibilities, 24-7 lifestyles—can compromise our efforts to fall asleep and stay asleep. If you toss and turn all night or wake up early or often, you may not be getting enough REM and non-REM sleep. Both types of sleep are necessary for the growth and repair of cells, including immune cells, as well as for learning and memory.

Today, more than one-third of American adults report that sleep deprivation adversely affects their work and social lives at least several days each month. It's estimated that sleep deprivation and sleep disorders such as sleep apnea affect up to 70 million Americans. The annual cost: an estimated $16 billion in health care expenses and $50 billion in lost productivity.

In our increasingly competitive global economy, work demands can wreak havoc on sleep. According to the latest US Census data, significantly more Americans leave for work between 5:00 and 6:30 a.m., spending more time—between 60 and 90 minutes—commuting. Between 1990 and 2000, the number of workers with commutes exceeding an hour rose by almost 50 percent.

To compensate for a chronic sleep deficit, many people rely on caffeinated beverages such as coffee, tea, and cola. This strategy may be effective in the short term, as caffeine tricks the body into thinking it isn't tired by blocking cell receptors that trigger sleep-inducing signals. Unfortunately, caffeine's effects can linger for 6 to 8 hours—so a late-afternoon cup could interfere with your ability to fall asleep at night. Many over-the-counter pain relievers also contain caffeine, which means they can disrupt sleep if taken near bedtime.

Many prescription medications can cause sleep problems, too. Among the offenders are beta-blockers, which help treat high blood pressure, and long- and short-acting beta agonists such as Serevent and albuterol, which help control asthma.

Other notorious sleep-robbers include stimulants such as nicotine, which causes lighter-than-normal sleep. Heavy smokers often wake up early from nicotine cravings. Alcohol may induce drowsiness, at least at first, but it prevents deep sleep and often leads to middle-of-the-night awakenings.

For a study published in September 2006 in the *Archives of Internal Medicine,* researchers from the National Center for Complementary and Alternative Medicine in Washington, DC, conducted a survey of 31,044 adults. They found that 96 percent of people with insomnia and sleep difficulties had other serious health issues such as high blood pressure, congestive heart failure, anxiety, or depression. Just 4 percent of those with insomnia identified it as their only significant medical problem.

Another study, this one by French researchers, concluded that people with allergic conditions such as hay fever and asthma are more likely to develop insomnia. As a result, they're more likely to experience daytime fatigue and sleepiness; impaired memory, mood, and sexuality; and increased reliance on alcohol and sedatives.

Because insomnia is such a common consequence of so many different medical conditions, these research findings suggest that doctors should focus on diagnosing and treating any underlying condition first to see if insomnia improves. If it doesn't, the next step may be to prescribe some sort of sleep aid. The results also suggest that patients need to be more proactive in seeking help for conditions that may compromise sleep.

Even if you don't have a chronic medical condition, you may be making lifestyle choices that sabotage your sleep, such as routinely eating large meals or exercising just before bedtime. Increased physical activity late at night suppresses melatonin, a hormone that's essential for promoting sleep. You also may be practicing poor sleep hygiene—going to bed and getting up at inconsistent times, for example, or sleeping in an environment that's too bright, noisy, or warm.

Sleep and the Single (Or Married) Woman

Although sleep deprivation affects everyone from school-age children to older adults, its strongest impact may be on women. After the National Sleep Foundation (NSF) found that women were more likely than men to experience sleep difficulties, it commissioned a survey of 1,003 women ages 18 to 64 to determine exactly who suffers most and why. Among the key conclusions, published in early 2007:

A GOOD NIGHT'S SLEEP IS HARD TO FIND. Sixty percent of respondents reported getting adequate sleep just three or fewer nights a week. For 43 percent, daytime sleepiness is serious enough to disrupt daily activities.

SLEEP ISN'T A PRIORITY. The respondents reported that when pressed for time, among the first things they sacrifice are sleep (52 percent) and exercise (48 percent). Even though they're tired, most will forgo an early bedtime in favor of watching television (87 percent), completing household chores (60 percent), surfing the Internet (36 percent), or doing job-related work (21 percent).

PERIMENOPAUSAL WOMEN GET THE LEAST SLEEP. On average, they spend only 7 hours 12 minutes in bed. Fifty-nine percent said that they experience insomnia at least several nights a week.

FIFTYSOMETHINGS HAVE THE MOST SLEEP PROBLEMS. Although 66 percent of these women reported spending at least 8 hours in bed on weeknights, they aren't getting good-quality sleep. Among their coping strategies are frequent naps (61 percent) and prescription, over-the-counter, or herbal sleep aids. Almost one-quarter of the respondents said they'd been told by their doctors that they have a sleep problem.

"Women who spend less than 7 hours in bed at night are more likely to doze off during the day, report symptoms of depression, drive drowsy, and use coping mechanisms just to make it through the day," says Kathryn Lee, PhD, a task force member of the NSF and chairperson of the School of Nursing at the University of California, San Francisco. "Furthermore, women tend to compromise the most important aspects of good health—diet, exercise, and sleep—when trying to juggle the day's ongoing responsibilities. Forgoing healthy lifestyle habits in favor of more time during the day is not the solution. In fact, it can be detrimental to optimum health and performance."

Tips for Better Sleep

According to research, the optimal amount of sleep for maximum immunity is 7 to 8 hours a night. But sleep needs vary from one person to the next. Some people thrive on only 7 hours, while others need 9 or more hours to feel up to snuff. In studies involving healthy adults who had the luxury of sleeping as much as they wanted, most chose between 8 and 8½ hours.

Of course, sleeping patterns change over the course of a lifetime. Babies typically sleep between 16 and 18 hours; school-age children, about 9 hours. By the prime of life, all stages of sleep tend to be lighter, and falling asleep and staying asleep may be more difficult. Middle-aged and older adults often complain of frequent and long nighttime awakenings, early morning awakenings, and daytime sleepiness.

To compensate for a sleep shortfall during the week, many people linger in bed on weekends. But depending on how much sleep you've lost, sleeping in on Saturdays and Sundays may not be enough to erase the debt. This strategy also can make falling asleep and staying asleep more difficult when you return to your regular schedule on Sunday night.

Another common way to compensate for short nighttime sleep is daytime naps. Some research suggests that a brief nap—no more than an hour—can help offset a poor night and improve alertness, mood, and work performance. A nap lasting longer than an hour, however, can have the opposite effect, leaving you feeling groggy and unable to perform at your best.

Further, napping is not a substitute for a good night's sleep. For example, it does not fully restore the healthy blood sugar fluctuations associated with 7 to 8 hours of quality sleep, which means that habitual napping in lieu of regular sleep could increase your risk of diabetes.

If you must take a nap, set a timer so that you don't sleep for more than an hour. Also, avoid napping after 3:00 p.m. because it can interfere with your ability to fall asleep that night.

So how can you ensure a good night's sleep? Try these tips to start.

Take stock of the amount of good-quality sleep you get each night. Keep a pad and a pencil by your bed, and write down when you go to bed, how long you're not able to sleep, and when you arise. If you see that you're getting far less than the recommended 7 to 8 hours a night, you need to make some lifestyle adjustments.

Set a regular sleep schedule. Go to bed and get up at the same time every day, even on weekends and vacations. A regular sleep schedule helps set your brain's circadian rhythm, which regulates your sleep-wake cycle. You'll have an easier time falling asleep, staying asleep, and waking up refreshed.

De-clutter your bedroom. Remove the TV, computer, stacks of bills, unfolded laundry, and anything else that reminds you of the stresses of the day. To strengthen the association between your bedroom and restful sleep, reserve the space for just two activities: sleep and sex.

Buy the best bed you can afford. If you've been sleeping on the same mattress for 9 or 10 years, it needs replacing. Choose a mattress that's comfortable and supportive. A less-expensive alternative may be to top your old mattress with a 3-inch memory-foam pad, which is made from the same material used in expensive Tempur-Pedic mattresses. Good memory-foam pads cost about $50 for a twin size and about $100 for queen or king.

Also choose a pillow that is comfortable and supportive. If you sleep on your side, you may need a thicker pillow to support your head and neck. If you encase your pillow in an inexpensive allergy-proof cover, you'll be less likely to develop allergy symptoms during the night, which can keep you awake.

Keep it cool. Most people sleep best when the bedroom temperature is on the cool side—70°F or less. Find the temperature that works best for you. During the winter, turn down the thermostat to promote sleep (and save on energy bills as a bonus). During the summer, consider cooling your bedroom with an energy-efficient window air conditioner.

Keep it quiet. Do everything you can to soundproof your bedroom. Heavy curtains can help block street noise, as can so-called white-noise devices. Even the gentle hum of a fan or humidifier can help. If your sleeping partner snores, wear earplugs. Some of the best are made from moldable silicone, which can reduce sound levels by up to 30 decibels. If they don't work, consider sleeping in separate bedrooms.

Keep it dark. Blackout shades can stop the sun from awakening you too early. An inexpensive pair of eyeshades can have a similar effect, fooling your body into thinking that it's still dark outside. To minimize light pollution from your alarm clock—as well as the stress that results from checking the hour each time you wake up—cover it with a dark cloth.

Keep it animal free. The National Sleep Foundation study found that 14 percent of women like to curl up with their dogs or cats. This same group also reported the most sleep disturbances. Invest in a comfy pet bed, and place it as far as possible from your bedroom.

Establish a regular, relaxing bedtime routine. Just as you need to set a regular sleep schedule, you need to set a regular wind-down schedule during the half hour or so before going to bed. For many people, a hot bath or a soak in a hot tub is just the ticket. (Be sure to give yourself enough time to cool down before you hit the hay.) Other people relax by listening to soothing music, reading a book, or engaging in meditation or prayer. The key is to choose a nonstimulating, relaxing activity and practice it in dim light. Unlike bright light, which alerts your brain and body to wake up, low light is the signal to go to sleep.

Avoid late-night distractions. During the half hour before bedtime, set aside rousing activities such as work, paying bills, playing competitive games, and attempting to solve family problems. Also avoid watching hyperactive TV programs or traumatic news coverage. Recent research shows that people who obsessively watched TV coverage of the 9/11 attacks—not just in America but in places as far away as Japan—experienced weeks of nightmares and disrupted sleep.

Consider your bedclothes. Obviously, this is a matter of personal preference. Some people like the feel of fluffy pajamas, while others prefer to sleep au naturel. According to a Swiss study, the warmer your hands and feet are, the sooner you may be able to fall asleep. This suggests that wearing socks—and even mittens—to bed may help improve your sleep.

Time your exercise. Although achieving maximum immunity requires 30 to 60 minutes of moderate physical activity every day, working out too close to bedtime raises body temperature and compromises sleep. Plan your exercise for at least 3 hours before your regular bedtime. For most people, a late-afternoon workout is the perfect way to prime the body for sleep.

Time your meals. As with exercising, eating a heavy or spicy meal too close to bedtime can affect your ability to fall asleep. It also may lead to nighttime heartburn and indigestion. Try to eat your evening meal no less than 3 hours before going to bed. Likewise, restricting fluids close to bedtime can reduce nighttime trips to the bathroom.

Time your alcohol consumption. Avoid drinking alcoholic beverages within 3 hours of your regular bedtime. Although alcohol is a central nervous depressant that may help you get to sleep, it robs you of deep and REM sleep. You might also wake up in the middle of the night, when its effects wear off.

Time caffeine consumption. The caffeine in coffee, tea, cola, and chocolate stays in your body for 3 to 5 hours, but its stimulating effects can linger up to 12 hours. Avoid consuming caffeine within 6 to 8 hours of your usual bedtime. The same advice applies for another commonly consumed stimulant: nicotine.

Get the right amount of sun exposure. Natural sunlight helps set your circadian rhythm and promote regular sleep and wake times. To keep this internal clock on schedule, try to get up to 30 minutes of morning sun exposure. For those who have trouble falling asleep, some experts recommend up to 60 minutes.

Pulling Out the Stops

If you try these tips but still can't get a good night's sleep, your problem may be psychological. Many people with insomnia are chronically anxious about not being able to fall asleep and stay asleep. They condition themselves to believe that they'll never get a good night's sleep again.

To break out of this pattern, some experts recommend what is known as reconditioning therapy. Here's how it works: If you can't fall asleep or go back to sleep within 20 minutes, get out of bed; engage in your usual, relaxing bedtime routine; and return to bed only when you feel sleepy. Other experts recommend progressive muscle relaxation, which involves tensing and then relaxing all of your major muscle groups in sequence.

For some people with insomnia, sleep restriction therapy is beneficial. Limit your first night's sleep to 4 or 5 hours, then gradually increase your sleep time until you establish a normal, restorative schedule. One caveat: If you try sleep restriction therapy, avoid driving a car or operating heavy machinery until you achieve adequate nighttime sleep.

If you continue to struggle with sleep, see your doctor. You may have an underlying medical condition that requires treatment. Or you may have a sleep disorder, for which you may need to see a sleep specialist. Depending on the diagnosis, your doctor may refer you to a psychologist or psychotherapist who practices cognitive behavioral therapy. Such therapy can help you replace negative thoughts (e.g., "I'm a bad person who's doomed to a lifetime of insomnia") with more positive ones ("I'm a worthwhile person who deserves the peaceful slumber that nature intended").

Key #4—Stress: Don't Let It Get the Best of You

Immune Rx: Try to Practice at Least One Stress-Busting Strategy Every Day

When our prehistoric ancestors found themselves face-to-face with a saber-toothed tiger, the stress hormones that lit up their brains and energized their muscles gave them the strength to either fight off the animal or flee into the woods.

We still rely on stress hormones such as *epinephrine* and *cortisol* to enable us to quickly react to everyday stressors. Epinephrine elevates blood pressure and heart rate, diverts blood to muscles, and speeds reaction time. Cortisol releases sugar to help fuel muscles and the brain.

Without these stress hormones, which are produced by the adrenal glands, we wouldn't have the wherewithal to roll out of bed each morning, brave our daily commutes, and work fast enough to satisfy our bosses. We certainly wouldn't have the moxie to respond to emergency situations. Ever wonder how ordinary people manage to gain the almost superhuman strength necessary to rescue others from raging rivers, burning buildings, and wrecked cars? It's because their bodies have literally been flooded with epinephrine.

The problem is that our prehistoric stress circuitry isn't designed to cope with the never-ending stresses of 21st-century life. After a danger has passed, the circuitry is supposed to switch off, allowing blood pressure, heart rate, and blood sugar levels to return to normal. In the face of unrelenting stress, however, the circuitry can become so sensitized that it never shuts down, leaving your body continuously awash in stress hormones.

Most experts agree that long-term stress is a serious threat to immune function and overall health. Also known as chronic stress and toxic stress, it often results from seemingly intractable problems such as a chronic illness, coping with a dead-end job or ongoing relationship or financial difficulties, or caring for a sick relative or friend. But it also can occur when seemingly inconsequential daily aggravations pile up and fester over a period of years.

No matter what its cause, long-term stress can put you in permanent fight-or-flight mode. This increases your risk of everything from minor bouts of colds and flu to major conditions such as weight gain, heart disease, high blood pressure, diabetes, cancer, depression, migraines, back pain, fatigue, and sleep disorders.

Chronically elevated cortisol levels suppress immune function by switching off disease-fighting white blood cells. They also may damage your thymus gland, spleen, and lymph nodes, all of which produce immune cells, according to James LaValle, RPh, ND, author of *Cracking the Metabolic Code*. His research points to a connection between elevated levels of cortisol and increased production of immature killer T cells, which crowd out the mature cells necessary to fight infections. The presence of excess cortisol also may step up production of interleukin-6, a protein that causes systemic inflammation and is associated with autoimmune diseases such as rheumatoid arthritis.

There may be a link between a high level of cortisol and a low level of serotonin, the brain chemical that helps regulate mood. Low serotonin can trigger carbohydrate cravings, overeating, and immune-damaging spikes in insulin, according to Dr. LaValle.

If stress continues for decades, it can exhaust your adrenal glands, leading to a decline in cortisol production. This blunting effect is most commonly seen in middle-aged and older people suffering from burnout. It also is common in rape victims, Holocaust survivors, and combat veterans suffering from post-traumatic stress disorder.

Too little cortisol hurts immune function, too. Your body needs the hormone not only to turn on the fight-or-flight response but also to turn it off. If you can't produce enough cortisol when you really need it, your immune system is less able to fight infections and respond appropriately in emergency situations. Insufficient cortisol also can disrupt your immune system's intricate balance, prompting it to become hyperactive and attack bodily tissues. This raises the risk of autoimmune conditions such as rheumatoid arthritis. By overactivating antibody-producing B cells, cortisol can aggravate existing autoimmune conditions such as lupus. It's no wonder that stress-related illnesses account for at least 75 percent of doctor visits in the United States each year.

When Stress Serves a Purpose

Despite its potential health effects, stress isn't always a bad thing. Actually, when it's acute or episodic—that is, it lasts for only a short time—it could enhance immune function.

A 2005 study published in the *American Journal of Physiology* illustrates this potential benefit. For the study, researchers at Ohio State University in Columbus injected 20 laboratory mice with keyhole limpet hemocyanin, a protein that triggers an inflammatory immune response. Two and a half hours before the injection, the researchers created a stressful situation for half of the mice by removing them from their regular cages and placing them in much smaller cages. All of the mice showed a similar immune response to the injection.

Nine months later, the researchers reinjected the mice with the same protein. This time, the stressed mice showed a much stronger immune response. According to the researchers, this suggests that short-term fear may positively influence immune function by boosting levels of disease-fighting T cells.

Another study found that short-term stress could enhance the effectiveness of the influenza vaccine. Two hours before administering the vaccine, researchers placed one group of mice in the same cage as an aggressive mouse. A second group stayed in their regular cages. The stressed mice produced significantly more influenza-specific antibodies than the control mice.

Of course, these are animal studies. How would short-term stress influence human immune function? It may depend on the nature of the stressor, according to the research to date.

In one study that appeared in the journal *Psychophysiology,* for example, Dutch researchers found significant differences between the immune impact of passive stress and active stress. (The phrase *passive stress* refers to a stressful situation over which we have no control. *Active stress* is the sort that allows us to respond in some way.) The researchers subjected 32 men between ages 18 and 34 to an especially gruesome passive stressor: a 12-minute surgical video. Then the men tried their hand at an active stressor—a memorization exercise followed by a 12-minute test. During each experiment, the researchers measured levels of immunoglobulin A (IgA), the primary antibody that protects mucous membranes from infection. They found that IgA dropped during the surgical video but increased during the memorization exercise.

This finding suggests that passive stress—the kind that leaves us simmering—is more harmful to the immune system than active stress, which engages our minds and forces us to complete a task. The research team even proposed that deliberately

What Worries Americans Most?

In late 2006, Mental Health America—formerly known as the National Mental Health Association—conducted a survey of 3,040 American adults ages 18 and over. Among their findings:

■ Forty-eight percent of Americans worry about finances. Other major stressors include health issues (34 percent) and employment issues (32 percent).

■ Parents, no matter what the age of their children, reported the most stress in all demographic groups. Some 40 percent of parents identified stress from at least three sources, including relationships with significant others or family, employment, and finances.

■ When faced with stress, 82 percent of Americans respond by watching TV, listening to music, or reading. Almost three-quarters (71 percent) rely on family and friends for support, while nearly two-thirds (62 percent) turn to meditation or prayer. Just over half (55 percent) report exercising to reduce stress.

■ Whites are more likely than other racial groups to engage in unhealthy behaviors to deal with stress. Some 30 percent of Native Americans and 28 percent of non-Hispanic whites said they turn to alcohol, tobacco, or drugs when feeling stressed out. Asian Americans were least likely to smoke, drink, or use drugs but most likely to rely on family members or friends or to exercise to manage stress.

■ Women (42 percent) were significantly more likely than men (31 percent) to eat as a coping mechanism.

"The majority of Americans struggle to find balance in the face of a multitude of challenges in our busy society," says David L. Shern, PhD, president and CEO of Mental Health America. "How they choose to cope—whether [through] distracting activities, exercise, talking through their troubles, or more harmful measures [such as] smoking and doing drugs—affects their mental health. If inappropriately or inadequately addressed, chronic stress and other mental-health problems jeopardize the health and well-being of Americans and of the nation as a whole."

pursuing active stressors such as bungee-jumping off a bridge or parachuting out of a plane might be beneficial to the immune system. The caveat is that in order for short-term stress to work to your advantage, you must have a sense of control over the situation and feel confident in your ability to respond to it. Otherwise, it can be just as harmful to your immune function as long-term stress.

When Stress Runs Amok

Modern life constantly challenges us with short-term stressors that activate the fight-or-flight response and leave us powerless to react. If your boss rejects your request for a raise, your kid gets in trouble with the law, or your spouse blows this month's mortgage at the racetrack, you can't pack your bags and run away from it all (though you might like to!). Similarly, when you're stuck in traffic, you can't drive over the cars in front of you even if you owned a vehicle that could accomplish such a feat.

As satisfying as such actions might be, you know in your heart that they wouldn't bode well for your future career or personal prospects (not to mention they could land you in jail). So you have no choice but to muddle through each crisis and annoyance the best you can, stewing in your own stress hormone–rich juices all the while.

Incidentally, positive experiences can trigger short-term stress, too. For example, getting married, starting a new job, or buying a new home can activate the fight-or-flight response and wreak as much hormonal havoc as getting a divorce, losing a job, or facing foreclosure.

Even remembering a stressful situation can trigger new stress by prompting the immune system to release a flood of inflammatory chemicals. When UCLA researchers asked a group of students to write essays about an experience that caused shame and anxiety, it produced much higher levels of inflammatory chemicals than when the students wrote essays about an emotionally neutral experience.

Some studies even suggest that short-term exposure to a passive stressor may raise cancer risk. For one 2004 study, published in the *Journal of the American Academy of Dermatology*, researchers from the Sidney Kimmel Comprehensive Cancer Center at Johns Hopkins in Baltimore exposed two groups of mice to cancer-inducing amounts of ultraviolet light. First, however, they subjected one group to an especially terrifying stressor: the smell of fox urine. The stressed mice—who could literally smell danger but not see it or respond to it—were twice as likely to develop skin cancer as the mice who smelled only their usual surroundings.

What's important to remember is that short-term stress appears to become troublesome only when it's beyond our control and continuously builds up without release. Then it turns into long-term stress, a chronic condition that leaves your body in a constant—and unhealthy—state of high alert.

Age and the Stress-Immunity Equation

As we've discussed elsewhere in this book, immune function naturally declines with age. So middle-aged and older adults may be especially vulnerable to the immune effects of stress, whether it's minor or major.

For a 2006 study published in the journal *Brain, Behavior, and Immunity,* British researchers measured IgA levels in the saliva of 640 middle-aged and 582 older adults and found that IgA was significantly lower in study participants who had experienced one or more major life stressors (such as illness, divorce, or job loss) during the previous 2 years than in those who hadn't. The results demonstrate how stress impairs immune function and increases the risk of developing upper respiratory tract infections.

With age, cortisol levels tend to rise while DHEA (dehydroepiandrosterone) levels fall—two strikes against immune function. DHEA is a steroid hormone with immune-stimulating effects. Typically, it peaks at about age 30, then declines 80 to 90 percent by age 80. The combination of higher cortisol levels and lower DHEA levels may account for the declining ability of older adults to resist infections such as influenza and pneumonia. The over-65 population accounts for 75 percent of the 10,000 to 40,000 flu-related deaths that occur in the United States every year. These people also are at high risk for developing pneumonia, the most common infection-related cause of death. Among those who experience trauma, an extreme form of stress, cortisol levels rise sevenfold in older adults but only twofold in younger patients. This may help explain why so many hospitalized elderly develop life-threatening infections. The combination of high cortisol and low DHEA, in addition to advanced age and trauma, reduces immunity to below the critical threshold at which these people become prone to infection.

Long-term stress not only magnifies the effects of aging on immune function, it also may contribute to premature aging. When researchers at the University of California, San Francisco, examined cells from women whose children had been born with a severe disability such as autism or cerebral palsy, they found that the long-term stress of caregiving had significantly shortened the women's telomeres. A telomere is a chunk of DNA at the end of a chromosome. Each time a cell divides, the telomere gets shorter, until eventually the cell dies. In some cases, this process was so advanced that the women's cells were 10 years older than their chronological age. The women also had higher levels of free radicals, which damage DNA and reduce levels of an enzyme that repairs injured telomeres.

Animal studies suggest that prolonged stress actually can shrink the brain by reducing the number of neurons in the hippocampus (the region associated with memory) and prefrontal cortex (associated with attention and decision making), according to Bruce McEwen, PhD, of the Rockefeller University in New York City, who presented these findings at the 2006 annual meeting of the American Psychological Association in New Orleans. But such adverse effects are not irreversible, Dr. McEwen adds. Because the human brain is more adaptable than animal brains, it can regain normal function with stress-busting interventions such as improved diet, increased exercise, psychotherapy, cognitive behavioral therapy, and—if necessary— medication.

How to Break the Stress Cycle

The lifestyle strategies for managing stress overlap to a degree with those for enhancing immunity. Healthy choices can help moderate your fight-or-flight response so that it activates only in the presence of real danger and not in response to the aggravations of everyday life. To naturally break your stress cycle, start with these basics.

Eat an abundance of immune-friendly foods. Nutrients such as B vitamins and omega-3 fatty acids are especially useful in counteracting stress because they help produce the neurotransmitters that regulate stress hormones.

Get active. Regular exercise has many positive effects on stress. Perhaps most notably, it helps break the stress cycle by restoring an appropriate balance of stress hormones.

Make time for sleep. Adequate sleep—at least 7 to 8 hours a night—allows your body and mind to recover from the stresses of the day. It also gives your immune system a breather to mop up any viruses and bacteria you might have picked up.

Incidentally, all three of these strategies are integral to the Immune Essentials Plan in Part III. By following the plan, you'll offset your body's stress response while strengthening your immune function.

How else can you manage short-term stress? These tips can help.

Take a deep breath. For on-the-spot relief, try this 30-second stress buster. Take three deep breaths, slowly inhaling and exhaling through your nostrils. If you wish, try whispering the word *peace* as you exhale. This 30-second time-out will help you calm down and collect your thoughts so you can respond appropriately to a stressful situation.

To get the maximum stress-relieving benefit from deep breathing, lie down in a comfortable spot, and place your hands on your stomach just below your ribs. If you are doing the exercise correctly, your abdomen should expand before your rib cage does. Just a single 5- to 10-minute session of deep breathing can switch off your body's stress circuitry, clear your mind, and refresh your spirit. Aim for two or three sessions per day.

As you become accustomed to the calming effects of deep breathing, you may notice an improvement in your normal respiration. Specifically, instead of reacting to stress with rapid, shallow breaths—which rob your body of oxygen—you might automatically respond with the slow, deep breaths that help reduce stress.

Inhale a soothing scent. Another quick fix for short-term stress is aromatherapy. Simply place a few drops of an essential oil on a handkerchief or cotton ball and inhale. Among the stress-busting scents are bergamot, chamomile, clary sage, cypress, frankincense, geranium, juniper, lavender, melissa, and sandalwood. When you have more time, you might try placing a few drops of your preferred essential oil into your bathwater before climbing in for a good long soak. Another option: Sprinkle a few drops on your pillow so you can enjoy the calming effects while you're sleeping.

Take a mental vacation. When you think about a stressful situation, it further activates your stress circuitry and contributes to tension and anxiety. But mentally switching gears by replacing negative thoughts with positive ones can deactivate your stress circuitry and instill calm. After relaxing your muscles and taking a few deep breaths, close your eyes and conjure up an image of a place where you feel at ease— perhaps a beach, the mountains, or an exotic locale. At first, give yourself a full 15 minutes to relish the imaginary sights, sounds, and smells. When you open your eyes, you may feel as refreshed as you would after taking an actual vacation. Once you become adept at taking a mental vacation, you may find that you need less and less time to realize its stress-busting benefits.

Try progressive relaxation. Begin by lying down in a comfortable place. Squeeze the muscles in your feet and lower legs as tightly as possible; feel the tension. Then gradually relax those muscles. Repeat the process with the muscles in your upper legs and hips, your hands and lower arms, your upper arms and shoulders, and your stomach. Finish by tensing your chest muscles while holding your breath, then gradually releasing the tension as you exhale. After 10 to 15 sessions, see if you can relax each muscle group without tensing them first.

Nurture your inner Pollyanna. When confronted with a short-term stressor, remind yourself of the many blessings in your life and be sure to count them. In the long run, you'll be much better equipped to cope with stress if you learn to live one day at a time, add a little love to everything you do, focus on understanding instead of being understood, and practice this corny-but-true maxim: It's better to give than to receive. It also helps to remember that most people—including you—are imperfect beings who are doing the best they can.

Although many short-term stresses are unavoidable, some of the most predictable ones can be circumvented with a little advance planning. Here's how to protect yourself from the sorts of everyday disasters that can send stress levels soaring.

Keep a to-do list. You're much more likely to keep appointments, return overdue library books, pick up the dry cleaning, and so on if the task is in writing and in a place where you can see it. An old Chinese proverb makes the point beautifully: "The palest ink is better than the most retentive memory."

Duplicate your house and car keys. If you've ever misplaced your keys, you know how quickly and easily it can send your blood pressure through the roof. Hide an extra house key in a secret spot in your yard or garden, and stow an extra car key in your wallet, apart from your key ring.

Practice preventive maintenance. If you put a little extra effort into maintaining your car and household appliances, they'll be less likely to break down at the least opportune moment. (Actually, this bit of advice applies to personal relationships, too.)

Coping with Stress: A Checklist

Mental Health America (formerly the National Mental Health Association) offers these additional tips to help counter the effects of stress.

■ Take one thing at a time. Pick one urgent task and work on it. When it's done, move on to the next.

■ Be realistic. If you're overwhelmed at home or at work, learn to say no.

■ Don't try to be Superman/Superwoman. No one is perfect, so don't expect perfection from yourself.

■ Take up or rediscover a hobby. Give yourself permission to do something you enjoy.

■ Be flexible! Arguing only increases stress. If you feel you're right, stand your ground, but do so calmly and rationally. Be prepared to make allowances for other opinions and to compromise.

■ Don't be overly critical. Remember, everyone is unique and has his or her own virtues and shortcomings.

If necessary, consider talking with your doctor, spiritual advisor, or someone with your employee assistance program. You may be referred to a mental health professional, who can offer additional tools and techniques for managing your stress.

Fix faulty goods. If an appliance is worn out or doesn't work properly, either repair it or replace it. The same goes for any other possession—such as a disintegrating wallet—that has outlived its usefulness and causes daily aggravation.

Be prepared. At home, stock a shelf of staple foods and bottled water that you can use during an emergency. On the road, always refill your gas tank when the gauge reaches the one-quarter mark. Apply this level of preparedness to other aspects of your life, too.

Organize, organize, organize. At work and at home, always return things to their proper storage places when you're done with them. You'll spare yourself the stress of wasting time looking for things that you've "lost."

The 3 Ms of Stress Management: Meditation, Massage, and Membership

If your short-term stresses have amassed and escalated into long-term, chronic stress, you probably need more than a few simple quick fixes to help break the cycle. To manage long-term stress, you need to integrate some long-term strategies into your everyday life. Among the most effective measures are the three Ms: meditation, massage, and membership.

■ Recent research shows that meditation—the ancient practice of taking regular time-outs to close your eyes, follow your breath, and dispassionately observe each fleeting thought and sensation—is a powerful technique for clearing and focusing your mind, reducing stress, and improving immune function.

■ Massage—which takes many forms—helps release stored stress in muscles and tendons. It, too, has important immune benefits.

■ The third M, membership, refers to your participation in the human race as well as your connections to other people. Studies offer convincing proof that social support from family, friends, and the larger community facilitates your ability to cope with stress while reducing your risk of acute and chronic illness.

Let's look at each of these in turn.

Meditation: Slow Down and Strengthen Your Immunity

Millions of people worldwide—from the most religious to the most agnostic—depend on meditation to help calm and focus a troubled mind. Meditation is a proven technique for alleviating stress as well as insomnia, chronic pain, depression, and even psoriasis. It helps supercharge immunity, too.

For a 2003 study published in *Psychosomatic Medicine,* meditation gurus Jon

Kabat-Zinn, PhD, of the University of Massachusetts Medical School, and Richard J. Davidson, PhD, of the University of Wisconsin, recruited 41 healthy employees (average age 36) from a biotechnology corporation in Madison, Wisconsin. The doctors randomly assigned 25 of the workers to practice a specific form of meditation called mindfulness-based stress reduction (MBSR). The remaining 16 served as a control group.

Developed at the University of Massachusetts Medical Center, MBSR is a widely accepted stress-reduction technique. During a session, patients focus their attention and objectively and nonjudgmentally acknowledge any stray thoughts, emotions, sensations, or perceptions. In this way, they're able to let go of past regrets, stop anticipating future difficulties, and fully experience the present.

During the study, the meditation group took an 8-week course consisting of weekly 2½- to 3-hour classes and one 7-hour retreat. On their own, they practiced meditation for an hour a day, 6 days a week, using guided audiotapes. After 8 weeks, both the meditators and the nonmeditators received a flu vaccine. Then, at the 4-week and 8-week marks, the researchers drew blood samples to evaluate immune response. Levels of flu-specific antibodies were twice as high in the meditation group as in the control group. Even 4 months after the conclusion of the meditation course, immune function remained higher in the meditators.

The reason? The meditation group showed significant increases in left-brain activity, which is associated with reduced stress and anxiety, positive mood, and enhanced immune function. The meditators with the most left-brain activity also had the highest levels of flu antibodies.

Other research demonstrates that MBSR can benefit people living with HIV, the virus that causes AIDS, which attacks and eventually destroys the immune system. In a 2003 study published in the *Journal of Alternative and Complementary Medicine,* researchers from Chicago's University of Illinois and Loyola University enrolled 24 HIV-positive patients—22 men and two women—in an 8-week MBSR class. After the conclusion, the immune function of the meditators was compared with that of 10 HIV-positive patients who served as controls. The researchers found that both the number and activity of natural killer (NK) cells more than doubled in the meditation group, while levels remained unchanged in the control group. The results suggest that MBSR helped dampen the stress-induced increase in cortisol, which tends to suppress the activity of NK cells.

A 2002 study, published in the *American Journal of Psychiatry,* assigned 25 HIV-positive men to either a 10-week training course or a control group. The course had a relaxation component, which covered meditation as well as progressive muscle relaxation and breathing exercises, plus a stress-management component. After 6 to 12 months, the University of Miami researchers found significantly higher T-cell counts in the relaxation/stress management group than in the control group. This prompted lead author Michael Antoni, PhD, and his colleagues to conclude that "stress management is associated with immunologic reconstitution in HIV-positive gay men" and may help protect them against opportunistic infections.

To get the most benefit from meditation, aim for daily practice. Some people meditate for an hour when they get up in the morning and another hour before going to bed. For others, it's more convenient to meditate for a few minutes each day while sitting at their desks, taking a walk, riding a bus, waiting in a doctor's office, or doing household chores.

How long you meditate is up to you. If a 3-minute session is enough to leave you feeling relaxed and calm, it's no less valuable than an extended practice. What's important is that you meditate every day. The more consistently you enter this state of contemplation, the more likely you are to fully experience its benefits to your emotional and physical well-being.

You can learn how to meditate at special meditation centers or in group classes led by instructors trained in forms of meditation such as yoga, tai chi, qigong, or guided meditation. But professional instruction isn't a requisite—you can also master meditation on your own. Just follow this advice to get started.

Focus on deep breathing. As you inhale and exhale deeply and slowly through your nostrils, concentrate on the simple act of breathing. If your mind wanders and stressful thoughts come crashing in, gently refocus your attention on the sounds and sensations of your respiration.

Tune in to your body. While continuing to breathe deeply, broaden your attention to your physical state. If you feel tense and anxious, imagine that each breath is transferring heat and relaxation to your tight muscles.

Recite a mantra. Many forms of meditation, including transcendental meditation (TM), rely on repeating a mantra either silently or aloud for several minutes or longer. In some traditions, a mantra is a sacred phrase or a deity's name. But any comforting name or phrase will do, even one you've made up. The repetition is meant to help clear your mind and create a sense of calm. Again, if distressing thoughts intrude, simply refocus your attention on your breathing and the relaxing rhythm of your mantra.

Give prayer a chance. As one of the oldest forms of meditation, prayer is an essential component of almost every major religion. Reciting a prayer, either silently or aloud, helps replace stress with a sense of spirit and a connection to the divine.

One of the best-known prayers, which is ecumenical enough to complement almost any belief system, is the Serenity Prayer.

> God grant me the serenity to accept the things I cannot change;
> courage to change the things I can;
> and wisdom to know the difference.

Massage: Hands-On Healing Touch

If you ever have received a massage from an expert therapist, you know how soothing it can be as it unties those knots in your neck, shoulders, and back. But massage offers many other therapeutic benefits, some of which have been recognized for centuries. As far back as 2000 BC, Chinese healers were singing the praises of this hands-on healing technique in medical texts that have survived to the present day. Massage can:

- Alleviate stress and anxiety
- Improve bloodflow and circulation
- Loosen tight or injured muscles
- Enhance the suppleness of skin
- Increase flow of lymph (the fluid that contains essential immune cells)
- Calm the central nervous system

In a comprehensive 2005 review published in the *International Journal of Neuroscience*, researchers from the University of Miami School of Medicine and Duke University Medical School found that massage reduces levels of cortisol—the hormone most strongly associated with stress and suppressed immune function—by up to 53 percent. It also raises levels of dopamine by 42 percent and serotonin by 38 percent. (Like serotonin, dopamine is a brain chemical with a strong connection to offsetting stress and enhancing immunity.) The researchers concluded that massage is beneficial in a wide range of circumstances, such as:

- Pregnancy depression, which affects 20 to 40 percent of moms-to-be. Two 20-minute massage sessions per week during the second and third trimesters resulted in lower levels of anxiety and depression, as well as reductions in leg and back pain.

- Postpartum depression, which affects 25 to 30 percent of new moms. Two 30-minute massage sessions per week effectively relieved anxiety and lowered levels of stress hormones, which helped the women form closer bonds with their newborns.

■ Chronic fatigue syndrome, which primarily affects women and can reduce physical activity levels by as much as 50 percent. Massage helped to boost energy while alleviating depressive symptoms, anxiety, and pain.

■ Breast cancer, which affects about one in nine American women. Three 30-minute massage sessions per week for 5 weeks eased feelings of anxiety, depression, and anger. Among the longer-term benefits were significant increases in the numbers of lymphocytes and NK cells.

■ Job stress, which affects almost everyone who works for a living. In one study of health-care workers, a single 15-minute chair massage reduced stress, anxiety, and depression while improving alertness and the ability to perform math computations.

According to the review article, massage may be especially effective at helping older people cope with the various emotional stresses of aging, such as loneliness and depression. One particularly poignant study involving elderly retirees showed that giving a massage—in this case, to hospitalized infants—enhanced the retirees' immunity and reduced their risk of infection even more than receiving a massage.

As is the case with meditation, some of the strongest evidence in support of massage comes from studies of people who are HIV-positive. In this population, regular massage sessions appear to lower immune-suppressing cortisol while raising infection-fighting T cells and NK cells.

Even a daily 15- to 20-minute back rub from a family member or friend can do wonders for your immune function. If you can afford to, though, you might consider a once- or twice-weekly session with a professional. Most states have licensing programs for massage therapists, though requirements vary from state to state. In general, look for someone who has been licensed by your state board and is recognized by the National Certification Board for Therapeutic Massage and Bodywork, which has certified about 80,000 therapists nationwide.

Make sure, too, that your massage therapist is a good communicator. He or she should be able to describe the type and purpose of the massage, the body parts that will and won't be manipulated, and the amount of pressure involved. The therapist also should ask about your medical history and current physical condition. This procedure, known as informed consent, is standard practice for all health professionals.

Membership: You Can Never Get Enough Loving Support

Membership completes the stress-reduction trifecta. The more you cultivate human contact through participation in anything from an informal circle of friends to organizations such as churches, clubs, and activist groups, the more likely you are to effectively cope with stress.

To assess the stress-busting benefits of social support, Hideki Ohira, PhD, of Nagoya University in Japan, recruited 24 college women—average age 20—and asked them to perform a task that strikes fear in most of us: speaking in public. All were given 10 minutes to prepare a 3-minute speech on a controversial topic. They could take any position on the topic, but they couldn't use notes during their presentations.

First, however, all of the students were assigned to one of three groups. The first group received emotional support from another female "participant" who actually was a member of the research team. Her task was to smile, be friendly, and empathize with the stress of giving a public speech. Those in the second group received informational support from another female "participant" who offered practical advice on how to relax and how to organize and present a speech but was otherwise neutral in her demeanor. The third group received no support.

As expected, all three groups showed a common effect of acute short-term stress: a spike in the concentrations of IgA antibodies in their saliva. But the spike wasn't as severe in either support group, suggesting that social support can help prevent the stress circuitry from overloading. Although the study did not measure levels of stress hormones, its findings "correspond to the evidence that social support can reduce the elevation of cardiovascular responses to stress," Dr. Ohira says.

Reaching out to the larger world—and making connections that matter—may have many positive effects on immunity. For a 2003 study published in the *Annals of Behavioral Medicine,* UCLA researchers recruited 43 women who had lost a close relative to breast cancer. Half of the women were asked to write about their losses every day for a month, while the rest wrote about an emotionally neutral topic. Both groups also answered a series of questions about their life goals.

The researchers expected that the women who wrote about the emotionally charged topic would experience relief and increases in NK cells. To the researchers' surprise, these women did not show enhanced immune function, compared with the women who wrote about a neutral topic. However, the women in both groups who reported a higher interest in personal development, relationship building, and "striving for meaning in my life" did show significant increases in NK-cell activity. According to these findings, people who place a high premium on building human connections and setting goals—even in the face of personal loss—are more likely to experience the benefits of maximum immunity.

To broaden your personal social circle, consider joining a church, a club, a recreational group, or another organization. Take a class at a library or community college. If you want to change the world, get involved with a charitable organization or an advocacy group, or sign up for a political campaign. Your local newspaper is a good source of listings for groups and organizations that are actively seeking members. You also can find people who share common interests by searching Web sites such as www.meetup.com.

As you form new relationships, make a point of seeking out people who are generally positive and upbeat. Spending time with worrywarts will only add to your own stress. If you find a friend to whom you can turn for clearheaded, helpful advice, that person is as good as gold. But don't panic if you can't find someone who fits the bill. Just the simple act of socializing with like-minded people will help take your mind off your troubles, reduce your stress, and boost your immunity.

Less Stress, Better Immunity

As you've seen, stress affects your immune system in myriad ways—some of them good, many others bad. Even short-term stressors can be harmful if they persist and accumulate over time.

Although you can't escape stress completely, you can manage it effectively. By experimenting with various stress-reduction techniques, you should be able to find at least one or two that work for you. Remember that these techniques are skills; the longer and more consistently you practice them, the more adept you'll become at creating your own island of calm in a world of chaos.

Key #5—Mood: Happiness Is Good Medicine

Immune Rx: Laugh at Every Opportunity

Until relatively recently, the idea that emotions could affect immune function wasn't taken all that seriously by the medical community. Most physicians and researchers agreed that the immune system was an automatic system, working independently of mind and mood.

This perspective began to shift in the 1970s, when animal experiments conducted by Robert Adler, PhD, of the University of Rochester in New York, showed that the immune system responded to psychological conditioning. In one of his experiments, Dr. Adler fed saccharine to rats while simultaneously giving them an immunosuppressive drug that caused stomach upset. The rats quickly learned to avoid saccharine because they associated it with digestive distress. When they continued to receive saccharine—even in the absence of the drug—they were more likely to die.

Because the rats had been psychologically conditioned, eating saccharine actually lowered their immunity, which in turn raised their risk of death from infectious disease. This led Dr. Adler to the then-novel conclusion that the mind and the immune system are inextricably linked. If animals can learn to alter immune function, he figured, people probably can do the same. "It never occurred to me that there might not be a connection between the brain and the immune system," Dr. Adler says. "You can't separate one from the other. There is only one integrated system." In 1980, he coined the term *psychoneuroimmunology* to describe the study of the relationship between the brain and the immune system.

Psychoneuroimmunology took another leap forward in 1985, when Candace Pert, PhD, and her colleagues at Johns Hopkins University in Baltimore discovered that chemical messengers called neuropeptides are present on the walls of brain cells as well as immune cells. This breakthrough demonstrated how the brain communicates with the immune system and vice versa. Further, it pointed to strong interactions between emotions, immune function, and overall health.

Dr. Pert also found that intense emotions unleash neuropeptides, which then travel to receptors in internal organs, muscles, and other tissues. This reaction may help explain the phenomenona that many people describe as "gut feelings." It also suggests the process by which intense emotions can disrupt immune function and increase the risk of infection and chronic illness. So far, researchers have identified about 100 different neuropeptides.

Since the 1980s, the field of psychoneuroimmunology has exploded, attracting researchers from specialties as diverse as neurology, immunology, physiology, rheumatology, infectious disease, pharmacology, psychology, psychiatry, and behavioral medicine. As researchers have learned more about how the brain communicates with the immune system, they've advanced the view that healing is a process not so much of "curing" but of regaining balance between mind and body. They believe that a positive attitude, strong social connections, and a healthy dose of laughter may be more important than drugs in achieving optimum health.

The Sunny Side: How a Positive Mood Affects Immunity

You may have noticed that you're less likely to get sick when you're calm and happy than when you're stressed and unhappy. You may even know some perpetually upbeat people who seemingly never get sick.

Your emotional style has a powerful impact on your immunity—for better or for worse. Most studies show that a positive emotional style is associated with enhanced immune function, while a negative emotional style is associated with suppressed immune function. In other words, if Mama (or Papa) ain't happy, the immune system ain't happy, either.

A generally positive mood may reduce your risk of getting the flu. For a 2003 study published in the *Proceedings of the National Academy of Sciences,* researchers from the University of Wisconsin–Madison conducted brain scans on 52 adults between ages 57 and 60. The researchers wanted to know if brain activity—as measured when the study participants recalled events that had made them either intensely happy or intensely sad, fearful, or angry—affected immune response to an influenza vaccination.

During the 6 months after the vaccination, the volunteers underwent three separate blood analyses to measure levels of influenza-specific antibodies. The researchers found that people with greater activity in the left side of the prefrontal cortex (an area of the brain associated with positive emotions) had higher concentrations of antibodies than those with greater activity on the right side (associated with negative emotions). "This study establishes that people with a pattern of brain activity that has been associated with a positive [attitude] also are the ones who show the best response to the flu vaccine," says lead researcher Richard Davidson, PhD. "It begins to suggest a mechanism for why subjects with a more positive emotional disposition may be healthier."

A generally positive mood also may offer some protection against the common cold. For a 2005 study published in *Psychosomatic Medicine,* researchers from Carnegie Mellon University in Pittsburgh recruited 334 healthy volunteers—159 men and 175 women—between ages 18 and 54. Their emotional styles ranged from happy, pleased, and relaxed to anxious, hostile, and depressed, with every shading in between. The study participants were treated with a nasal spray containing two cold viruses, after which they were quarantined for 5 days.

The researchers found that the people with higher positive emotional scores were less likely to develop colds and less likely to report cold symptoms when they weren't actually sick. This group also had lower levels of stress hormones such as epinephrine, norepinephrine, and cortisol.

In those with higher negative emotional scores, the researchers identified the opposite pattern. This downbeat group not only was more likely to come down with colds, they also were more likely to imagine having a cold in the absence of clinical evidence. Their stress hormones were higher, too.

From research like this, it's clear that the psychoneuroimmunologists are on to something. A positive mood is a state of mind *and* body, one that balances and boosts your immune system and reduces your risk of disease.

The Downside of Negative Thinking

A chronically negative outlook, on the other hand, appears to give the immune system a license to run amok, as it floods your body with inflammatory substances. In a 2007 study published in the *Archives of Internal Medicine,* researchers from the University of Michigan explored the connection between a negative mood and the immune system's production of the inflammatory substances interleukin-6, C-reactive protein, and fibrinogen. There's a strong association between high levels of these markers and an increased risk of cardiovascular disease, heart attack, and stroke.

The researchers analyzed data collected from the Multi-Ethnic Study of Atherosclerosis, involving 6,814 men and women between ages 45 and 84. For the original study, participants answered questionnaires that assessed three psychosocial factors: cynical distrust, chronic stress, and depression. The researchers found that people with high levels of chronic stress tended to have high blood levels of interleukin-6 and moderately high levels of C-reactive protein. Likewise, people with high levels of depression also had high levels of interleukin-6.

But people with high levels of cynical distrust had the worst results of all, with high levels of all three inflammatory markers: interleukin-6, C-reactive protein, and fibrinogen. The correlation was strongest in those who were overweight or obese or had diabetes. According to the researchers, these findings suggest that people with negative emotional styles may be more likely to overeat, be physically inactive, and adopt unhealthy behaviors such as smoking and excessive alcohol consumption.

Some long-term research suggests that a chronically negative mood just might shorten a person's life expectancy. Back in 1975, Yale University researchers surveyed 660 people over age 50 about their attitudes toward aging. The participants were asked to agree or disagree with statements such as "Things keep getting worse as I get older," "I have as much pep as I did last year," and "I am as happy now as I was when I was younger."

In 1998, the researchers checked back to see which participants still were alive. They also collected data on those who had died. They found that the positive thinkers—those who viewed aging in an optimistic light—had outlived the negative thinkers by an average of 7½ years.

For a separate study, researchers at the Mayo Clinic conducted psychological tests of more than 800 people in the 1960s, then followed their subjects for another 30 years. The researchers found that in any given year, the negative thinkers were 19 percent more likely to die from any cause than the positive thinkers.

From this and other research, it's safe to conclude that negative thinking—especially chronic negative thinking—is harmful to your immunity. It suppresses the production of antibodies that protect against infection, increases the production of inflammatory substances that can cause chronic disease, and could shorten life span.

How Your Personality Type Affects Immunity

The latest research into mood and immunity suggests that the relationship between the two is not so much black-and-white as shades of gray. This appears especially true when assessing the effects of a positive attitude and outlook on immune function.

In a study with 1,041 participants, Harvard University researchers found that all-out optimists—the sort of people who are convinced they can succeed no matter what—were more likely to catch colds and flu and develop high blood pressure and diabetes than those who were more guardedly optimistic. This latter group included people who are hopeful—generally optimistic yet realistic—as well as people who are curious and skeptical, who educate themselves about health issues and pepper their doctors with lots of questions. It's possible that the all-out optimists have perfectionist tendencies that impair their immune function.

This conclusion seems to be corroborated by researchers at the University of Kentucky in Lexington, who conducted a study in which they gave both optimists and pessimists a complicated arithmetic problem. The optimists showed declines in immune function because they persisted in trying to solve the problem even after it had become apparent that they couldn't. The pessimists were more likely to shrug, say "Oh, well," and pronounce the problem unsolvable—which actually enhanced immune function.

Both of these studies suggest that a rigid personality type—even one that's essentially upbeat—may be worse for immunity than a more flexible type.

Researchers long have known that people with a particularly rigid personality type—the classic example is a type A personality, characterized by high levels of impatience, anxiety, and hostility—are much more likely to develop cardiovascular disease and heart attacks than the calmer and happier type B. Now there appears to be an even riskier type, which researchers have newly identified as type D. Although type Ds are as hostile and cynical as type As, they seldom express these feelings to others. They keep their emotions as tightly contained as the explosives in a hand grenade. Eventually, type Ds are likely to blow.

When Belgian researchers explored the health effects of various personality types, they found that type Ds were even more likely than type As to experience heart attacks. Type Ds also were more likely than others to develop congestive heart failure and four times more likely to die from the condition. The reason: Type Ds have dangerously high levels of tumor necrosis factor, an inflammatory substance produced by the immune system that's associated with the rupture of plaques in the coronary arteries. They also have depleted levels of infection-fighting killer T cells.

What does all this mean? Although a positive mind-set is more beneficial to immune function than a negative one, maintaining some degree of flexibility in your perspective also is important. Being rigidly optimistic can lead to disappointment and frustration, which undermines immunity over time.

Further, if you tend to be more hostile and cynical in your worldview, it's better to express those emotions—even if they're negative—than keep them bottled inside. Otherwise, you could raise your risk of cardiovascular disease and impair your immune function in the process.

The Benefits of Friendship, Intimacy, and Humor

Around 500 BC, the Greeks built temples to Asclepius, the god of healing, which became forerunners to our modern hospitals. Although patients had their own rooms, where they received nutritious food and fresh water, they weren't isolated from other patients as is typical today. The Greeks believed it was just as important for patients to interact with each other as it was for them to eat healthfully, exercise regularly, and pray.

As the ancient Greeks understood, social connectedness is essential for health and healing. It also helps cultivate a positive mood. In this section, we'll explore the health benefits—and especially the immune benefits—of three of the cornerstones of human interaction: friendships, intimacy, and humor. Just as important, you'll learn how you can incorporate more of this emotional medicine into your everyday life.

Socializing Is Good Medicine

Research at the Children's Hospital of Pittsburgh offers a fascinating glimpse into the effects of social interaction on immune function. For one study, researchers sprayed cold viruses into the noses of volunteers, then sequestered them in a hotel for a week. The so-called loners were more likely to come down with a cold.

In another study, this one involving 276 adults between ages 18 and 55, the same researchers found additional evidence that social wallflowers have suppressed immune function. Their conclusion: Those who interact with three or fewer people at least once every 2 weeks are four times more likely to develop colds than social butterflies who interact with at least six people over the same time frame.

If you're an introvert, you may be thinking, "Oh, great—now I'm supposed to get out and mingle more." Not necessarily. Although research confirms that social support from anyone—including spouses, children, parents, friends, and colleagues—appears to enhance immunity, it's not just the size of your social network that counts. It's also the quality of those relationships. Some people are perfectly content to have only a few close confidantes. Others are most comfortable surrounded by a crowd of 100 casual acquaintances.

For a 2005 study published in the journal *Health Psychology,* Carnegie Mellon researchers recruited 83 college freshmen—37 men and 46 women—mostly between ages 18 and 19. After completing health behavior questionnaires, the students received influenza vaccinations and then carried palm computers that prompted them to log in four times a day and assess their moods, as well as their levels of stress and loneliness.

After 1 month and again after 4 months, the researchers drew blood samples to measure influenza-specific antibodies. At 1 and 4 months, antibody levels in students with a small social network (four to 12 members) that interacted at least once a month were about half the levels of those with medium (13 to 18 members) or large social networks (19 to 20 members). Similarly, antibody concentrations in students who reported a high level of loneliness were only half of those who reported a low level of loneliness.

When the researchers combined these two variables—size of social network and level of loneliness—the results were quite interesting. The antibody levels of students who had small social networks but didn't feel lonely were almost as high as those of students with medium networks and actually higher than those of students with large networks. Conversely, students with small social networks who reported feeling lonely were more likely to have lower antibody concentrations than those with medium or large networks who felt lonely.

So if you have a small circle of friends—and you have enough social interaction to avoid feeling lonely—you may be just as resistant to colds, flu, and other infections as people whose personal e-mail accounts are bulging with addresses. "You can have very few friends but still not feel lonely," says Sarah Pressman, MS, the study's lead author. "Alternatively, you can have many friends yet still feel lonely."

High-quality friendships—regardless of their quantity—are important to immune function and general health, Pressman adds, because "they may encourage good behaviors such as eating, sleeping, and exercising well, and they may buffer the stress response to negative events." On the other hand, a total absence of social interaction—even for short periods—may suppress immune function.

A 2004 study published in the *Journal of Applied Physiology* seems to bear this out. Japanese researchers tracked the effects of a 10-day confinement on the immune systems of 10 men between ages 20 and 27. The researchers found that forced isolation caused several adverse changes in immune function.

It's clear that social interaction is vital to optimal immune function. The more friendships you cultivate, the stronger your immune system will be. That said, if you're content having a small number of close friends, you may be just as likely to reap the benefits of social connectedness.

How do you broaden your social circle? Start by reconnecting with existing friends and acquaintances—perhaps by organizing a get-together such as a picnic or hike. Encourage your friends to bring along other people. It's always easier to establish a new relationship with someone who's a friend of a friend.

To meet more of your neighbors, consider joining a Neighborhood Watch group or organizing a block party. Your local library or community center can put you in touch with clubs and organizations that are actively seeking members. You also can meet new people at gyms and recreational centers, especially if you sign up for classes in yoga, tai chi, water aerobics, and other group activities. (See page 113 for more tips on expanding your social network.)

Intimacy and Immunity

A solid relationship with your significant other—especially one full of love, affection, and occasional frolicking between the sheets—can have a powerful effect on your immunity.

Even deep into old age, a happy marriage can help overcome the increased susceptibility to infection that commonly occurs with the passage of time. For proof, consider a 2005 study conducted by researchers at the University of Birmingham in the United Kingdom, in which they examined the immune function of about 180 people age 65 and older. The researchers determined that couples in happy marriages had significantly higher levels of influenza-specific antibodies than those in troubled marriages. Those who were recently bereaved also had lower levels of antibodies.

This isn't to say that an absolutely placid marriage is the key to optimal immune function. For a 2006 study conducted at UCLA, researchers asked 41 middle-aged couples to discuss a troublesome issue for 15 minutes. According to the researchers, an open airing of differences caused surges in blood pressure and heart rate but also increased production of infection-fighting white blood cells.

Interestingly, the same study found that couples who fought foul—frequently using sarcasm, insults, and put-downs in their disputes—had lower levels of natural killer (NK) cells and higher levels of stress hormones. This directly affected their ability to heal from muscle injuries and other injuries (unrelated to the spats, fortunately). Recovery time was 40 percent longer for them than for those couples who engaged in more constructive criticism.

If you're in an intimate relationship—preferably one in which you fight fair—amorous activity can be quite beneficial for immune function. This was the conclusion of a 2006 study for which Japanese researchers recruited volunteers who had pollen, dust mite, and latex allergies. After the volunteers paired off for a 30-minute kissing session, the researchers measured their levels of immunoglobulin E (IgE), an antibody that's elevated in people with allergies and is associated with allergic symptoms. (Although high levels of some antibodies—such as immunoglobulin A, or IgA—usually indicate a properly functioning immune system, high levels of IgE actually are a sign of a hyperactive immune system.) The study participants showed a 40 percent decline in IgE production, suggesting that smooching helped balance their hyperactive immune systems. Interestingly, a tamer form of amorous expression—hugging—did not improve immune function.

Sexual intercourse in a loving relationship appears to have immune-enhancing effects as well. For example, researchers at Wilkes University in Wilkes-Barre, Pennsylvania, found that couples who engage in sex once or twice a week have significantly higher levels of IgA—the antibody that protects mucous membranes from infection—than couples who indulge their passion less frequently. Considering that the average American woman has sex less than once a week, this research suggests that couples would do themselves—and their immune systems—a lot of good if they made a little more time for canoodling.

Paging Dr. Groucho Marx

Both friendships and intimate relationships are essential to maximum immunity. But they may have even greater benefit when a healthy dose of humor is added to the mix.

It's been said that laughter is the shortest distance between two people. And it's true: The more we can laugh together with our families, friends, and co-workers, the less life's stresses seem to overwhelm us. Do you notice how people who are having a good time in a social setting make stronger eye contact with each other, touch more often, and just seem to connect in a different way? This is because humor is a uniting force—the glue that binds us, lightens our burdens, and helps us maintain a measured perspective on our problems.

At the very least, humor is a distraction from distressing emotions. When something tickles your funny bone, it's hard to remain angry or depressed. And the stress-busting benefits of a prolonged tickling are delightful, as you may have noticed at parties that reach their heights of hilarity. The sound of roaring laughter is far more contagious than the latest bug that's going around.

As a bonus, humor can help us to expand our social networks. We are naturally attracted to those around us who have a keen sense of humor and a cheerful disposition.

In terms of physical health, laughter has a real, measurable effect on immune function. It unleashes a cascade of immune cells—including NK, B, and T cells—that fight infection and cancer. It also increases production of gamma-interferon, a disease-fighting protein, while reducing production of stress hormones.

Multiple studies have demonstrated that humor is good for overall health. For starters, it helps lower blood pressure. When you have a good chuckle, your blood pressure rises at first, but then it falls to a lower level. People who laugh regularly tend to have lower resting blood pressure readings than people who don't. Laughter also enhances deep breathing, which speeds the circulation of oxygen and nutrients throughout the body.

A good sense of humor could help protect against heart disease. According to a study at the University of Maryland Medical Center in Baltimore, people who don't have heart disease are 40 percent more likely to laugh in a variety of situations than people of the same age who have heart disease.

There's no question that laughter helps exercise your diaphragm as well as your abdominal, respiratory, back, leg, and facial muscles. It also massages your abdominal organs, which may improve digestion. And because it stimulates both sides of the brain, laughter might improve cognitive function.

SERIOUSLY, WHY AREN'T WE LAUGHING?

Most American adults don't take full advantage of the healing power of humor. Preschoolers laugh about 300 times a day; grown-ups, just 17, on average. It seems that we've become so overwhelmed by our 24-7 lifestyles, which are dominated by family and job responsibilities, that we simply have forgotten how to laugh. As life's disappointments pile up, it's easy to become as jaded as England's Queen Victoria, who now is most remembered for her famous rejoinder: "We are not amused."

Certainly there is nothing more subjective than humor. One person's gut-buster is another person's groaner. But if you want to reconnect with your sense of humor, start by remembering what once made you laugh, and laugh often. Maybe you responded to gentle humor, such as this joke.

> While walking through a forest, a little girl and her dog fall into a pit. Try as they might, they can't crawl to the top. No one answers the little girl's cries for help or her dog's plaintive barks. As darkness falls, wolves begin howling as they edge closer and closer to the pit. The little girl hugs the dog and says, "This looks like the end for us, Muffy." When the dog says, "Yeah, we're history," the little girl is flabbergasted. "I didn't know you could talk!" she gasps. "Well," says the dog, "I was just waiting for the right time to tell you."

If jokes like that one don't tickle your funny bone, maybe you're the sort who appreciates one-liners, such as this one from Woody Allen.

> I don't want to achieve immortality through my work. I want to achieve immortality by not dying.

Then again, maybe you're the sort who prefers the dark humor of TV programs such as *Desperate Housewives.*

As far as your immune system is concerned, it really doesn't matter what gets you guffawing. What's most important is that you indulge your sense of humor at every opportunity. The more frequently you activate your inner laugh track, the better it is for your immune function.

Even anticipating a comedy break can boost your immune system, according to researchers at the University of California, Irvine. They tracked mood changes in 10 male volunteers before and after the men watched a 60-minute humor video. A full 2 days before the men watched the tape, which was of their choosing, their depression ratings had declined by 51 percent. They also were significantly less angry, tense, tired, and confused. Immediately after watching the show, their moods improved even more. They also reported significant boosts in energy.

"We've demonstrated that watching a funny video can stimulate the body's ability to manage stress and fight disease," says lead author Lee Berk, MD. "But this is the first time we've seen that just anticipating such an event can change the body's responses. We believe this 'biology of hope' underlies recovery from many chronic disorders. Treatments that take advantage of the effects of this hope may go a long way toward stimulating immune response and hastening recovery."

For a separate study, researchers at Loma Linda University School of Medicine in California asked 10 healthy male volunteers to watch an hour-long comedy. The men showed significant increases in gamma interferon, a chemical that activates infection- and tumor-fighting NK cells.

Are you seemingly impervious to humor? A study by researchers at Pennsylvania State University in University Park involved 40 volunteers who resolutely disliked most aspects of conventional comedy. When these serious-minded souls had the opportunity to narrate a serious film in an irreverent manner, they loosened up—and subsequently showed signs of enhanced immune function.

As you may be noticing, most studies of the relationship between humor and immunity have involved male volunteers. That's unfortunate, because men and women don't always agree on what is funny and what is not.

One exception is a 2003 study published in *Alternative Therapies,* in which researchers from Indiana State University College of Nursing in Terre Haute tested the effects of humor in a group of 33 women. The researchers measured each volunteer's immune cell levels before and after she watched both a humorous video and a ho-hum tourism video. To help ensure that the women watched a humorous video that they actually would find funny, they were given a choice: *Bill Cosby: Himself, Tim Allen: Men Are Pigs,* or *Robin Williams: Live at the Met.* Most of the women chose the Bill Cosby video. The women who responded with what the researchers described as mirthful laughter showed significantly greater NK cell activity. But this wasn't the case for the women who were not amused by the humorous video. They actually showed declines in NK cell activity.

"Because of the role of natural killer cells in viral illness and various types of cancer, the ability to increase natural killer cell activity in a brief period of time using a noninvasive method could be clinically important," lead researcher Mary P. Bennett, DNSc, RN, and her colleagues concluded. "The use of humor to stimulate laughter could be an effective complementary therapy to decrease stress and improve natural killer cell activity in persons with viral illness or cancer."

Another study published in 2006 by researchers from the University of Maryland in College Park bolstered the theory that watching the right video can have a beneficial effect on immune function. The study showed that watching a funny video can increase blood circulation—along with immune cell circulation—by 22 percent. By the same token, watching a stressful video—such as the battle scenes from *Saving Private Ryan*—had a constricting effect on blood vessels, which actually reduced blood circulation by 35 percent.

HOW TO INCREASE YOUR HUMOR QUOTIENT

Like driving a car, humor is a skill that can be improved with practice. Even if you've convinced yourself that you cannot tell a joke, the truth is you probably can. All you need is good material. Start collecting jokes, cartoons, anecdotes, and stories—either in a notebook or on your computer—and practice retelling them. You'll have a wealth of material at your disposal with which to amuse those around you in social situations.

What if you don't want to be the life of the party? Try these tips for incorporating humor into your everyday life.

Remind yourself to have fun. Nature intended for you to be a fun-loving person. So adopt a fun-loving, even irreverent attitude. Life is crazy. Be okay with that. Foolishness (within limits) is no sin. Be okay with that, too.

Home in on homegrown hilarity. If you look for it—and can groove on it—every day is a collection of ridiculous, absurd, incongruous events that can split your sides.

Learn from the masters. Rent or collect movies featuring your favorite comedians. All of the best comedy is available on video, from Charlie Chaplin to Chris Rock. Watch how the comedians set up a joke or comedic routine and then deliver a killer punch line. For more pointers, read joke books, visit comedy Web sites, or patronize a comedy club.

If Nothing Else, Fake a Smile

What if you're the sort who simply doesn't find anything amusing? Here's a hint: Crack a smile. It doesn't matter one whit to your immune system if it's genuine or not.

For a study published in the *Journal of Personality and Social Psychology*, researchers at the University of California, Berkeley, looked at college yearbook photos and tracked down the grads 30 years later. They found that the women with the widest smiles in the photos were most likely to be in happy marriages and careers—and to have experienced fewer setbacks—than the women with more taciturn expressions.

When you smile, you engage at least three major muscle groups. This not only increases bloodflow to your face—which gives you a more vibrant complexion—it also enhances the circulation of immune cells.

If you aren't naturally inclined to put on a smiley face, it's okay to fake one. If you force yourself to open your lips, raise your cheeks, and assume a Miss America smile, it fools your body into thinking that it's the real thing. Smiling simultaneously enhances your immune function, lifts your spirits, and gives you the silent satisfaction of knowing that you've gotten something for nothing.

Channel surf for topical humor. You always can find the most au courant topics—and the most amusing takes on them—on late-night TV shows featuring comedians such as David Letterman, Jay Leno, and Conan O'Brien. For an edgier view, check out the faux news shows hosted by Jon Stewart and Stephen Colbert on Comedy Central.

Rediscover your inner child. Spend a little time with infants and young children, and watch what gets them giggling. Usually they're delighted and amused by the most ordinary things. They can help you remember why such things are funny.

Learn to laugh at yourself. Although it's important to take your work and other responsibilities seriously, it's emotionally healthy to not take yourself so seriously. Laugh at yourself and your life—in a way that's not self-degrading—and the world will laugh with you. Everyone loves a self-deprecating sense of humor.

Schedule a regular silliness check. If you work standard hours, about 4:30 p.m. is an ideal time to make the rounds and cheer up your co-workers with a joke, a smile, or some witty banter. Think of it as a "day cap" to a hard day's work.

Are You in the Mood for Maximum Immunity?

As you've seen, your mood has a profound effect on your immune function. But your mood is malleable. If you strive to develop and enhance your social network, strengthen your intimate relationship with your significant other, and leaven all of your relationships with a healthy dose of humor, you not only will boost your immunity but also add immeasurable joy and pleasure to your life.

For more advice on improving your mood, see Immune Essentials: The 4-Week Plan, beginning on page 149. The plan shows how you can integrate mood-boosting techniques with the rest of the keys to maximum immunity—nutrition, exercise, sleep, stress reduction, sun exposure, and environmental controls—to protect yourself against infection and chronic disease.

Key #6—Sunlight: A Small Amount Is a Great Source of Vitamin D

Immune Rx: Get 10 to 15 Minutes of Sun Exposure 2 or 3 Days a Week

Among the essential vitamins and minerals, vitamin D is unique because it's the only one your body manufactures with help from sunlight. When a short-wavelength form of the sun's ultraviolet rays—UVB—reaches your unprotected skin, it triggers vitamin D synthesis.

Vitamin D may be best known for supporting healthy bones and helping to prevent bone diseases such as osteoporosis. Its importance first came to light in the early 20th century, when many children suffered from rickets, a disease of extreme vitamin D deficiency in which bones mineralize improperly and fail to develop normally. Because so few foods naturally contain vitamin D, the dairy industry began fortifying milk with the vitamin in the 1930s, all but eliminating rickets in children in the United States. This measure also helps prevent another disease of extreme vitamin D deficiency: osteomalacia, which causes weak bones and muscles in adults.

But vitamin D's benefits extend beyond bone health. Researchers now recognize its importance in regulating the immune system's response to infectious and chronic diseases. A growing body of evidence suggests that vitamin D may help lower the risk of autoimmune conditions such as multiple sclerosis, type 1 diabetes, rheumatoid arthritis, and inflammatory bowel disease. It also may help protect against certain cancers, including those of the colon, breast, and prostate.

In part because of these benefits, vitamin D has become the focus of growing debate within the medical and scientific communities: Just how much does the human body need? And where should it come from? Though no more prestigious an organization than the National Institutes of Health (NIH) recognizes sun exposure as "the most important source of vitamin D," spending too much time outdoors without adequate protection is a known risk factor for skin cancer.

In this chapter, we'll explore the effects of vitamin D on immune function, the ongoing controversy over the risks and benefits of sun exposure—and how an occasional walk in the sun might enhance your immunity by boosting your body's vitamin D supply.

The Relationship between Vitamin D and Infectious Disease

Because large amounts of vitamin D appear to suppress autoimmune diseases (in which the immune system attacks healthy tissues) and reduce the chances of organ rejection after transplants, some researchers surmised that vitamin D would inhibit the immune system's response to infection. Recent studies have not borne out this theory. In fact, many suggest just the opposite: that vitamin D can enhance resistance to many common infectious diseases.

As far back as 1981, researchers noted that influenza epidemics occur when people are getting the least sun exposure and, therefore, have the lowest vitamin D levels: during the winter months. New research has found that vitamin D stimulates production of potent antimicrobial peptides in many types of immune cells—including neutrophils, monocytes, and natural killer (NK) cells—as well as in the epithelial cells that line the respiratory tract and help protect the lungs from infection.

In a 2006 review article published in the journal *Epidemiology and Infection,* the authors noted that children with low vitamin D levels were more likely to develop respiratory infections and that supplemental vitamin D can help reduce this risk. The authors concluded, "Ultraviolet radiation—either from artificial sources or from sunlight—reduces the incidence of viral respiratory infections, as does cod liver oil, which contains vitamin D."

Also in 2006, a study published in *Science Express* explored the relationship between vitamin D and tuberculosis. The research team behind the study—with members from UCLA and Harvard School of Public Health—wanted to know why African Americans are eight times more likely than whites to develop tuberculosis. They found that vitamin D simulates production of an antimicrobial peptide called cathelicidin, which has been shown to kill the tuberculosis bacterium in a test tube. When the researchers examined cell cultures, they found that those from African Americans produced 63 percent less cathelicidin than those from whites. The reason? African Americans have large amounts of melanin, a skin pigment that blocks ultraviolet rays, so they're more likely to have low levels of vitamin D. When the researchers added vitamin D to the cell cultures, it significantly increased cellular production of cathelicidin.

"Tuberculosis is a devastating disease that strikes vulnerable populations particularly hard," says study coauthor Barry Bloom, PhD, of Harvard. "It is exciting to consider the possibility that innate immunity to tuberculosis and other infections in vulnerable populations might be enhanced by providing a simple vitamin that would cost only pennies a day."

The evidence that vitamin D could help prevent a wide range of infectious diseases continues to mount. In a 2007 study published in the *Journal of Clinical Investigation,* researchers from the University of California, San Diego, School of Medicine found that a wound prompts surrounding skin to increase production of vitamin D. The vitamin, in turn, stimulates production of infection-fighting cathelicidin. "Our study shows that skin wounds need vitamin D to protect against infection and begin the normal repair process," says Richard Gallo, MD, the study's lead author. "A deficiency in active vitamin D may compromise the body's innate immune system, which works to resist infection, making a patient more vulnerable to microbes."

The Relationship between Vitamin D, Immunity, and Asthma

Researchers long have been aware of another correlation between limited sun exposure and illness: Populations at northern latitudes are at greater risk for autoimmune diseases such as multiple sclerosis, type 1 diabetes, rheumatoid arthritis, and inflammatory bowel disease than populations in sunny regions near the equator. For example, the risk of multiple sclerosis—in which the immune system attacks the protective myelin sheath surrounding nerve fibers—is five times higher in North America and Europe than in the tropics. People who live at northern latitudes also are more prone to allergies and asthma.

According to the latest research, the higher disease risk may be due at least in part to low vitamin D levels associated with limited sun exposure. Vitamin D appears to balance two types of immune cells: T-helper 1 cells and T-helper 2 cells. During a normal immune response, these cells work in concert, ordering B cells to produce antibodies against an invader and killer T cells to attack it. If the T-helper 1 response predominates, the immune system becomes disorganized and can mistake healthy tissue for a virus, bacterium, or tumor. Then it goes on the attack, setting the stage for autoimmune disease. If the T-helper 2 response predominates, the immune system can mistake harmless intruders such as pollen grains and mold spores for deadly threats, prompting the release of inflammatory chemicals that cause the characteristic symptoms of allergies and asthma. Because vitamin D regulates the development and function of T cells, it helps harmonize the activities of these two types of T cells to orchestrate proper immune response to real threats.

For a 2006 study published in the *Journal of the American Medical Association*, Harvard researchers compared blood samples from 257 people with multiple sclerosis (MS) and 514 people without the condition. Those with the highest vitamin D levels were 62 percent less likely to have MS than those with the lowest levels.

In another 2006 study, Australian researchers examined the relationship between sun exposure and allergic asthma in laboratory mice. The mice treated with ultraviolet light for 15 to 30 minutes before exposure to an allergen were significantly less likely to develop inflamed airways than untreated mice. "This research clearly shows that controlled exposure to ultraviolet light markedly limits the development, incidence, and severity of asthma symptoms in mice," says Prue Hart, PhD, the study's lead author. "It appears that sunlight can suppress specific immune reactions. . . . We are now working to better understand that mechanism with the aim of generating new ways to prevent and treat this chronic disease."

The Relationship between Vitamin D and Cancer

Since the 1940s, population studies have consistently shown that cancer rates are significantly lower in the southernmost regions of the United States than in more northern latitudes. According to one 1990 study, women living in the sunny Southwest were half as likely to die from breast cancer as women living in the cloudy Northeast. A 2001 study, published in the *Lancet,* found that British boys who spent a lot of time in the sun were 66 percent less likely to develop prostate cancer later in life than their peers who spent less time in the sun. Further, if these men did develop prostate cancer, they did so almost 5 years later (at age 72.1 versus 67.7).

In 2004, researchers from the University of Sydney in Australia conducted a survey of 700 adults between ages 20 and 74 with non-Hodgkin's lymphoma and 700 adults of similar age who didn't have this common blood cancer. The researchers asked the participants to estimate their sun exposure at ages 10, 20, 30, 40, 50, and 60, expecting to find a correlation between greater exposure and increased risk of non-Hodgkin's lymphoma. But the results suggested exactly the opposite: Those who spent the most time in the sun actually were 35 percent less likely to develop the disease than those who spent the least time in the sun, regardless of age.

Sun exposure may have much more general anticancer activity. A study published in a 2006 issue of the journal *Anticancer Research* by University of California at Santa

Cruz researchers linked sun exposure to reduced risk of 16 common cancers. Studies like this one suggest that vitamin D helps strengthen the immune system's ability to identify and destroy cancer cells before they can form life-threatening tumors. "Enhancing vitamin D status appears to be the single most important thing that people can do to reduce their risk of cancer, apart from avoiding tobacco and [moderating their] intake of alcohol," says the study's coauthor, Cedric Garland, DrPH.

A trio of more recent studies, all published in 2007, offers further proof of the relationship between vitamin D status and cancer risk—specifically colon, breast, and prostate cancers.

■ A study published in the *American Journal of Preventive Medicine* tracked the health status of 1,448 people for up to 25 years. Those with the highest vitamin D levels were least likely to develop colon cancer, prompting the researchers to conclude that increasing vitamin D intake could prevent up to two-thirds of colon cancers.

■ For another study, researchers analyzed the health records of 1,760 women enrolled in the Harvard Nurses Health Study and the St. George's Hospital study. The women with the highest vitamin D levels had the lowest breast cancer risk.

■ The third study—an analysis of data collected from 14,916 male health professionals over 17 years—found that the men with below-median vitamin D levels were more than twice as likely as men with above-median levels to develop aggressive prostate cancer. "Vitamin D insufficiency is a common problem," concluded lead researcher Haojie Li, MD, and colleagues from Harvard Medical School. "Improving vitamin D status through moderate sun exposure and vitamin D supplements, in particular, is essential for optimal health."

Our Love-Hate Relationship with Sunlight

Amid mounting evidence of the health benefits of vitamin D, physicians and public health organizations alike are reevaluating their stances on what constitutes adequate vitamin D intake and how people should go about shoring up their supplies. Adding fuel to the debate is the decidedly mixed opinion about whether sun exposure is a necessary and appropriate solution for those concerned about vitamin D deficiency.

The body's ability to manufacture its own vitamin D with help from the sun's rays evolved over thousands of years. Scientists trace the first of our human ancestors to sunny, equatorial regions, where dark, melanin-rich skin offered protection from the sun's burning rays. As certain groups migrated north, their skin became lighter, so they could better absorb vitamin D from the weaker, more intermittent sunshine. By the time humans reached the frigid Arctic, the only way for them to get enough vitamin D was to eat lots of fish and animal blubber.

Although our early ancestors didn't realize how vitamin D helped to build bones and immune systems, they seemed to know intuitively that sunlight was good for them. As long as 6,000 years ago, ancient Egyptian and Greek healers—including Hippocrates, the father of modern medicine—noted the role of sunlight in maintaining health and treating a wide range of conditions.

For the better part of its early existence, the human population remained largely agrarian. With most people working outdoors and getting plenty of sunshine, vitamin D deficiency was rare. That changed in the 1800s, when the Industrial Revolution forced more people to congregate in cities and work in offices and factories. By the late 19th century, diseases associated with vitamin D deficiency had become epidemic. Indeed, scholars have speculated that rickets was responsible for crippling Tiny Tim, the character in the Charles Dickens classic *A Christmas Carol*.

In the early 20th century, Americans and Europeans began heading back outdoors in deliberate search of the sun. Before long, millions of regular folks were sunning themselves in their backyards or heading to beaches in ever-skimpier swimsuits. The sun-worshipping craze probably reached its apogee in the 1960s, when beach movies such as *Where the Boys Are* were all the rage, and their stars sported rich brown tans.

The proverbial pendulum took yet another swing in the late 20th century, when researchers identified a strong relationship between *overexposure* to sunlight and increasing rates of skin cancer—including melanoma, the most serious form of skin cancer—and cataracts. In 2001, the US Department of Health and Human Services Report on Carcinogens identified solar ultraviolet radiation as a known carcinogen, effectively putting sunshine in the same category as tobacco among cancer-causing agents.

Over the course of a few decades, public sentiment seemed to shift from worshipping the sun to fearing it. While many refused to throw in their beach towels, many more either shunned the sun altogether or ventured outdoors only after donning long-sleeved shirts, long pants, and wide-brimmed hats and coating every square inch of exposed skin with sunblock. In a 2005 American Academy of Dermatology survey of 1,016 men and women, 62 percent of men and 77 percent of women reported that they were either very careful or somewhat careful to protect their skin from the sun. Similarly, 64 percent of men and 74 percent of women stayed in the shade when they were outdoors for long periods of time. (Interestingly,

Are You Vitamin D Deficient?

If you suspect you may have a vitamin D deficiency, your doctor can order a blood test that measures 25 vitamin D levels. The optimal level is in the range of 30 to 50 nanograms per milliliter of blood; below 20 indicates a deficiency. According to the National Institutes of Health, certain populations are especially likely to run low on vitamin D. They include:

PEOPLE AGE 50 AND OLDER. Deficiency becomes more common with age because the skin is less efficient at synthesizing vitamin D and the kidneys lose some of their ability to convert vitamin D to its active form.

PEOPLE WHO DON'T GET MUCH SUN. At risk are residents of northern latitudes, office workers and others with indoor occupations, the homebound, and people who wear robes and head coverings for religious reasons.

PEOPLE WITH DARKER SKIN. The darker your skin, the less able you are to produce vitamin D from sunlight. That's because dark skin contains a large amount of melanin, a pigment that protects against the sun's harsh effects. Dark-skinned people who live in a temperate region like the United States—where the sun's rays are relatively weak—are especially likely to be vitamin D deficient.

PEOPLE WHO ARE OVERWEIGHT OR OBESE. Fat cells absorb vitamin D that the body would use to enhance bone and cellular health.

---

60 percent of men and 54 percent of women said that people look better and healthier with a tan.)

Is the pendulum set to swing yet again? It seems likely, given the current state of the research into the complex relationship between sunlight, vitamin D, and disease prevention. Though no one is recommending hours of unprotected sun exposure, some researchers are arguing that a little bit is healthy. At the forefront of this pro-sun movement is Michael F. Holick, MD, author of *The UV Advantage*. "Today, we face what is in fact a 'medically significant' epidemic of vitamin D [deficiency]," Dr. Holick contends. "Forty to 60 percent of Americans are seasonally or chronically vitamin D deficient."

The Ongoing Debate over Vitamin D, Sun Exposure, and Skin Cancer

To be sure, Dr. Holick's views have generated considerable controversy among his peers. They also have prompted public health policy makers to try to formulate consensus guidelines for safe sun exposure.

In 2006, researchers from around the world convened in Toronto for a conference with the ambitious objective of reconciling the latest research findings about the health effects of vitamin D, the best sources of the vitamin, and the benefits and risks of sun exposure. Among the conference's key conclusions:

■ Sun exposure raises the risk of melanomas, nonmelanoma skin cancers, and cataracts. Sun protection is essential when the sun's rays are strongest, between 10:00 a.m. and 4:00 p.m.

■ Vitamin D is important for maintaining musculoskeletal health and preventing bone fractures in the elderly. It also may help protect against certain types of cancer, especially colorectal cancer. In the general population, however, vitamin D status may be too low to achieve these benefits.

■ People can obtain vitamin D through sun exposure, diet (especially fortified foods), and supplementation.

■ The sun's known risks must be weighed against its potential benefits. A few minutes a day of unprotected exposure may improve vitamin D status in some people, but it could raise the risk of skin damage in others. Because so many factors influence the manufacture of vitamin D from sunlight—including age, diet, skin pigmentation, geographical location, and sun intensity—more research is necessary in order to formulate guidelines for sun exposure.

The researchers went on to say that the current Daily Value for vitamin D—400 IU—is too low to achieve optimal health. "The most appropriate supplementation level is likely to be above this but below the safe upper [limit] of 2,000 IU per day for adults," the consensus statement says. "More research is needed to determine the optimal amount of vitamin D . . . required to prevent health problems."

Until further research produces more precise guidelines, the conference participants propose that people improve their vitamin D status with a combination of supplements and very limited unprotected sunshine. "If you are concerned about adequate vitamin D levels, discuss supplementation with your health care provider," the consensus statement suggests.

Although the American Cancer Society (ACS) endorsed the findings of the vitamin D conference and acknowledged the impracticality of completely avoiding sun exposure, the organization cautioned that the evidence in favor of moderate exposure is not conclusive enough to advise people to actually seek out sunlight. For now, the ACS stands by its recommendations to protect the skin for any amount of time spent in the sun.

Echoing the ACS's more conservative position, the World Health Organization warns that *over*exposure actually can suppress immune function and increase the risk of infection and certain cancers. "The harmful effects of exposure to UV radiation usually far outweigh [the] benefits," WHO says. "Overexposure to UV radiation affects your skin, your eyes, and probably your immune system. Many people forget that the effects of exposure to UV radiation accumulate over a lifetime. Your sun exposure behavior now determines your chances of developing skin cancer or cataracts later in life. [The incidence of] skin cancer is strongly correlated with the duration and frequency of sun exposure."

Yet even WHO acknowledges that the relationship between sun exposure and skin cancer may be more complex than once thought. There's much more to study and learn, particularly with regard to melanoma. "The causes of malignant melanoma are not fully understood," WHO says. "Exposure during childhood is thought to be more important than exposure later in life. Tumor development may be linked to occasional exposure to short periods of intense sunlight, such as [over] weekends or on holiday. The higher incidence of malignant melanoma in indoor workers compared to outdoor workers supports that notion."

Paradoxically, the very form of solar radiation that causes skin cancer—UVB— also seems to help protect against the disease. In a 2007 study published in *Nature Immunology,* researchers from Stanford University showed how sun exposure strengthens the immune system. They found that vitamin D stimulates T-cell activity in the skin, helping to protect against infection and skin cancer.

What's the Bottom Line on D?

The search for definitive answers on the optimal dosage and best sources of vitamin D is far from over. As additional studies produce new and perhaps contradictory findings, it's important to remember one simple fact: Vitamin D is an essential nutrient, vital for optimal health and specifically for optimal immune function. For this reason alone, you need to make sure that you're getting at least the Daily Value of 400 IU but no more than 2,000 IU (unless you're under a doctor's close supervision).

Vitamin D is fat-soluble, which means that unused amounts accumulate in the body's tissues. Over time, excessive consumption can cause vitamin D toxicity, with symptoms of nausea, vomiting, poor appetite, constipation, weakness, and weight loss. It also can produce abnormally high blood levels of calcium, leading to mental confusion, heart rhythm abnormalities, and calcinosis, a condition in which calcium and phosphate are deposited in soft tissues and organs such as the kidneys.

Because vitamin D isn't all that plentiful in food sources, the chance of getting too much from diet alone is relatively low, unless you consume large amounts of cod

Dietary Sources of Vitamin D

To avoid exceeding the safe upper limit of 2,000 IU of vitamin D per day, you may want to keep track of how much you're getting from both foods and supplements on a daily basis. The following chart highlights some of the best food sources.

FOOD	SERVING	VITAMIN D
Salmon, cooked	3½ oz	360 IU
Mackerel, cooked	3½ oz	345 IU
Sardines, canned in oil, drained	1¾ oz	250 IU
Tuna, canned in oil	3 oz	200 IU
Vitamin D–fortified milk (all types)	1 c	98 IU
Vitamin D–fortified margarine	1 Tbsp	60 IU
Vitamin D–fortified ready-to-eat cereals	¾–1 c	40 IU
Whole egg (yolk contains vitamin D)	1 egg	20 IU
Beef liver, cooked	3½ oz	15 IU
Swiss cheese	1 oz	12 IU

liver oil. According to the NIH, vitamin D toxicity is much more likely to occur with excessive doses of supplements.

A typical multivitamin supplies 400 IU of vitamin D, consistent with the Daily Value. So does a typical calcium-plus-D caplet, which also contains 640 milligrams of calcium. This is important because studies involving laboratory animals suggest that the immune-boosting benefits of vitamin D may depend on an adequate intake of calcium.

Both the ACS and the National Council on Skin Cancer Prevention favor supplementation over sun exposure as a source of vitamin D. Other experts take the opposing view, advocating exposure but allowing for supplementation in certain circumstances—for example, when sun exposure isn't possible or convenient. They note that because the body makes only as much vitamin D from sunlight as it needs, there's no risk of toxicity as there is with supplementation.

Beyond vitamin D, sun exposure offers another immune-boosting benefit: It triggers the release of feel-good brain chemicals such as beta-endorphins and serotonin. As we've discussed previously, a positive mood plays an important role in optimal immune function.

Until further research suggests otherwise, perhaps the best bet is to follow the sensible guidelines for sun exposure issued by the NIH: "Ten to 15 minutes of sun exposure at least two times per week to the face, arms, hands, or back without sunscreen is usually sufficient to provide adequate vitamin D. [This] allows time for vitamin D synthesis and should be followed by application of a sunscreen with an SPF of at least 15 to protect the skin." The NIH also advises those with limited sun exposure to include good sources of vitamin D in the diet.

The caveat about protecting your skin when you're out in the sun beyond those 20 to 30 minutes per week is absolutely critical. Too much sun can raise your risk of skin cancer and contribute to premature skin aging.

For a 2007 review article published in *Lancet,* researchers from Triemli Hospital in Zurich, Switzerland, summarized the findings from 200 recent studies on how best to protect against skin cancer and photo-aging. Among their conclusions: Avoiding direct sunlight and wearing protective clothing may be better preventive strategies than using sunscreen because people tend to apply sunscreen too thinly, then use it as an excuse to bake in the sun for hours on end. The researchers acknowledge that duck-and-cover measures may not be practical or socially acceptable and that sunscreens could remain the "predominant mode of sun protection." Nevertheless, they caution, "Sunscreens should not be abused in an attempt to increase time in the sun to a maximum."

In their article, the researchers explain that sunscreens fall into two major categories: inorganic, which contain zinc or titanium oxides that scatter UV light, and organic, which contain compounds that actually absorb UV light. "The application of a liberal quantity of sunscreen is by far the most important factor for [the] effectiveness of the sunscreen, followed by the uniformity of application and the specific absorption spectrum of the agent used," the researchers conclude. "Application of organic sunscreens to exposed sites should be done 15 to 30 minutes before going out into the sun. Waterproof or water-resistant sunscreens should be used to diminish the need for reapplication after swimming followed by toweling, friction with clothing or sand, and sweating."

Although sunscreens with SPFs higher than 15 have not been proven to offer additional protection against UVB radiation, the researchers determined that the overall data favor high-SPF products over low-SPF products. They also recommend broad-spectrum sunscreens that offer adequate protection against both UVA and UVB radiation.

As for protective clothing, the researchers found that denim, wool, and polyester fabrics offer the best protection, while cotton, linen, and acetate are much more porous. In addition, dry fabric is more effective than wet fabric because it's denser.

Key #7—Environment: How You Can Outsmart Germs

Immune Rx: Wash Your Hands Often

Your environment is overflowing with viruses, bacteria, and other organisms that can cause a host of infectious diseases, including colds and flu. Your home can be an especially problematic place—and not just because you share the same quarters with sometimes-sick family members. Potentially harmful food-borne microorganisms can hitch a ride from the supermarket to your kitchen counters, refrigerator, stove, and sink. Other bad bugs can thrive in leftover food or proliferate in dishrags, towels, sponges, and brushes.

Environmental toxins and pollutants—both inside and outside your home—also can increase your susceptibility to acute and chronic disease. Long-term exposure to even low levels of certain chemicals in many household products can damage your immune system and increase your risk of developing serious conditions such as cardiovascular disease and cancer.

By adopting the immune-boosting strategies recommended in previous chapters—including good nutrition, exercise, sleep, stress reduction, mood enhancement, and moderate sun exposure—you should be able to offset many of these threats to your immunity. You can further protect yourself by taking commonsense precautions and implementing sound environmental controls. Essentially, this means targeting the primary sources of contaminants in your immediate surroundings.

■ Surfaces. Be wary of anything that other people—especially those who carry infectious diseases—have touched.

■ Foods. It's essential to rigorously observe recommendations for safe food handling, preparation, and storage.

■ Air. Although you can't do anything about the air outside your home, you can take steps to improve air quality inside.

■ Household products. Hundreds of cleaners, disinfectants, and other products contain chemicals that may impair your immunity. You can replace them with nontoxic products that will do the job just as effectively.

Let's look at each of these in turn.

It's on the Surface: A Major Threat to Your Immunity

At some point during your schooling, it's likely you were shown those infamous stop-action photos of a human sneeze in progress. You may have been amazed at how a single sneeze can shower a room with germ-laden droplets at the same speed that a major-league pitcher can throw a blazing fastball. So now you may have an instinctive reaction to people who cough and sneeze anywhere near you: "Get out of my face!"

It certainly is possible to get infected from a cough or sneeze, especially if you're trapped with a sick person in an enclosed space such as an office, bus, or elevator. But the fact is, you're much more likely to pick up the latest bug that's going around by touching a contaminated surface than by inhaling an airborne virus or bacteria.

Think of all the surfaces that you—and the people around you—touch each day. From the moment you awaken, your hands are constantly busy.

Let's say one of your co-workers has a sinus infection and pours a cup of coffee from the communal coffeepot. He does so with the same hand that's been catching sneezes and blowing a runny nose for up to 10 days. Fifteen minutes later, you grab yourself a cup of coffee from the same pot and head back to your office or cubicle. If you brush your fingers against your lips, scratch your nose, or rub your eyes, you can unknowingly infect yourself with the same bug that caused your co-worker's sinus infection—and suffer the same fate a few days later.

Viruses and bacteria love the mucous membranes in your eyes, nose, mouth, and respiratory tract because they are your body's most vulnerable points of entry. Once these bugs establish a foothold there, it's easy for them to launch an attack on the rest of your body.

Almost any surface within reach of the human hand can become contaminated. You can pick up germs wherever people congregate: at work, in restaurants and other public places, and at home. Though you can't wash other people's hands, you can do the next best thing: Wash your own.

What to Do When a Family Member Gets Sick

If your spouse, your child, or another family member comes down with a nasty cold or flu, how can you avoid the same fate? According to the Centers for Disease Control and Prevention (CDC), it's more important than ever to follow the recommended rules of hand washing. The following tips also may reduce your risk of infection.

■ Substitute disposable paper towels for community cloth towels in your bathrooms and kitchen.

■ Sleep apart from the infected person.

■ Separate toothbrushes. Most experts recommend that you replace your toothbrush after you've had a cold, the flu, a mouth infection, or a sore throat to reduce the risk of reinfection. (Even when you're not sick, it's a good idea to replace your toothbrush every 3 months because the bristles wear out.)

■ Avoid contact with possibly contaminated surfaces, including counters, utensils, telephones, and computer keyboards.

When a family member is sick, some experts recommend using a commercial disinfectant on everything from toilet seats, faucets, door handles, and light fixtures to telephones, remote controls, and kitchen appliances. The CDC recommends an old standby: a solution of ¼ cup chlorine bleach to 1 gallon warm water. When using this potent disinfectant, wear rubber gloves and ventilate the area. If you're sensitive to bleach, wear a protective mask as well. Allow the solution to stand on the surface for 10 minutes before rinsing.

Your Mother Was Right: Wash Your Hands Often

Hand-to-hand contact spreads many common infectious diseases, including colds, the flu, and gastrointestinal diseases such as diarrhea. Although colds seldom are serious, the flu can be life-threatening—especially if it progresses to pneumonia, which often happens in older people with weakened immune systems. Pneumonia is the seventh-leading cause of death in the United States.

Respiratory infections tend to spread like wildfire in populations that share close quarters, such as the military. Such was the case between 1918 and 1919, when thousands of soldiers who had survived World War I were struck down by the worst influenza pandemic in recorded history.

In a study published in 2006, researchers from the Naval Health Research Center in San Diego examined the effects of a new policy aimed at reducing the spread of respiratory infections among new recruits. Under the policy, recruits were required to attend monthly lectures on the importance of hand washing, soap dispensers were made more widely available, and all military personnel were strongly encouraged to wash their hands five times a day. As a result, the new crop of 45,000 recruits developed 45 percent fewer respiratory infections than the previous years' recruits.

Regular hand washing would have the same effect if adopted in workplaces, schools, and homes, says William Schaffner, MD, chair of the preventive medicine department at Vanderbilt University School of Medicine in Nashville. "I'm not talking about just before dinner," he emphasizes. "We have a rule in my house: Anytime you walk in the door, you hang up your coat and march to the sink to wash your hands."

Unfortunately, many Americans are not so committed to scrubbing up, even after using public restrooms in airports, train stations, bus stations, and restaurants. As a rule, you always should wash your hands before:

- Eating meals at home or in restaurants
- Inserting or removing contact lenses

You always should wash your hands after:

- Using a private or public restroom
- Touching animals or animal waste
- Blowing your nose
- Coughing or sneezing into your hands
- Handling garbage

Be Careful with Pet Treats

In a 2006 issue of the Centers for Disease Control and Prevention (CDC) journal *Morbidity and Mortality Report,* researchers documented nine cases between 2004 and 2005 in which people developed salmonella poisoning after handling pet treats. The reason: As frozen raw beef and salmon were dehydrated to make the treats, the temperatures weren't high enough to kill infectious organisms.

Until manufacturers adopt more rigorous quality-control standards, the CDC advises consumers to thoroughly wash their hands with soap and water after handling pet treats. The agency also recommends that the following groups avoid handling the treats altogether: children under age 5, older adults, and those with immune system disorders.

■ Shaking hands with other people

■ Changing a diaper—and be sure to wash the diaper wearer's hands, too.

You always should wash your hands before *and* after:

■ Preparing food, especially raw meat, poultry, or fish

■ Treating wounds or cuts

■ Touching a sick or injured person

Proper hand washing before and after treating wounds is not the only strategy that you should employ. Whenever you get a cut or scrape, clean it and cover it with antibiotic ointment and a bandage. The wound should stay covered until you see pink, healthy tissue. This can help prevent the development of a scab, which is an open invitation to infection because a scab is a bacterial culture medium. It's one of the primary reasons that so many eczema patients develop recurring staph infections and so many burn victims die from infection.

Hand Washing 101

Hand washing certainly seems like a simple, straightforward exercise. But there is a right way to do it, especially if your objective is to scrub away disease-causing germs.

Wet your hands with warm running water, then apply enough liquid or bar soap to work up a good lather. For at least 15 seconds, vigorously scrub your palms, the backs of your hands, and between your fingers. Take special care to clean under your fingernails. According to some research, this is where 90 to 95 percent of the germs on your hands hide out. So dig into bar soap with your fingernails—which you ideally should keep short—to remove as many pathogens as possible.

After thoroughly rinsing your hands, dry them with a clean cloth towel or disposable paper towel. To prevent transmission of germs that may be lingering on the faucet, use the towel to turn off the water.

Studies show that plain soap and water kill and remove germs just as effectively as antibacterial soaps. Old-fashioned hand washing has an added benefit: It doesn't promote the development of germs that are resistant to antibacterial agents.

If you don't have access to soap and water, use a commercial hand-washing product to help wipe away viruses and bacteria. These include antimicrobial hand washes, alcohol-based hand rubs, and waterless hand wipes. When using a hand wash or rub, squeeze about ½ teaspoon onto your palm and rub it all over your hands—again taking extra care to clean under your fingernails—until both hands are dry. When using a hand wipe, scrub for at least 15 seconds and properly dispose of the wipe.

Which Way Is Best?

Although experts say that the optimal hand-washing routine takes at least 15 seconds, few people scrub for that long. Even health care workers average about 10 seconds.

To assess how various hand-washing techniques perform in the real world of 10-second scrubs, researchers from the University of North Carolina at Chapel Hill designed an intriguing study that appeared in a 2005 issue of the *American Journal of Infection Control.* They recruited 62 volunteers who weren't squeamish about having their hands smeared with two harmless microorganisms—the virus MS2 bacteriophage and the bacterium *Serratia marcescens,* both of which mimic the activity of more harmful germs. After being "infected" with these microorganisms, the volunteers were randomly assigned to scrub their hands for 10 seconds using an array of antibacterial soaps, antimicrobial hand washes, alcohol-based hand rubs, and waterless hand wipes. For the sake of comparison, some volunteers were assigned to scrub with regular soap and water or just plain tap water.

After each scrubbing, the researchers measured how many microorganisms remained on the volunteers' hands. "Our study showed that at a short exposure time of 10 seconds, all agents, with the exception of hand wipes, demonstrated a 90 percent reduction of bacteria on the hands," says lead researcher William Rutala, PhD, MPH. But not all of the hand-washing routines were equally effective. The best bacterium removers were antimicrobial hand washes containing chlorhexidine gluconate (CHG), triclosan, or benzethonium chloride, followed by tap water alone and plain soap and water. Compared with these methods, alcohol-based hand rubs (such as Purell) and waterless hand wipes were less effective at combating *S. marcescens.*

CHG is found in products such as Prima-Kare and BactoShield. Triclosan is the active ingredient in Prevacare, among other products. The PureWorks line of products contains benzethonium chloride.

The best virus removers were—surprise—regular soap and water and just plain tap water. These old standbys were just as effective as antimicrobial hand washes containing CHG, triclosan, or benzethonium chloride, as well as an alcohol-based hand rub containing silver iodide. Other alcohol-based hand rubs—and all of the waterless hand wipes—were less effective at combating MS2 bacteriophage.

Although the most popular hand rubs—the alcohol-containing variety—didn't perform quite as well as some of the other interventions, the researchers say they still play an important role in stopping the spread of viruses and bacteria. Dr. Rutala and his colleagues conclude, "The use of alcohol-based hand rubs will continue to be an important addition to our existing infection control [options] to improve hand hygiene compliance in those locations at which sinks are not available."

Alcohol-based hand rubs also may prevent irksome infections caused by so-called stomach bugs. In a 2006 study of 292 families by researchers at Children's Hospital Boston, those who used an alcohol-based hand rub for 5 months developed 59 percent fewer gastrointestinal infections than those who didn't.

Kitchen Safety: Stop Food-Borne Illnesses

Improper food handling and preparation can spread serious food-borne illnesses such as salmonella and *Escherichia coli* infection. Each year, up to 75 million Americans develop food-borne illnesses, resulting in about 350,000 hospitalizations and 5,000 deaths, according to the Centers for Disease Control and Prevention (CDC).

One bacterium in particular—*E. coli* 0157:H7—periodically causes serious health scares. In late 2006, for example, almost 200 Americans became sick—and three died—after eating contaminated bagged spinach. *E. coli* O157:H7 can contaminate raw vegetables such as spinach, lettuce, alfalfa sprouts, tomatoes, and green onions, as well as raw fruits, particularly melons. It also contaminates unpasteurized milk, apple juice and apple cider, and dry-cured sausage and salami. But most cases of infection result from eating undercooked ground meat.

E. coli bacteria naturally exist in animal intestines. During the slaughtering process, some meat can become contaminated. Ground meat is more likely to be contaminated than whole cuts because it's made from many different animals. In addition, harmful bacteria can be spread throughout the meat during the grinding process.

If you cook ground meat at a high enough temperature to kill any lurking bacteria—not just on the meat's surface but also at its center, so there's no "pink"—

Your Secret Weapon: The Microwave Oven

Even the cleanest-looking kitchen can be crawling with nasty germs such as *Escherichia coli* and *salmonella.* It's easy to unwittingly spread these pathogens by using the same sponges and dishcloths to wipe down counters, stove tops, tabletops, and other surfaces. Because sponges and dishcloths contain the two essential elements to sustain microbial life—water and nutrients— they're ideal habitats for viruses, bacteria, and other microorganisms.

You can disinfect dishcloths by regularly laundering them with hot water. But what can you do about sponges and plastic scrubbers?

To find out, researchers from the University of Florida, Gainesville, conducted a novel experiment, the results of which were published in a 2006 issue of the *Journal of Environmental Health.* The researchers soaked sponges and scrubbing pads in raw wastewater containing a witch's brew of viruses, fecal bacteria, protozoan parasites, and bacterial spores, including one especially hard-to-kill spore: *Bacillus cereus.* Then they tested the ability of the common microwave oven to destroy these pathogens.

The results were unambiguous: Just 2 minutes of microwaving damp sponges and scrubbing pads at full power was enough to inactivate more than 99 percent of the pathogens. But 4 minutes of microwaving was required to inactivate *Bacillus cereus,* which is similar to the protozoan cysts and oocysts that cause giardiasis, a common gastrointestinal infection.

"People often put their sponges and scrubbers in the dishwasher, but if they really want to decontaminate them and not just clean them, they should use the microwave," says lead researcher Gabriel Bitton, PhD. "The microwave is a very powerful and inexpensive tool for sterilization." He recommends microwaving sponges according to how often you cook, with every other day being a good rule of thumb.

After the study was published, some consumers complained that microwaving caused sponges and scrubbers to catch fire, which ruined their microwave ovens and stunk up their homes for several hours. As it turned out, the consumers had nuked sponges and scrubbers when they were *dry.* This prompted the University of Florida to issue the following advisory: "To guard against the risk of fire, people who wish to sterilize their sponges at home must ensure [that] the sponge is completely wet. Two minutes of microwaving is sufficient for most sterilization. Sponges should have no metallic content."

it significantly reduces your risk of infection. That's why you should order meat cooked either medium-well or well done when eating out.

Although 80 percent of food-borne illnesses originate in public eateries—fast-food restaurants and cruise ships being two of the most notorious examples—that still leaves 20 percent occurring at home. Since this is the only environment that's completely within your control, it's especially important to strictly adhere to food-safety guidelines when preparing and storing food.

Start by washing all produce, even fruits and vegetables that are sold as "prewashed." Firm produce such as carrots, apples, and peaches should be thoroughly scrubbed by brush or hand under running water. It's best to soak berries in several changes of water. For leafy produce such as lettuce and cabbage, remove the outer leaves and swish the remainder in a colander under running water.

Exercise even greater caution when handling raw meat. You should thoroughly wash everything that touches the meat—including your hands, any utensils, and countertops—with hot, soapy water; a disinfectant solution made from ¼ cup bleach in 1 gallon water; or disinfecting wipes. Although you probably already know this cardinal rule, it bears repeating: Never place cooked burgers on the same plate that held the uncooked patties.

To ensure that meats and other foods are cooked at a high enough temperature to reduce the risk of food-borne illness, buy an inexpensive meat thermometer. Remember that most contaminated food looks and smells normal, so rely on your

How to Interpret Dates on Food Products

Contrary to popular belief, the dates stamped on food products are not an indicator of safety. Rather, they show you how long a food will remain at peak freshness, based on the manufacturer's good-faith promise, according to the US Department of Agriculture.

Currently, there is no uniform or universally accepted dating system for food products in the United States. Federal regulations require dating only for infant formulas and some baby foods. Any other dating is strictly voluntary.

Here's how to interpret the expiration terminology that you're most likely to see on food products.

SELL BY: This tells the store how long to display the product. You should not buy it after this date.

BEST IF USED BY OR BEFORE: This tells you how long the product will retain its flavor and quality.

USE BY: This is the latest date—as determined by the manufacturer—that the product will retain its peak quality.

CLOSED OR CODED: This date is for use by the manufacturer to track inventory, rotate stock, or locate the product in the event of any kind of problem.

The bottom line: In the absence of a uniform dating system, it's safest to buy, use, or freeze products before the stated expiration dates.

thermometer, not your nose. The Food Safety and Inspection Service of the US Department of Agriculture recommends the following cooking temperatures to destroy food-borne contaminants.

- Ground beef, pork, veal, and lamb: 160°F

- Ground poultry: 165°F

- Whole cuts of beef, veal, and lamb: medium rare, 145°F; medium, 160°F; well done, 170°F

- Poultry: 180°F (either whole birds or parts)

- Pork (fresh): medium, 160°F; well done, 170°F

- Ham: fresh, 160°F; cooked, 140°F; leftover cooked, 165°F

- Fish and shellfish: 145°F

- Egg dishes: 160°F

- Casseroles, combination dishes, stuffing, stews, and leftovers: 165°F

To reduce your risk of food-borne illness, handle leftovers with lots of TLC. Throw out perishable foods such as meat, poultry, fish, eggs, and casseroles if they've been sitting at room temperature for more than 2 hours or at temperatures above 90°F for more than 1 hour. Only refrigerate leftovers if you plan to eat them within 3 to 4 days; otherwise, freeze them immediately. Frozen leftovers stored at 0°F can be kept indefinitely, though over time they can lose flavor and become dry. Here are the maximum time frames for safely refrigerating or freezing certain commonly prepared foods.

- Ground beef: Refrigerate 1 to 2 days; freeze 3 to 4 months.

- Fish: Refrigerate 1 to 2 days; freeze 3 to 6 months.

- Chicken parts: Refrigerate 1 to 2 days; freeze 9 months.

- Pork chops or roasts: Refrigerate 3 to 5 days; freeze 4 to 6 months.

- Milk: Refrigerate 5 days; freeze 1 month.

- Ice cream: Freeze 2 to 4 months.

- Fresh eggs in shell: Refrigerate 3 weeks; do not freeze.

Before eating leftovers, reheat them in your oven at a setting of at least 325°F. Because quick reheating is essential for killing harmful microorganisms, avoid using slow cookers or chafing dishes to reheat food. Before eating leftover sauces, soups, and gravies, reheat them to boiling.

How Pollution Affects Your Immune System

Researchers have long known that exposure to the tens of thousands of synthetic industrial chemicals, pesticides, metals, and other substances in the environment—even at low levels—can adversely affect immune function and increase cancer risk. Some experts have suggested that such toxins suppress the immune system by either killing immune cells or impairing their function. Another possibility is that toxins generate higher levels of cell-damaging free radicals.

Until recently, however, researchers haven't understood exactly how toxins affect health. It has been difficult to determine if a specific chemical is toxic or associated with certain diseases. Advances in molecular biology, genetics, and stem-cell biology have provided researchers with a new understanding of how toxic substances impact human health on a cellular and molecular level.

For a 2007 study published in the online journal *Public Library of Science—Biology*, researchers from the University of Rochester in New York conducted a laboratory experiment involving a specific group of brain cells called glial cells. These advanced-stage stem cells are essential to the growth, development, and normal function of the central nervous system. The researchers exposed the glial cells to low levels of lead, mercury, and paraquat, one of the world's most widely used herbicides. They found that all three toxins triggered a chain reaction that caused the glial cells to shut down and stop dividing.

"We have discovered a previously unrecognized regulatory pathway by which chemically diverse [toxins] converge and disrupt normal cell function," says lead researcher Mark Noble, PhD. Because lead, mercury, and paraquat are very different substances with similar effects on glial cells, this discovery could pave the way for a simple and effective way to determine if other chemicals pose a health threat, Dr. Noble says.

The Air You Breathe May Not Be So Healthy

Every day, you take about 20,000 breaths and inhale about 3,000 gallons of air into your body. Unfortunately, the air may contain not only life-giving oxygen but also high levels of metals such as cadmium, nickel, and manganese, as well as large amounts of particulates, the microscopic bits of carbon particles produced by motor vehicles, power plants, and factories. All of these pollutants may impair immune function by increasing oxidative stress on immune cells.

More than a decade ago, researchers identified higher death rates among people who reside in areas with high concentrations of fine particulate matter. But a 2007 study published in the *New England Journal of Medicine* by researchers from the University of Washington in Seattle sheds new light on the association between particulate exposure and an increased risk of heart disease, particularly in women. The researchers analyzed data from the Women's Health Initiative, a landmark study involving 65,893 postmenopausal women living in 36 metropolitan areas nationwide with varying levels of particulates. Between 1994 and 1998, none of the women had cardiovascular disease. After a median of 6 years, however, 1,816 had suffered a nonfatal or fatal cardiovascular event such as a heart attack or stroke.

The researchers found a strong link between the women's level of particulate exposure and subsequent risk of disease or death. For every 10-microgam increase in particulates per cubic meter of air, there was a corresponding 24 percent increase in the risk of a cardiovascular event and a 76 percent increase in the risk of death from cardiovascular disease—substantially higher than risks reported in previous studies conducted by the American Cancer Society and Harvard.

"The mechanisms by which fine particulate air pollution influence the risk of cardiovascular disease are still under investigation," say Douglas W. Dockery, ScD, and Peter H. Stone, MD, in an accompanying editorial in the *New England Journal of Medicine*. "There is evidence that inhalation of particulate air pollution creates and exacerbates both pulmonary and systemic inflammation and oxidative stress, leading to direct vascular injury, atherosclerosis, and autonomic dysfunction. The findings of the Women's Health Initiative Study strongly support the recommendations for tighter standards for long-term fine particulate air pollution."

Safeguard Your Home against Environmental Toxins

Aside from lobbying your lawmakers, there isn't a lot that you can do to reduce your exposure to particulate matter and other pollutants when you're outside. But there are steps you can take to limit your exposure to environmental toxins inside your home, where concentrations can be even higher than outdoors.

A first and necessary step is to prohibit indoor smoking. Tobacco smoke contains more than 4,000 chemicals, many of which cause cancer. As many as 3,000 non-smoking Americans die each year from lung cancer associated with exposure to secondhand smoke.

Another essential strategy is to check for toxic chemicals in the multitude of products you bring into your home—everything from disinfectants and cleaning supplies to paints, insecticides, and herbicides. Before buying any product, read the label. A word such as *danger* or *poison* is a red flag that the product is highly toxic.

Choosing the Best Air and Water Filters

You can significantly reduce your exposure to indoor airborne and waterborne toxins by using air and water filters.

The best air cleaners utilize a high-efficiency particulate air (HEPA) filter or an electrostatic filter. Either type will help rid the air of pollen, mold, and particulate matter. When choosing an air cleaner, here are some factors to keep in mind.

- The appliance's speed (Be sure its capacity is compatible with the room in which you intend to use it.)
- Its efficiency at removing particles from the air
- Its noise level
- The cost of replacement filters

Be wary of ion generators. This type of air cleaner is not only ineffective at controlling indoor pollution, it also produces ozone, which can aggravate symptoms in people with allergies and asthma.

Before installing a water filter, find out what's in your water by obtaining a Consumer Confidence Report (CCR) from your local water supplier. You also can find your CCR on the Environmental Protection Agency's Web site: www.epa.gov.

When looking for a water filter, be sure it's certified by the National Sanitation Foundation. Also consider the pros and cons of these various types.

- A point-of-use filter attaches to your water main to treat all water that enters your home, including what goes into your sinks, showers, and toilets.

- Activated-carbon filters can be installed at various points of entry. They effectively remove chlorine, radon, some volatile organic compounds, pesticides, and trihalomethanes. But they must be replaced on a regular basis.

- Reverse osmosis filters, in which water passes through a cellophane-like membrane, effectively reduce levels of bacteria, metals such as cadmium and chromium, and some pesticides. But these filters waste a lot of water for each gallon they treat and are less effective than activated-carbon filters at removing volatile organic compounds and trihalomethanes.

- Distillers boil water into steam and condense it back to water. Although they effectively remove arsenic and some pesticides, they can leave other contaminants behind.

- Water softeners—also known as ion exchangers—neutralize and replace contaminants with safer chemicals such as sodium or chloride. Although they help reduce water levels of heavy metals, they also leave high amounts of sodium in drinking water.

If the label says "Warning" or "Caution," the product is somewhat less toxic but still potentially hazardous.

In either case, try to avoid buying and storing such products in your home unless you have an absolutely compelling reason to do so. If you must use such products, follow the label instructions to the letter, and make sure that your home is properly ventilated.

Whenever possible, find nontoxic, biodegradable substitutes for toxic chemicals. Instead of a noxious oven cleaner, for example, try using steel wool with baking soda and water. You also can use baking soda to scrub your toilets.

Another helpful nontoxic ingredient is undiluted white vinegar, which makes a great household disinfectant. Instead of using a toxic drain cleaner, try a weekly drain-cleaning regimen that combines ½ cup of white vinegar with ½ cup each of baking soda and hot water.

If you live in a standard single-family dwelling or an apartment below the third floor, you may be exposed to radon, a radioactive gas that is the second-leading cause of lung cancer after cigarette smoking. Although many commercial radon test kits are available, look for those that are state-certified or say "Meets EPA Requirements." If radon levels are too high, you can get assistance with radon remediation from the Consumer Federation of America Foundation's National Radon Fix-It hotline at 800-644-6999.

PART III
Immune Essentials: The 4-Week Plan

4 Weeks to Maximum Immunity

If you use a computer, you know that cyberspace is filled with viruses, worms, Trojans, and spyware that can infect and disable your computer. So you probably have been careful to protect your computer with a reliable, up-to-date antivirus and anti-spyware program.

Give yourself the same attention! As a being made of flesh and blood instead of bits and bytes, you're vulnerable to a multitude of biological threats—viruses, bacteria, parasites, and fungi—that can infect and disable you. Since you're a magnificent machine that's infinitely more complex than any computer and designed to last about 30 times longer, you need to do everything you can to fortify your body's first line of defense: your immune system.

In previous chapters, you learned how your immune system works and how various lifestyle choices can help or hinder your immune function. You know that your immune system is exquisitely sensitive to what you eat, how often and how intensely you exercise, how much you sleep, and whether you get any sunlight. You've seen how immunity can be compromised by stress, negative mood, and environmental toxins.

Perhaps you've noticed that you're getting more colds each year and that they're hanging on longer. Or you're concerned that skin wounds, which once seemed to heal almost overnight, now take weeks to fade away. Changes like these could be early signs of an immune system in need of a boost.

Now you're ready to put what you've learned into action. Think of this 4-week plan as a "downloadable," personalized antivirus program that provides step-by-step instructions for achieving maximum immunity.

The Maximum Immunity Menus

In this plan, you'll find 4 weeks' worth of immune-friendly menus, developed by Kim Galeaz, RD, CD, an Indianapolis–based nutrition and culinary consultant. Each day's menu includes a hearty breakfast, lunch, and dinner, with an emphasis on whole grains, fruits and vegetables, beans, and lean pork and fish. You'll also enjoy satisfying snacks such as oatmeal cookies, which supply a generous amount of immune-boosting beta-glucan; chocolate milk, which doubles as an effective postexercise recovery drink; and dark chocolate and almonds, both rich in antioxidants. Other delicious extras include yogurt and its drinkable kissing cousin, kefir, which comes in flavors such as blueberry and peach and contains large amounts of immune-enhancing probiotic bacteria.

Each day's menu supplies roughly 1,800 calories. This is just the right amount of energy for a healthy 55-year-old woman who engages in at least 30 minutes a day of moderate physical activity and wants to maintain her current weight. Although this is not meant to be a weight-loss plan, it can be turned into one. By judiciously cutting 250 calories per day from the menu plan—not from just one food group—and continuing to exercise 30 minutes per day, you should be able to lose a sensible ½ pound per week.

For extra nutritional insurance, Galeaz suggests taking a daily multivitamin that supplies no more than 100 percent of the Daily Values for the essential vitamins and minerals. This is important, she says, because it's difficult to get the recommended intake for certain nutrients—such as vitamin E (30 IU)—from diet alone.

Is it wise to take supplements that exceed the Daily Values? "I don't believe in megadoses of vitamins and minerals," Galeaz says. "I know a lot of experts out there say that maybe you should get a little bit more of this or that nutrient. But the government sets its nutritional standards for good reasons, based on the best current evidence."

Serving Up Success

If you don't already have one, you might want to invest in a good set of measuring cups before starting the Immune Essentials Plan. "People often underestimate the true amount of a serving, so you need to get a handle on how much food equals a half cup or cup," says Kim Galeaz, RD, CD, an Indianapolis-based nutrition and culinary consultant. "Once you recognize exactly what constitutes a serving, you'll be able to accurately eyeball it."

The Maximum Immunity Workout

Each week of the plan has an exercise component, complete with simple stretches to begin and end each workout; an easy walking routine to improve cardiovascular fitness; and resistance-training exercises to tone the muscles in your upper body, core, and lower body. During weeks 2, 3, and 4, the exercise component becomes just a bit more ambitious.

For the walking routine, all that's necessary is a pair of good-quality walking shoes, which are better than running shoes because they stabilize your foot through the heel-to-toe movement of each stride. If you need extra cushioning, opt for cross-training shoes, which are appropriate for both walking and running. When you buy a new pair, write the date on the inside of your shoes with a magic marker. Replace them every 500 to 700 miles.

For the resistance training, you'll need one pair of adjustable-weight dumbbells or four pairs of fixed-weight dumbbells. If you haven't lifted weights before, start with 3-, 5-, 8-, and 10-pound dumbbells.

Remember that your goal is to work up to 30 to 60 minutes of moderate aerobic activity every day. This is the single best fitness strategy for strengthening your defenses against viruses, bacteria, and parasites, as well as rogue cancer cells. For general health, though, you'll get the most benefit from a well-rounded fitness program that includes 10 minutes of resistance-training exercises most days of the week. Resistance training builds muscle and bone, improves posture and balance, and boosts metabolism. Because muscle tissue burns more calories than fat, a regular resistance-training regimen can help melt away extra pounds—including dangerous intra-abdominal fat, which makes its home around your midsection and raises your risk of developing chronic conditions such as heart disease and diabetes.

Think of the resistance-training exercises in this plan as more of a workout buffet than a structured program: You can pick and choose which routines you want to do. How you mix them is a matter of personal preference, as long as you're spending about 10 minutes on resistance training almost every day. It may be most beneficial to perform upper-body, core, and lower-body exercises on alternate days, giving the muscle groups more time to recover and grow stronger before you challenge them again.

If you're new to resistance training, it helps to understand the terminology. A *repetition*—or *rep*—is one complete exercise (i.e., one pushup). A *set* is a specific number of repetitions. For most of the exercises presented here, we recommend 2 sets of 8 to 12 repetitions each.

When using dumbbells, it's simple to choose the right weight for any given exercise. If you aren't able to lift a weight eight times using good form, it's too heavy. If you can easily lift a weight more than 12 times, it's too light. Pick an intermediate weight that works your muscles without overstraining them.

A similar rule applies when you perform exercises that use your own body weight as resistance, such as pushups and abdominal crunches. Start with 2 sets of 8 to 12 repetitions. If that's too easy, increase the number of repetitions, but be careful not to overexert yourself.

You'll find that as you gain strength, you'll be able to work up to heavier dumbbells—or, in the case of pushups and crunches, to do more reps. It's a measurable and motivational sign of your progress.

The Rest of the Plan

As you'll see, the plan offers daily and weekly tips and tools for addressing the remaining keys to maximum immunity: sleep, stress, mood, and environment. Each week begins with a series of strategies targeting each of these areas, along with room to write down the challenges you anticipate in the days ahead, the steps that you can take to overcome them, and the goals that you've set for yourself.

Each daily entry includes the day's menu along with a journal page for tracking your physical activity, stress level, sun exposure, and what you did to improve your sleep, stress, mood, and environment. You also will find a fresh "Tip of the Day" focusing on one of the 7 Keys to Maximum Immunity. (Feel free to refer back to previous chapters for additional tips.)

At the end of each week, you'll have room to record and acknowledge your accomplishments. Take this time to pause and reflect on what you've achieved. Making even modest lifestyle adjustments is no small feat, so give yourself a much-deserved pat on the back! You also will find space to identify areas that may require more attention the following week. You can use this information to help tweak the plan until it's just right for you.

Please don't leave the journal pages blank! Whenever the spirit moves you, grab a pencil, pen, marker, stray crayon, or whatever you can find, and jot down what's on your mind—positive or negative. You don't need to confine your comments to the plan. If you want to express random or off-the-wall thoughts, that's okay, too.

Studies consistently show that people who keep journals are most likely to follow through with a lifestyle-improvement plan. It's rewarding to have a written record of the progress you've made and the hurdles you've overcome. So feel free to make notes in the "official" spaces—or anywhere else in the book that you like. It will help you stick with the plan—not just for the next 4 weeks but for life.

Get Set for Week 1

Date ....

Maximum Immunity Success Strategies

EXERCISE

Walking/aerobic: beginner, 15 minutes a day; veteran, 30 minutes a day minimum
Resistance training: 10 minutes most days

SLEEP

If you're like most Americans, you sleep less than the recommended 7 to 8 hours a night. In fact, you may be so fatigued that you don't realize how it has been affecting your immune function and overall health. Take control of your sleep habits by creating a "sleep diary." Keep track of when you go to bed, how long you sleep, how well you sleep, and how energized—or fatigued—you feel the next day. Make special note of daily and nighttime activities and bedtime routines that seem to enhance—or interfere with—your sleep quality.

STRESS

A major source of stress is the sense that you don't have enough time to do all of the things that you need or want to do. Manage your time in the same way that you manage your finances: with a budget. To create a "time budget," start by making a detailed list of everything you do during the day, from the moment you get up until the moment you turn in for the night. Seeing exactly how you spend your time is an essential first step toward making better use of one of your most precious resources.

MOOD

Nobody is purely happy or unhappy. But how do you know where you fall on the positive-negative spectrum? Take control of your mood by keeping a "mood diary" that lists the events—both positive and negative—that trigger powerful emotions. If the balance tilts too much toward the negative side, start considering how you can work more mirth or joy-inducing events into your daily schedule.

ENVIRONMENT

Germ-proof your personal space, starting with your hands, teeth, and mouth. Make a conscious effort to wash your hands before preparing and eating food, after using the toilet, and after visiting possibly germ-laden public places such as malls, movie theaters, and gyms. To reduce the risk of gum disease, which studies have linked to heart disease, resolve to brush your teeth at least twice a day—even better, after every meal—and floss at least once a day.

Challenges I anticipate this week:

....

....

....

....

Strategies I can use to overcome them:

....

....

....

....

My goals for this week:

....

....

....

....

Your Maximum Immunity Workout

GET LOOSE

Stretching loosens your muscles, tendons, and ligaments so they stay flexible. It's an important, if often overlooked, step that reduces your risk of injury during any form of sustained cardiovascular or resistance-training exercise. It doesn't matter if your workout is light, moderate, or vigorous; if you engage in 5 to 10 minutes of stretching before and after, you'll be much less likely to become one of those sorry souls who watch from the sidelines and lament, "I used to exercise before I hurt my _____ [insert body part here]."

Before you start exercising, limber up with this light stretching routine. (During weeks 2, 3, and 4, we'll show you other stretches that you can add.) Remember to move slowly. Don't strain or bounce, and avoid stretching to the point of discomfort.

Side stretch. Stand with your feet shoulder-width apart and your hands on your hips. Slowly reach one arm over your head and toward the opposite side, keeping your hips steady and your shoulders straight. Hold for 10 seconds before returning to the starting position. Repeat to the opposite side.

Knee pull. Stand with your back against a wall. Keeping your head, hips, and feet in a straight line, pull one knee toward your chest and grasp it with your hands. Hold for 10 seconds before returning to the starting position. Repeat with the other knee.

Wall push. Stand 3 to 4 feet from a wall and place your hands against it. Slide one foot forward, bending your knee. Keep your back leg straight, with your foot flat on the floor and your toes pointing straight ahead. Hold for 10 seconds before returning to the starting position. Repeat with the other leg.

Lying quadriceps stretch. Lie on your left side with your legs straight, one on top of the other. Bend your left elbow and support your head with your left hand. With your right hand, grab your right foot and pull your right heel toward your right buttock. Hold for 10 seconds before returning to the starting position. Then roll over and repeat with the other leg.

GET FIT

Walking is an easy, pleasurable activity that's safe for most everyone at any age. As little as 15 minutes of walking a day burns calories and improves cardiovascular fitness while boosting mood and reducing stress. To get the optimal immune-enhancing benefit, your goal is to work up to at least 30—and ideally, 60—minutes of walking (or another aerobic activity) most days.

If you haven't been exercising regularly, or if you have an existing medical condition, please be sure to check with your doctor before launching a walking routine. The following tips can help you get the most from your daily constitutional.

If you're a beginner, aim for 15 minutes to start. Go slow for the first 5 minutes, then a little faster for the next 5 minutes. Downshift for the final 5 minutes, which will help you cool down. (You'll gradually build the duration and intensity of your walks during weeks 2, 3, and 4.)

Try to make walking a daily habit. While it's beneficial to exercise most days, you'll notice faster improvement in cardiovascular fitness and endurance by making your workouts a daily event. That said, if you miss a day, don't try to make up for it by walking twice as fast or twice as long during your next workout. Slow, steady progress is key.

Put your whole body into it. To make each step shorter and quicker, roll from your heel to the outside of the foot to the ball of the foot. Then push off with your toes. More effort equals more burned calories.

Pump your arms. Bend your arms at 90-degree angles, holding them close to your sides and making loose fists. During each upswing, your thumb should brush against a spot just beneath your waistband as your fist continues in an arc toward your breastbone. During each downswing, move your fist behind the side seam of your shorts or pants.

Think brisk. Aim for a moderate pace at which you break a sweat without busting your lungs. On a physical activity scale of 1 to 10—with 1 being TV watching and

10 being all-out exertion—aim for about a 7. You should be breathing harder than usual but also able to carry on a simple conversation.

GET STRONG

For the resistance-training portion of your workout, here are three time-tested exercises—one each for your upper body, core, and lower body. (During weeks 2, 3, 4, we'll introduce more moves, which you can add to your workout at your discretion.)

UPPER BODY: MODIFIED PUSHUP

Lie facedown on an exercise mat or another padded surface. Place your palms flat on the floor just outside your shoulders, with your fingers pointing forward and your elbows pointing upward. Bend your knees so that your lower legs are perpendicular to the floor.

Push up your torso with your body weight resting on your knees. Tighten your abdominal muscles and keep your head, neck, back, buttocks, and thighs in a straight line. Your shoulders should be directly above your hands, but avoid locking your elbows. Hold for 1 second, then lower your torso and repeat.

According to the American Council on Exercise, a woman between ages 50 and 59 who can perform at least 21 modified pushups without resting is in excellent physical condition. If you can't do that many, no matter what your age or gender, don't despair! Do as many as you can. By making modified pushups a regular part of your resistance-training routine, you'll gradually build enough upper-body strength to perform the suggested 2 sets of 8 to 12 repetitions with ease.

CORE: CURL-UP

Put two long pieces of masking tape on the floor so that they're parallel but 3½ inches apart. Lie on your back across the pieces of tape with your feet flat and your knees bent at 90-degree angles. Rest your arms at your sides, with your palms down and your fingers touching the closest piece of tape. Using your upper-abdominal muscles, lift your torso and extend your fingers until you touch the second piece of tape. Return to the starting position, then repeat.

As with push-ups, do as many curl-ups as you can to start. Gradually work up to the suggested 2 sets of 8 to 12 repetitions.

LOWER BODY: THIGH-SCULPTING MOVES INSPIRED BY TAI CHI

You can use these exercises for gentle lower-body toning or to help cool down after a workout. Like other tai chi movements, they help enhance immunity.

Empty step. Keeping your body relaxed, stand up straight but with your knees slightly bent, arms at your sides with palms facing each other. Now take a step with your right foot, lifting it as though you are about to start walking. Hold your heel a few inches above the floor for 30 seconds as you practice deep breathing. Return to the starting position, then repeat with your left foot. Continue alternating feet until you've done 6 reps on each side.

Rooster pose. Keeping your body relaxed, stand up straight, with your feet hip-width apart. Hold both hands in front of your chest as though grasping a softball. Raise your left knee to hip height, with your toes pointed out slightly. Breathe deeply as you extend the leg forward slightly. Hold for 30 seconds, then lower your leg and repeat with your right leg. Perform the exercise twice on each side.

Note: Skip this exercise if you don't feel steady enough to balance on one foot, because it could lead to a fall.

Crouch step. Stand with your feet more than shoulder-width apart and your toes angled outward slightly. Bend your elbows in front of you so that your lower arms are at chest height, parallel to each other but about 10 inches apart. Your palms should be facing each other.

Keeping your right leg straight, bend your left knee and let your body sink toward the floor. Hold for 30 seconds, breathing deeply as you do. Then return to the starting position and repeat with your right leg. Perform the exercise twice to each side.

Your Maximum Immunity Menu

Week 1/Day 1

BREAKFAST

1 whole wheat bagel, toasted and topped with 1½ tablespoons peanut butter and 1 sliced banana

1 cup 1% milk

LUNCH

Chicken Spinach Strawberry Salad: 3 cups fresh spinach leaves, 3 ounces cooked chicken strips, ¾ cup strawberries, and 2 tablespoons honey-roasted almonds with 3 tablespoons light raspberry vinaigrette dressing

6 multigrain crackers

1 cup 1% milk

SNACK

1-ounce piece dark chocolate

DINNER

Savory Salmon: 3 ounces grilled or baked salmon cooked with 1 teaspoon honey, 1 teaspoon lime juice, and ¼ teaspoon salt-free garlic-and-herb seasoning

¾ cup cooked whole wheat couscous sprinkled with parsley

1 cup cooked asparagus spears

1 whole wheat dinner roll with 1 teaspoon light margarine

1 plum

1,815 calories; 19% protein (87 g); 52% carbohydrate (236 g); 29% fat (58.5 g); 8% saturated fat (16 g); 159 mg cholesterol; 35 g dietary fiber; 11,087 IU vitamin A; 116 mg vitamin C ; 12.5 mg vitamin E ; 443 IU vitamin D ; 3 mg vitamin B$_6$; 517 mcg folate; 6.4 mcg vitamin B$_{12}$; 1,413 mg sodium; 3,536 mg potassium; 1,134 mg calcium; 17 mg iron; 11 mg zinc

FOOD FACTS

■ Whole grains, like the whole wheat bagels and couscous in today's menu, are easy to find in supermarkets. Whole grains typically provide more protein, vitamins, minerals, and fiber than refined grains. Couscous cooks in 5 minutes in boiling water, making it a perfect whole grain choice for busy lifestyles.

■ Light margarine in the tub is your best bet for watching fat and calories. Most available brands are trans fat free. Choose a light margarine with no more than 5 grams of fat per tablespoon.

Best food choice(s) today:

....

....

....

EXERCISE RECORD

Walking or other aerobic activity: .... *minutes*

Resistance training: Upper body ....
                       Lower body ....
                            Core ....

STRESS RECORD

Today my stress level is: Yellow .... *Orange* .... *Red* .... *Flashing red* ....

SUN DIARY

Today I got .... *minutes of sun exposure.*

THIS IS WHAT I DID TODAY TO IMPROVE . . .

My sleep:

....

....

....

My stress level:

....

....

....

My mood:

....

....

....

My environment:

....

....

....

 TIP OF THE DAY Move your sad DVDs to the back of the shelf and watch comedies instead. Funny movies can improve your mood, boost your immunity, and—happy news for dieters—diminish your desire to stuff yourself with comfort food, according to a 2007 study published in the *Journal of Marketing*. Researchers at Cornell University in New York, recruited 38 administrative assistants to watch one of two movies—*Sweet Home Alabama* or *Love Story*. The volunteers were offered an unlimited supply of hot, buttery, salty popcorn and seedless grapes. Those who watched *Sweet Home Alabama* ate 36 percent less popcorn than those who watched *Love Story* and were more likely to pop grapes. The study's authors suspect that happy people want to extend their mood in the short term but favor more nutritional snacks because they also consider the long term. Sad people, on the other hand, feel a pressing need to "jolt themselves out of the dumps" with a quick, high-calorie snack that gives them a "bump of euphoria."

Week 1/Day 2

BREAKFAST

2 cups fat-free vanilla yogurt mixed with ⅓ cup crunchy barley-nugget cereal

1 cup pomegranate juice

LUNCH

Turkey and Cranberry Sandwich: 2 slices whole grain cinnamon-swirl bread, 3 ounces honey-roasted turkey slices, 2 tablespoons whole cranberry sauce, and 3 large leaves romaine lettuce

1 cup red, yellow, orange, and green bell pepper strips

1 red Anjou pear

1 cup 1% milk

SNACK

1 whole wheat English muffin, toasted and topped with 1 tablespoon unsalted creamy almond butter

DINNER

3 ounces broiled or grilled sirloin steak

1 medium sweet potato, baked and topped with 2 teaspoons light margarine and ½ teaspoon ground cinnamon

1 cup cooked broccoli spears, tossed with 1 teaspoon light margarine and a sprinkle of garlic

1 cup mixed berries (blackberries, blueberries, raspberries, and strawberries)

1,798 calories; 22% protein (100 g); 61% carbohydrate (275 g); 17% fat (35 g); 6% saturated fat (12 g); 132 mg cholesterol; 31 g dietary fiber; 25,438 IU vitamin A; 430 mg vitamin C; 6.4 mg vitamin E; 154 IU vitamin D; 2 mg vitamin B_6 ; 423 mcg folate ; 6.3 mcg vitamin B_{12} ; 2,484 mg sodium; 4,217 mg potassium; 1,681 mg calcium; 22 mg iron; 15 mg zinc

FOOD FACTS

■ Choose yogurt with no added sugar, like those with noncalorie sweeteners, to save unnecessary empty calories. Fat-free or low-fat yogurt will save total fat and saturated fat as well.

■ Almond, cashew, sunflower seed, or soy nut butter is a nice change from peanut butter. All nut butters are extremely nutrient-dense and contain heart-healthy fat.

Best food choice(s) today:

....

....

....

EXERCISE RECORD

Walking or other aerobic activity: .... *minutes*

Resistance training: Upper body ....
Lower body ....
Core ....

STRESS RECORD

Today my stress level is: Yellow .... *Orange* .... *Red* .... *Flashing red* ....

SUN DIARY

Today I got .... *minutes of sun exposure.*

THIS IS WHAT I DID TODAY TO IMPROVE . . .

My sleep:

....
....
....

My stress level:

....
....
....

My mood:

....
....
....

My environment:

....
....
....

 TIP OF THE DAY For under $200, you can turn any room of your house into a home gym. For $35 to $55, you can buy four pairs of lightweight dumbbells (3-, 5-, 8-, and 10-pounders are best for beginners). For another $20, you can buy a foam pad for floor exercises, stretches, pushups, and crunches. For another $75 or so, you can buy a sturdy weight bench, which is useful for dozens of different exercises with either dumbbells or barbells.

Week 1/Day 3

BREAKFAST

1½ cups cooked oatmeal (made with 1% milk) topped with 2 table-spoons chopped dates, 1 tablespoon dried sweet cherries, and 2 tea-spoons brown sugar

1 cup orange juice

LUNCH

2 cups lentil and ham soup

Tossed Vegetable Salad: 2½ cups mixed greens, 6 grape tomatoes, ¼ cup sliced mushrooms, ¼ cup chopped cucumber, and 8 whole grain crou-tons with 3 tablespoons light Italian vinaigrette dressing

1 cup papaya chunks

SNACK

1 Fuji apple

1 ounce string cheese

DINNER

4 ounces cooked pork tenderloin seasoned with salt-free lemon-pepper seasoning

1½ cups cooked whole wheat penne tossed with 2 teaspoons light margarine and a sprinkle of basil

1 cup sugar snap peas cooked with 2 tablespoons shallots and 1 tea-spoon light margarine

1 cup 1% milk

1,827 calories; 23% protein (105 g); 56% carbohydrate (255 g); 21% fat (43 g); 8% saturated fat (16.5 g); 162 mg cholesterol; 28 g dietary fiber; 13,160 IU vitamin A; 265 mg vitamin C; 8 mg vitamin E; 140 IU vitamin D; 1.7 mg vitamin B$_6$; 413 mcg folate; 3.4 mcg vitamin B$_{12}$; 4,189 mg sodium; 3,988 mg potassium; 1,221 mg calcium; 15 mg iron; 12 mg zinc

FOOD FACTS

▓ Bored with chicken? Enjoy more pork tenderloin. It's just as lean as boneless, skinless chicken breast, with only 3 grams of fat in a 3-ounce serving. Keep it flavorful and don't overcook; 150° to 160°F is perfect.

▓ Using salt-free seasoning blends and other spices, whether dried or fresh, is an easy and healthy way to add flavor without all the sodium to meats, poultry, fish, pasta, and vegetables.

◼ Canned soup contributes to the high sodium value of today's menu. However, it's balanced by lower sodium on other days. All bean soups—lentil, split pea, black bean, and navy bean—are extremely nutrient-dense. Choose lower-sodium versions when possible.

Best food choice(s) today:

....

....

....

EXERCISE RECORD

Walking or other aerobic activity: .... *minutes*

Resistance training: Upper body ....
Lower body ....
Core ....

STRESS RECORD

Today my stress level is: Yellow .... *Orange* .... *Red* .... *Flashing red* ....

SUN DIARY

Today I got .... *minutes of sun exposure.*

THIS IS WHAT I DID TODAY TO IMPROVE . . .

My sleep:

....

....

....

My stress level:

....

....

....

My mood:

....

....

....

My environment:

....

....

....

A little walking goes a long way toward improving your sleep. When researchers studied more than 700 men and women, they found that those who walked at least six blocks a day at a moderate pace were one-third less likely to have sleeping problems than those who walked shorter distances. Those who walked at a brisker pace were most likely of all to enjoy sound sleep. Other studies show that a regular walking program is as effective at improving sleep as medication—but without the risk of side effects and dependence.

Week 1/Day 4

BREAKFAST

Better Breakfast Sandwich: 1 toasted whole wheat English muffin, 2 ounces Canadian bacon, and 1-ounce slice reduced-fat Cheddar cheese

1 cup ruby red grapefruit juice

LUNCH

Roast Beef Sandwich: 2 slices whole grain bread with 3 ounces lean deli roast beef, ¼ cup fresh spinach leaves, 2 slices tomato, and 1 teaspoon zesty mustard

10 baby carrots

1 cup green seedless grapes

1 cup fat-free vanilla yogurt

SNACK

2 tablespoons *each* chocolate-covered almonds and chocolate-covered raisins

DINNER

Teriyaki Shrimp Stir-Fry: 3 ounces shrimp cooked with 1 cup snow pea pods, ½ cup edamame, ¼ cup sliced onion, 2 tablespoons teriyaki stir-fry sauce, and ½ tablespoon olive or canola oil

1 cup cooked brown rice

1 cup mandarin oranges packed in light syrup or water

1 fortune cookie

1 cup 1% milk

1,810 calories; 21% protein (96 g); 59% carbohydrate (266 g); 20% fat (41 g); 7% saturated fat (14.5 g); 264 mg cholesterol; 26 g dietary fiber; 18,623 IU vitamin A; 245 mg vitamin C;

9.5 mg vitamin E; 127 IU vitamin D; 1.3 mg vitamin B_6; 214 mcg folate; 3.7 mcg vitamin B_{12}; 3,138 mg sodium; 3,578 mg potassium; 1,327 mg calcium; 16 mg iron; 11 mg zinc

FOOD FACTS

▪ Canadian bacon and ham are the two best breakfast-meat choices, saving on calories and fat but providing nutrient-dense protein.

▪ Choose 100 percent fruit juices with no sugar added.

▪ Increase the nutritional value of sandwiches (and get more veggies) by adding sliced tomatoes and dark leafy lettuces. Use spinach leaves instead of lettuce for an even greater vitamin and mineral boost.

▪ Edamame (ed-a-MAH-may)—also known as green soybeans—are a crunchy, sweet, nutrient-dense protein. You can buy them frozen or fresh. Toss them into stir-fries and salads, or serve them as a side dish.

Best food choice(s) today:

....

....

....

EXERCISE RECORD

Walking or other aerobic activity: .... *minutes*

Resistance training: Upper body ....
                   Lower body ....
                        Core ....

STRESS RECORD

Today my stress level is: Yellow .... *Orange* .... *Red* .... *Flashing red* ....

SUN DIARY

Today I got .... *minutes of sun exposure.*

THIS IS WHAT I DID TODAY TO IMPROVE . . .

My sleep:

....

....

....

My stress level:

....

....

....

My mood:

....

....

....

My environment:

....

....

....

 TIP OF THE DAY Shoo away stress in 6 minutes with *Savasana,* a yoga posture also unflatteringly known as Corpse Pose. Lie on your back on a firm, flat surface with a small pillow or cushion beneath your head. Your arms should be 6 to 8 inches from your sides, palms facing up. Draw your shoulder blades away from your ears to open your chest. Close your eyes, relax your abdomen, and surrender to the stillness. With each breath, feel the rise and fall of your abdomen. Relax your chest muscles and take increasingly deeper breaths. Slowly inhale and exhale, imagining that each exhalation is releasing another bit of stored stress into thin air.

Week 1/Day 5

BREAKFAST

Super Blueberry Smoothie: 1½ cups blueberry kefir, ¾ cup blueberries, and ¼ teaspoon vanilla or almond extract

1 slice whole grain cinnamon-swirl bread

2 teaspoons apple butter

LUNCH

Fiesta Bean Wrap: 1 whole wheat tortilla (8 to 9 inches) with ½ cup pinto beans, ¼ cup shredded reduced-fat Mexican-blend cheese, and ¼ cup chopped avocado

1 ounce baked tortilla chips

⅓ cup chunky salsa

1 kiwifruit

SNACK

2 tablespoons roasted-garlic hummus spread on 4 whole wheat crackers and topped with ¼ cup roasted red pepper slices

DINNER

3 ounces tuna steak, grilled or broiled with 2 teaspoons lemon juice and salt-free onion-herb seasoning

1 small acorn or butternut squash, cooked with 2 teaspoons light margarine and a sprinkle of ground cinnamon

Apple Walnut Salad: 2 cups mixed greens (romaine, radicchio, spinach; and/or arugula), ½ sliced Gala apple, and ¼ cup toasted walnuts with 2 tablespoons light raspberry vinaigrette

1 whole wheat dinner roll with 1 teaspoon light margarine

1 cup 1% milk

1,813 calories; 18% protein (82 g); 58% carbohydrate (264 g); 24% fat (48 g); 6% saturated fat (12 g); 92 mg cholesterol; 41 g dietary fiber; 6,550 IU vitamin A; 180 mg vitamin C; 9.3 mg vitamin E; 127 IU vitamin D; 2.3 mg vitamin B$_6$; 404 mcg folate; 3.4 mcg vitamin B$_{12}$; 3,064 mg sodium; 4,050 mg potassium; 1,427 mg calcium; 12 mg iron; 7 mg zinc

FOOD FACTS

■ If you like yogurt, you probably will like kefir (KEE-fur). Basically, it's a drinkable yogurt, chock-full of good-for-you bacteria that help keep your digestive system healthy. Look for kefir—both plain and flavored varieties—in the refrigerated dairy case at your supermarket.

■ Canned beans—such as pinto, black, red, and kidney—are packed with immune-boosting nutrients. Rinse them before using, and you'll cut the sodium content significantly.

■ Keep jars of roasted red peppers on hand in your pantry to use in entrées, salads, and snacks. They're low calorie, fat-free, and packed with antioxidants.

Best food choice(s) today:

....

....

....

EXERCISE RECORD

Walking or other aerobic activity: .... *minutes*

Resistance training: Upper body ....
Lower body ....
Core ....

STRESS RECORD

Today my stress level is: Yellow .... *Orange* .... *Red* .... *Flashing red* ....

SUN DIARY

Today I got .... *minutes of sun exposure.*

THIS IS WHAT I DID TODAY TO IMPROVE . . .

My sleep:

....

....

My stress level:

....

....

My mood:

....

....

My environment:

....

....

TIP OF THE DAY Divide your shoe collection into "outside" and "inside" footwear. Throughout the world—but not so much in the United States—people routinely remove their shoes and park them by the door when they enter a home. They also ask visitors to do likewise. This custom doesn't just keep carpets cleaner—it's a great way to protect yourself and your family from the germs, toxins, and crud that everyone steps in during their daily rounds. Studies show that about 80 percent of the dirt on floors is tracked in from outside. Invest in doormats for all of your entrances, a comfy pair of "inside" shoes for everyone in your family, and a couple pairs of one-size-fits-all slippers to offer to visitors who can't bear the thought of padding around your home in their stocking (or bare) feet.

Week 1/Day 6

BREAKFAST

2 whole grain pancakes (made from packaged mix, using fat-free milk and egg) topped with 1 cup pureed or mashed peaches and ½ teaspoon ground cinnamon

1 cup 1% milk

1 cup orange juice

LUNCH

Smoked Salmon Caesar Salad: 3 cups chopped romaine lettuce, 3 ounces smoked salmon, ⅓ cup marinated artichoke hearts, 8 whole grain croutons, and 2 tablespoons shredded Parmesan cheese with 3 tablespoons light Caesar dressing

1 cup fresh pineapple chunks

SNACK

3 cups light butter-flavor microwave popcorn

DINNER

Easy Chicken Parmesan: 3 ounces cooked boneless, skinless chicken breast topped with 1-ounce slice Mozzarella cheese, served over 1½ cups whole wheat angel-hair pasta with 1 cup tomato basil pasta sauce

1 cup fresh spinach sautéed with 1 teaspoon olive oil and ½ teaspoon minced garlic

1 cup 1% milk

1,818 calories; 24% protein (110 g); 51% carbohydrate (235 g); 25% fat (51 g); 7% saturated fat (15 g); 224 mg cholesterol; 30 g dietary fiber; 32,406 IU vitamin A; 257 mg vitamin C; 15 mg vitamin E; 257 IU vitamin D; 2.6 mg vitamin B$_6$; 703 mcg folate; 6 mcg vitamin B$_{12}$; 3,775 mg sodium; 4,811 mg potassium; 1,723 mg calcium; 20 mg iron; 11 mg zinc

FOOD FACTS

■ You won't need empty-calorie pancake syrup if you puree or mash fresh, canned, or frozen fruits for a nutrient-dense pancake, waffle, or French toast topping.

■ Smoked salmon, typically found in thin slices in the refrigerated meat/seafood case of the supermarket, now can be purchased in convenient shelf-stable pouch packs in the canned seafood aisle. All salmon is rich in heart-healthy omega-3 fatty acids.

■ Whole grain croutons add crunch, vitamins, and minerals to your salad. Look for boxes or bags of the new whole grain versions in the salad dressing or bread aisle.

Best food choice(s) today:

....

....

....

EXERCISE RECORD

Walking or other aerobic activity: .... *minutes*

Resistance training: Upper body ....
                    Lower body ....
                          Core ....

STRESS RECORD

Today my stress level is: Yellow .... *Orange* .... *Red* .... *Flashing red* ....

SUN DIARY

Today I got .... *minutes of sun exposure.*

THIS IS WHAT I DID TODAY TO IMPROVE . . .

My sleep:

....

....

....

My stress level:

....

....

....

My mood:

....

....

....

My environment:

....

....

....

 TIP OF THE DAY Love dark chocolate but don't know which brands contain the most immune-boosting antioxidants? In general, chocolates with the highest cocoa content—70 percent and above—offer the largest amounts of flavanols, which protect immune cells from free radical damage and enhance immune function. Good choices include Dove Dark chocolate, El Rey Gran Saman Dark Chocolate, and Scharffen Berger Bittersweet. The recommended "dosage" is 1 ounce, about the amount used in scientific studies.

Week 1/Day 7

BREAKFAST

2 extra-large eggs, scrambled with milk

2 slices whole wheat toast with 2 teaspoons light margarine and 1 tablespoon sugar-free orange marmalade

½ cup strawberries

1 cup 1% milk

LUNCH

Ham Sandwich: 2 slices hearty whole grain bread, 3 ounces extra-lean deli ham, 3 romaine lettuce leaves, 2 slices tomato, and 1 teaspoon zesty mustard

1 cup shredded coleslaw mix tossed with 1 tablespoon light coleslaw dressing

1 tangerine or tangelo

1 cup 1% milk

SNACK

¾ cup light vanilla ice cream topped with 1 tablespoon chocolate syrup

DINNER

Beef and Bean Fajitas: 3 ounces cooked lean beef sirloin strips sprinkled with chili powder and cumin, ½ cup drained and rinsed Cuban-style black beans, ¼ cup shredded reduced-fat Mexican-blend cheese, ¾ cup cooked bell pepper strips, and ¼ cup cooked onion slices, divided between 2 whole wheat or multigrain flour tortillas

¼ cup chunky salsa

1 cup mango chunks

1,840 calories; 23% protein (107 g); 52% carbohydrate (240 g); 25% fat (51 g); 8.5% saturated fat (17.5 g); 574 mg cholesterol; 29 g dietary fiber; 6,238 IU vitamin A; 234 mg vitamin C; 8 mg vitamin E; 289 IU vitamin D; 2.3 mg vitamin B_6; 404 mcg folate; 6 mcg vitamin B_{12}; 3,565 mg sodium; 3,469 mg potassium; 1,420 mg calcium; 13 mg iron; 14 mg zinc

FOOD FACTS

■ Save unnecessary calories by using sugar-free jellies, jams, and marmalades or spreadable 100 percent fruit blends.

■ Cabbage is just one of the cruciferous vegetables with immune-boosting, disease-fighting nutrients. You can make a healthier, lower-fat version of coleslaw by picking up one of those convenient preshredded mixes at the supermarket and stirring in a little low-fat coleslaw dressing.

■ Add even more nutrients to coleslaw by topping it walnuts, pecans, almonds, or any dried fruit.

■ Yes, you *can* have a little ice cream even if you're trying to lose weight. Just choose wisely. Look for light or reduced-fat versions with no more than 4.5 grams of fat in a ½ cup serving. And measure your ice cream so you'll know how much is in your bowl!

Best food choice(s) today:

....

....

....

EXERCISE RECORD

Walking or other aerobic activity: .... *minutes*

Resistance training: Upper body ....
Lower body ....
Core ....

STRESS RECORD

Today my stress level is: Yellow .... *Orange* .... *Red* .... *Flashing red* ....

SUN DIARY

Today I got .... *minutes of sun exposure.*

THIS IS WHAT I DID TODAY TO IMPROVE . . .

My sleep:

....

....

....

My stress level:

....

....

....

My mood:

....

....

....

My environment:

....

....

....

TIP OF THE DAY

Bang a drum. When researchers randomly assigned 111 volunteers to one of six groups—four of which performed drumming exercises together, while the other two either listened to the drums or did nothing at all—the drummers not only had a great time but also had significantly higher levels of infection- and cancer-fighting natural killer (NK) cells. To find a drumming group in your area, check with your local music store. If you can't find one, you may get the same benefit by digging an old drum kit, a tambourine, or bongos out of storage and turning your family circle into a drum circle. Bonus: Drumming burns 281 calories an hour!

Week 1 Review

Date ....

I'M MOST PROUD OF MEETING THE FOLLOWING GOALS:

Diet:

....

....

....

Exercise:

....

....

....

Stress reduction:

....

....

....

Sleep improvement:

....

....

....

Mood improvement:

....

....

....

Sun exposure:

....

....

....

Environmental improvement:

....

....

....

AREAS I NEED TO IMPROVE:

....

....

....

Get Set for Week 2

Date ....

Maximum Immunity Success Strategies

EXERCISE

Walking/aerobic: beginner, 20 minutes a day; veteran, 40 minutes or more a day
Resistance training: 10 minutes most days of the week, perhaps combining two or more routines and taking the next day off

SLEEP

Review the sleep diary you created last week. You may find that you need to either establish or reinforce your bedtime rituals—the comforting things you do in the 45 minutes to an hour before turning in to help you unwind from the pressures of the day and prepare your body for sleep. These rituals vary from person to person. For some, it's taking a warm, 20-minute bath. For others, it's curling up with a book or engaging in prayer or meditation. What's important is that you find a ritual that works for you and perform it every night before you go to bed.

STRESS

Look back at the time budget you created last week. Make a list of the really important things you need or want to do, assigning each a priority level. You may see that you're spending too little time on what really matters and too much time on activities that do nothing to enhance your immunity, health, or quality of life.

MOOD

Read through the mood diary you created last week. If your balance sheet shows that negative moods prevail, make a list of the things that give you pleasure. Again, this will vary from person to person. For some, it's a weekend getaway with a spouse or friend—or perhaps alone. For others, it's engaging in a hobby, sport, or social activity or simply watching a favorite DVD. Find ways in which you can reconnect with activities that get you to your "happy" place.

ENVIRONMENT

Last week, you took steps to germ-proof your personal space. Now take action to germ-proof your kitchen. Wash your hands before preparing food, and rinse and scrub fresh produce. When working with raw meat and fish, be sure to disinfect contaminated surfaces, and always follow recommended cooking temperature guidelines to ensure that your meals are free of pathogens.

Challenges I anticipate this week:

....

....

....

....

Strategies I can use to overcome them:

....

....

....

....

My goals for this week:

....

....

....

....

Your Maximum Immunity Workout

GET LOOSE

People have good reason to complain that the weight of the world rests on their shoulders. Considering the amount of time that many of us spend hunched and immobile in front of computer screens, we probably store more tension in our shoulders and necks than in any other body part. When we further stress these muscles by lugging groceries, bags, and other heavy items, it's no wonder they feel sore. The following three stretches can help provide relief.

Seated shoulder/wrist stretch. Sit close to the edge of a chair with your spine erect and your hands resting on your thighs. Slowly make a large circle with your right arm, raising your arm in front of you and then continuing up and dropping it behind you. Start a second circle, but stop when your hand is directly overhead. Rotate your hand in a clockwise circle two times to relieve any soreness in your wrist. Then lower your arm behind you to complete the circle.

Make another large circle with your right arm, this time raising your arm to the back and then dropping it toward the front. Again, start a second circle, but stop while your hand is directly overhead. Rotate your hand in a counterclockwise circle two times before lowering your arm to complete the circle.

Repeat the sequence with your left arm.

Standing shoulder stretch. Stand with your feet shoulder-width apart and your arms at your sides. Extend your arms straight out behind your body, stretching back and upward as far as you can without straining. If possible, clasp your hands. Hold the stretch for 30 seconds. This loosens the deltoid muscles in your shoulders, as well as the biceps and triceps in your upper arms.

Bowing shoulder stretch. Kneel on all fours on an exercise mat or another padded surface. Your hands and knees should be about shoulder-width apart. Keeping your back flat, neck straight, and eyes focused on the floor, sit back on your heels and extend your arms in front of you. Push lightly on the mat with your hands. Hold for 20 to 30 seconds. This loosens your deltoids, biceps, and triceps, as well as the latissimus dorsi in your middle and lower back.

GET FIT

Walking on a treadmill is ideal for those bad-weather days when you just don't want to be outside. If you don't own a treadmill, you might consider joining a gym where you can use one year-round.

By Week 2, you should be ready for a slow-paced 20-minute treadmill workout on a level surface. If you're accustomed to walking outside, you can simulate outdoor conditions by programming the treadmill for a 1 or 2 percent incline. At higher inclines, you work not only your leg muscles but also your abs and glutes (the buttock muscles). By increasing the incline just a degree or two, you can burn up to 60 percent more calories.

To get the most from your treadmill workout, heed this advice.

■ Maintain an upright posture. Keep your shoulders over your hips and your hips over your ankles.

■ Start with a 5-minute slow walk, followed by a 5-minute brisk walk. Then you're ready for your first "hill."

■ Depending on the duration of your workout, try alternating 5-minute hills with 5 minutes of level walking. Finish up with another 5-minute slow walk.

■ Maintain the same speed on hills as on a level surface. Start at 3.5 miles per hour, with a moderate incline. Over time, you can increase the incline to 5 percent. Don't go above 7 percent, which can strain your back, hips, and ankles.

■ Between hill workouts, allow your muscles to rest and recover for 48 hours.

GET STRONG

UPPER BODY: BICEPS CURL

Stand with your feet about shoulder-width apart and hold a pair of dumbbells at your sides, palms facing inward. In one smooth motion, bend your elbows and rotate your forearms as you raise the dumbbells to shoulder height. Remember to keep your wrists and back straight. Slowly lower the dumbbells back to the starting position. Work up to 2 sets of 8 to 12 repetitions.

CORE: ABDOMINAL CRUNCH

Unlike the curl-up described in Week 1, the abdominal crunch is an exercise-industry standard. Lie on your back on an exercise mat or another padded surface, with your knees bent and your feet flat on the floor. Your lower back should be relaxed against the mat. Then, instead of resting your arms at your sides, bend your elbows and place your hands behind your neck. Slowly lift your chest and shoulders off the mat without arching your lower back. Be careful not to pull your head forward with your hands, which can cause neck strain. Hold for a count of 5, then slowly return to the starting position. Work up to 2 sets of 8 to 12 repetitions.

Note: If you have lower-back pain, you might try this exercise with your feet and lower legs resting on the seat of a chair.

Holding a pair of light dumbbells at your sides, stand with your feet slightly more than shoulder-width apart and your toes pointing forward or slightly outward. Keeping your back straight, heels flat on the floor, and eyes focused straight ahead, lower your body in a smooth, controlled motion, as though sitting down into a chair. Sit back over your heels instead of squatting straight down. Your knees should be directly above your toes. Briefly hold this position, then return to the starting position by pushing up from your heels and straightening your legs. Squeeze your buttock muscles and repeat. Work up to 2 sets of 8 to 12 repetitions.

Week 2/Day 1

BREAKFAST

1½ cups frosted mini shredded-wheat squares with 1 cup 1% milk

1 cup raspberries

LUNCH

1 cup minestrone soup

Italian Bean Salad: 3 cups chopped romaine lettuce, ½ cup chickpeas (garbanzo beans), ⅓ cup shredded Italian-blend cheese, 8 grape tomatoes, 2 tablespoons chopped red onion, and 6 black olives with 4 tablespoons light balsamic vinaigrette dressing

1 whole wheat dinner roll with 2 teaspoons light margarine

SNACK

Cinnamon-Sugar Pecan Rollup: 1 whole wheat flour tortilla (8 inches) topped with 1 tablespoon light margarine, 1 teaspoon sugar, ½ teaspoon ground cinnamon, and 1 tablespoon chopped pecans, heated in the microwave and rolled up

DINNER

3 ounces broiled scallops sprinkled with lemon juice and chopped fresh parsley

Savory Roasted Sweet Potato Wedges: 1 large sweet potato cut into wedges, tossed with 1½ tablespoon light Italian salad dressing, and oven roasted

1 cup whole green beans, cooked with 2 teaspoons honey-roasted almonds

¾ cup tropical fruit canned in light juice

1 cup 1% milk

1,813 calories; 16% protein (73 g); 60% carbohydrate (272 g); 24% fat (49 g); 6% saturated fat (12 g); 79 mg cholesterol; 46 g dietary fiber; 34,588 IU vitamin A; 136 mg vitamin C; 19.3 mg vitamin E; 254 IU vitamin D; 2.3 mg vitamin B_6; 740 mcg folate; 6 mcg vitamin B_{12}; 3,649 mg sodium; 3,664 mg potassium; 1,330 mg calcium; 35 mg iron; 11 mg zinc

FOOD FACTS

▪ Choose whole grain cereals as often as possible. The word *whole* should appear at the start of the ingredient list. Varieties include toasted O-shaped cereal, raisin bran and other bran flakes, low-fat granola, and shredded wheat (frosted or unfrosted).

▪ Full-fat cheese, although rich in protein and calcium, contains a little too much total and saturated fat. Reduced-fat versions save fat but still provide calcium and protein. They melt well, too.

Best food choice(s) today:

....

....

....

EXERCISE RECORD

Walking or other aerobic activity: .... *minutes*

Resistance training: Upper body ....
Lower body ....
Core ....

STRESS RECORD

Today my stress level is: Yellow .... *Orange* .... *Red* .... *Flashing red* ....

SUN DIARY

Today I got .... *minutes of sun exposure.*

THIS IS WHAT I DID TODAY TO IMPROVE . . .

My sleep:

....

....

....

My stress level:

....

....

....

My mood:

....

....

....

My environment:

....

....

....

TIP OF THE DAY Put more spring into your walking routine by:

Pushing off with the toes of your back foot to propel yourself forward. With each step, smoothly roll your foot from heel to toe. For an extra-powerful push-off, raise the heel of your back foot to show off the sole of your new walking shoe.

Pumping your arms with your elbows bent at 90 degrees. With each step, pull back your elbow so that your hand is by your hip, and swing it forward until it's about chest-high. Avoid swinging your arms out to the sides, which will slow you down.

Focusing on extending the leg of your back foot and pulling the leg forward after you push off. If you overstride by reaching forward with your front foot, it can slow you down and increase your risk of a back or hamstring injury.

Week 2/Day 2

BREAKFAST

½ pita, filled with 1½ tablespoons unsalted almond butter and ½ apple, sliced

1 cup cranberry juice cocktail

1 cup 1% milk

LUNCH

Veggie Cheeseburger: 1 soy veggie burger, 1-ounce slice reduced-fat Cheddar cheese, 6 fresh spinach leaves, 2 tomato slices, and 1 teaspoon zesty mustard on a whole grain hamburger bun

12 baked ruffled potato chips

1 cup blueberries

SNACK

1 brownie (2-inch square)

1 cup 1% milk

DINNER

3 ounces roasted or grilled chicken breast topped with 1 tablespoon barbecue sauce

1 large ear corn on the cob with 1 tablespoon light margarine

1 cup cooked turnip or collard greens seasoned with 1 teaspoon light margarine and ¼ teaspoon salt-free onion seasoning

1½ cups watermelon chunks

1,766 calories; 21% protein (94 g); 49% carbohydrate (225 g); 30% fat (59 g); 8% saturated fat (15.5 g); 134 mg cholesterol; 27 g dietary fiber; 18,822 IU vitamin A; 219 mg vitamin C; 17.6 mg vitamin E; 255 IU vitamin D; 1.6 mg vitamin B_6; 553 mcg folate; 3 mcg vitamin B_{12}; 2,026 mg sodium; 3,571 mg potassium; 1,397 mg calcium; 15 mg iron; 8 mg zinc

FOOD FACTS

▪ This week's menu showcases meatless soy-based alternatives, which provide protein and nutrients with less total fat, saturated fat, and cholesterol than typical meat products. Look for them in the refrigerated or freezer case and start adding them to your breakfast, lunch, and dinner meals.

▪ If fresh corn on the cob isn't available, buy frozen cobettes or sweet kernels. All corn is rich in fiber, vitamins, and minerals.

▪ Green leafy vegetables such as collard, mustard, turnip, and kale greens are power-packed with antioxidants and other valuable nutrients. Bags of prewashed cut greens are available in the produce area near the salad blends. Frozen or canned greens are great options, too; just rinse them to get rid of some of the sodium.

Best food choice(s) today:

....

....

....

EXERCISE RECORD

Walking or other aerobic activity: .... *minutes*

Resistance training: Upper body ....
Lower body ....
Core ....

STRESS RECORD

Today my stress level is: Yellow .... *Orange* .... *Red* .... *Flashing red* ....

SUN DIARY

Today I got .... *minutes of sun exposure.*

THIS IS WHAT I DID TODAY TO IMPROVE . . .

My sleep:

....

....

....

My stress level:

....

....

....

My mood:

....

....

....

My environment:

....

....

....

TIP OF THE DAY Recover from a poor night's sleep with a midday power nap. In a study of 12 sleep-deprived college students, Australian researchers analyzed the effects of 5-minute, 10-minute, and 30-minute naps. They found that a 5-minute nap wasn't long enough to have any rejuvenating effects, while 30 minutes was too long—students entered deep sleep and experienced grogginess after they woke up. The 10-minute nap was just right—it immediately improved the students' alertness, mood, and performance scores.

Week 2/Day 3

BREAKFAST

1½ cups fat-free cherry vanilla yogurt mixed with 1 tablespoon wheat germ and 1 tablespoon ground flaxseed

1 red or pink grapefruit half

LUNCH

Super Spaghetti and Meatballs: 1½ cups cooked whole wheat spaghetti topped with 1 cup pasta or marinara sauce, 5 Italian-style meatless soy meatballs, and 1 tablespoon grated Parmesan cheese

1 cup cooked broccoli florets

Garlic Mozzarella Toast: 1 slice Italian bread, toasted and topped with 1 teaspoon light margarine, ⅛ teaspoon garlic powder, and a ½-ounce slice mozzarella cheese

SNACK

1 cup red seedless grapes

DINNER

3 ounces grilled or baked salmon, cooked with a sprinkle of lemon juice, minced garlic, and fresh chopped dillweed

1 cup cooked brown wild rice blend

1 cup cooked green peas with pearl onions with 1 teaspoon light margarine

1 cup 1% milk

1,781 calories; 25% protein (110 g); 56% carbohydrate (249 g); 19% fat (37 g); 5% saturated fat (9.5 g); 86 mg cholesterol; 39 g dietary fiber; 7,477 IU vitamin A; 207 mg vitamin C; 11 mg vitamin E; 129 IU vitamin D; 2.6 mg vitamin B_6; 782 mcg folate; 5.4 mcg vitamin B_{12}; 2,688 mg sodium; 4,511 mg potassium; 1,434 mg calcium; 16 mg iron; 15 mg zinc

FOOD FACTS

■ Flaxseed is a top-notch source of fiber, antioxidants, and omega-3 fatty acids, but it must be ground for the nutrients to be absorbable. Look for bags of preground flaxseed, often called flaxseed meal, in the baking aisle or specialty food section. Add it to cereal, yogurt, or virtually any baked goods.

■ Add crunch to cereal, yogurt, and smoothies with a couple of tablespoons of wheat germ. It's chock-full of vitamin E and other valuable nutrients, as well as fiber.

■ Look for meatless meatballs in the freezer case; they're available in several flavors, such as Italian, mushroom, and traditional. Simply heat, serve, and save calories, fat, and cholesterol on that family-favorite spaghetti.

Best food choice(s) today:

....

....

....

EXERCISE RECORD

Walking or other aerobic activity: .... *minutes*

Resistance training: Upper body ....
                                   Lower body ....
                                          Core ....

STRESS RECORD

Today my stress level is: Yellow .... *Orange* .... *Red* .... *Flashing red* ....

SUN DIARY

Today I got .... *minutes of sun exposure.*

THIS IS WHAT I DID TODAY TO IMPROVE . . .

My sleep:

....

....

....

My stress level:

....

....

....

My mood:

....

....

....

My environment:

....

....

....

TIP OF THE DAY Brighten your morning mood by placing some citrus, vanilla, or rosemary potpourri in a covered jar on your nightstand. Before you get out of bed, open the jar, take a deep whiff, and imagine that you're in a field of fresh flowers. The scent helps produce a burst of feel-good endorphins and also communicates (in a good way) with areas of the brain that control memory, emotion, body temperature, and appetite.

Week 2/Day 4

BREAKFAST

1½ cups raisin bran with 1 cup 1% milk

1 cup apricot nectar

LUNCH

Turkey Veggie Wrap: 1 multigrain tortilla filled with 2 ounces smoked deli turkey meat, 1 ounce provolone cheese, 2 tablespoons chopped roasted red bell pepper, 2 tablespoons chopped marinated artichoke hearts, 2 tablespoons chopped soft sun-dried tomatoes, and 2 teaspoons light Italian dressing

1 cup fresh sugar snap peas

1 banana

SNACK

½ cup light chocolate ice cream

DINNER

1½ cups chunky ham-and-bean soup

1 piece (3-inch square) corn bread (made with whole grain cornmeal) with 2 teaspoons light margarine

Mixed Greens and Fruit Salad: 1 cup fresh spinach leaves, 1 cup spring mixed greens, ½ cup mandarin oranges (drained), and 2 tablespoons pomegranate seeds with 2 tablespoons light poppy-seed or raspberry vinaigrette

1,824 calories; 15% protein (68 g); 61% carbohydrate (278 g); 24% fat (49 g); 8.5% saturated fat (17.5 g); 141 mg cholesterol; 44 g dietary fiber; 20,709 IU vitamin A; 348 mg vitamin C; 15.5 mg vitamin E; 192 IU vitamin D; 3 mg vitamin B₆; 648 mcg folate; 6.5 mcg vitamin B₁₂; 4,223 mg sodium; 3,830 mg potassium; 1,140 mg calcium; 35 mg iron; 14 mg zinc

FOOD FACTS

▓ Apricots are extremely high in vitamin A. Choose fresh apricots when in season; canned, packed in natural juices or light syrup; or apricot nectar.

▓ Ham-and-bean soup from a can is convenient, but homemade is easy, too. Just use canned navy or great Northern beans and add ham cubes.

▓ Pomegranate seeds and juice are among the newest fruit products to go mainstream. Only the seeds are edible from the actual fruit; they're used to make the juice. Look for juice with no added sugar.

Best food choice(s) today:

....

....

....

EXERCISE RECORD

Walking or other aerobic activity: .... *minutes*

Resistance training: Upper body ....
Lower body ....
Core ....

STRESS RECORD

Today my stress level is: Yellow .... *Orange* .... *Red* .... *Flashing red* ....

SUN DIARY

Today I got .... *minutes of sun exposure.*

THIS IS WHAT I DID TODAY TO IMPROVE . . .

My sleep:

....

....

....

My stress level:

....

....

....

My mood:

....

....

....

My environment:

....

....

....

De-stress with progressive muscle relaxation. Lie down on a comfortable surface, close your eyes, and take three deep breaths. Now inhale deeply as you slowly tighten the muscles in your face. Hold the tension for several seconds, then exhale deeply as you slowly relax your facial muscles. Savor the sensation of calm and stillness. Repeat this process with every major muscle group, moving from your neck, arms, chest, and abdomen to your buttocks, legs, and feet. Progressive muscle relaxation increases your awareness of how much tension you store in your body during the course of a busy day and helps you release it in a natural, healthy way.

Week 2/Day 5

BREAKFAST

Mushroom and Cheddar Omelet: 2 extra-large eggs, ⅓ cup sliced shiitake mushrooms, 2 tablespoons chopped green bell pepper, 1 tablespoon chopped onion, and ¼ cup shredded reduced-fat Cheddar cheese

1 veggie sausage-style patty

1 multigrain English muffin, toasted and topped with 2 teaspoons light margarine and 1 tablespoon sugar-free strawberry jelly

1 cup grapefruit juice

LUNCH

Crunchy Tuna Salad Pocket: ½ whole wheat pita filled with 4 spinach leaves and 3 ounces canned water-packed albacore tuna mixed with 1 tablespoon light mayonnaise, 2 tablespoons diced celery, 1 tablespoon diced onion, and 1 tablespoon chopped honey-roasted almonds

1 cup mango chunks

1 cup 1% milk

SNACK

6 ounces tomato or vegetable juice

4 whole wheat crackers

DINNER

3 ounces grilled beef tenderloin

1 large baked potato topped with 2 teaspoons light margarine, 1 tablespoon light sour cream, and 1 tablespoon chopped chives

1 cup cooked asparagus spears

1 cup sliced fresh strawberries

1 cup 1% milk

1,786 calories; 25% protein (112 g); 50% carbohydrate (225 g); 25% fat (50 g); 8% saturated fat (16 g); 564 mg cholesterol; 24 g dietary fiber; 7,178 IU vitamin A; 306 mg vitamin C; 11.9 mg vitamin E; 301 IU vitamin D; 3 mg vitamin B$_6$; 423 mcg folate; 9.3 mcg vitamin B$_{12}$; 2,703 mg sodium; 4,684 mg potassium; 1,172 mg calcium; 18 mg iron; 14 mg zinc

FOOD FACTS

■ Mushrooms are filled with immune-boosting nutrients. Be adventurous and try new varieties, such as shiitake and enoki, along with the standard white button and portobello mushrooms.

■ Choose water-packed tuna and skip the unnecessary calories and fat from the oil-packed version. Look for albacore white and light chunk tuna for more omega-3 fatty acids.

■ Chives, a member of the onion family, are rich in disease-fighting phytonutrients. Use liberal amounts of chives; garlic; and red, yellow, white, or green onions in your cooking.

Best food choice(s) today:

....

....

....

EXERCISE RECORD

Walking or other aerobic activity: .... *minutes*

Resistance training: Upper body ....
Lower body ....
Core ....

STRESS RECORD

Today my stress level is: Yellow .... *Orange* .... *Red* .... *Flashing red* ....

SUN DIARY

Today I got .... *minutes of sun exposure.*

THIS IS WHAT I DID TODAY TO IMPROVE . . .

My sleep:

....

....

....

My stress level:

....

....

....

My mood:

....

....

....

My environment:

....

....

....

 TIP OF THE DAY Frequent, satisfying sex improves your mood and balances your hormones, which enhances immunity. Using a code word that only you and your partner know, schedule regular sex breaks into your weekly calendar. If possible, rendezvous at a time when you're both wide enough awake to enjoy yourselves (not at midnight on a work night!).

Week 2/Day 6

BREAKFAST

1½ cups cooked oatmeal (made with 1% milk) topped with 2 tablespoons walnuts and ¼ cup chopped dried figs

1 cup pomegranate juice

LUNCH

Southwest Salad: 3 cups chopped romaine lettuce, ½ cup black beans, ⅓ cup sweet-corn kernels, ¼ cup reduced-fat shredded Mexican-blend cheese, and 2 tablespoons chopped avocado with 3 tablespoons light creamy ranch dressing

1 ounce multigrain or baked tortilla chips

¼ cup salsa

1 cup mixed cantaloupe and honeydew melon chunks

SNACK

1 cup hot chocolate made with 1% milk

DINNER

3 ounces cooked boneless pork loin seasoned with a small amount of coarse ground pepper and minced garlic

1 cup cooked whole wheat couscous sprinkled with fresh basil

1 cup baby carrots cooked with 1 tablespoon maple syrup

1 kiwifruit

1,856 calories; 19% protein (90 g); 58% carbohydrate (269 g); 23% fat (47 g); 6.5% saturated fat (13.5 g); 128 mg cholesterol; 36 g dietary fiber; 28,103 IU vitamin A; 197 mg vitamin C; 10.5 mg vitamin E; 156 IU vitamin D; 1.5 mg vitamin B$_6$; 565 mcg folate; 3.6 mcg vitamin B$_{12}$; 2,239 mg sodium; 4,669 mg potassium; 1,483 mg calcium; 13 mg iron; 12 mg zinc

FOOD FACTS

■ If you like that tasty filling in fig bars, you'll love adding dried figs to your meals for a sweet, nutrient-dense, fiber-filled boost. Look for figs in the raisin aisle, and choose either the Black Mission or Calimyrna variety.

■ Dried beans, legumes, and lentils count as both a protein and a vegetable serving—the only foods to belong to two groups! All kinds—from black, red, and white beans to split peas, lentils, and pinto beans—are packed with vitamins, minerals, phytonutrients, and fiber.

Best food choice(s) today:

....

....

....

EXERCISE RECORD

Walking or other aerobic activity: .... *minutes*

Resistance training: Upper body ....
Lower body ....
Core ....

STRESS RECORD

Today my stress level is: Yellow .... *Orange* .... *Red* .... *Flashing red* ....

SUN DIARY

Today I got .... *minutes of sun exposure.*

THIS IS WHAT I DID TODAY TO IMPROVE . . .

My sleep:

....

....

....

My stress level:

....

....

....

My mood:

....

....

....

My environment:

....

....

....

TIP OF THE DAY Do you drink five or more sodas a day but hate the idea of switching to plain water? Gradually switch to no-cal tea—black, green, or oolong. All three contain large amounts of an antioxidant called epigallocatechin gallate, which increases insulin activity and lowers blood sugar levels. You can drink up to 5 cups of green, black, or oolong tea per day.

Week 2/Day 7

BREAKFAST

3 whole grain blueberry pancakes (made from packaged mix, using fat-free milk and egg) with 1 tablespoon light margarine and 2 tablespoons sugar-free pancake syrup

1 cup blueberries (⅔ cup for pancake batter and ⅓ cup for topping)

1 cup 1% milk

1 cup orange juice

LUNCH

2 slices Homemade Hearty Sausage and Pepperoni Pizza: ⅓ cup favorite pasta sauce, 2 tablespoons meatless sausage-style crumbles, 6 slices

turkey pepperoni, ⅓ cup mozzarella cheese, ¼ cup chopped mushrooms, and 1 tablespoon chopped onion divided between 2 slices whole wheat pizza crust (each one-sixth of a 12-inch crust)

1 fresh peach or nectarine

SNACK

1 Asian pear

DINNER

Thai Peanut Sauce Penne and Chicken: 1½ cups cooked whole wheat penne tossed with 2 ounces cooked chicken breast strips, 3 tablespoons prepared Thai peanut satay sauce, ⅓ cup shredded carrot, ½ cup chopped broccoli, 1 tablespoon chopped red bell pepper, 2 tablespoons chopped green onions, and a sprinkle of crushed red pepper

1 cup 1% milk

1,819 calories; 20% protein (93 g); 62% carbohydrate (282 g); 18% fat (36 g); 6% saturated fat (12 g); 106 mg cholesterol; 30 g dietary fiber; 10,483 IU vitamin A; 199 mg vitamin C; 11.1 mg vitamin E; 340 IU vitamin D; 1.7 mg vitamin B₆; 244 mcg folate; 4.3 mcg vitamin B₁₂; 3,630 mg sodium; 3,825 mg potassium; 1,338 mg calcium; 13 mg iron; 9 mg zinc

FOOD FACTS

■ There's no excuse for not adding whole grains to your eating plan—your supermarket likely stocks a whole grain version of practically every bread item. Find whole grain pancake and baking mix in the baking aisle or specialty foods section. Whole wheat pizza crust is available either as precooked crust or as refrigerated dough.

■ Keep that whole grain pizza healthy by using plenty of lycopene-rich tomato/pizza sauce and lower-fat pizza toppings. Soy sausage crumbles and turkey pepperoni provide lots of spicy flavor with a fraction of the total fat, saturated fat, and cholesterol of their meat-based counterparts.

■ Make blueberry pancakes and muffins more nutritious by adding extra fresh or frozen blueberries to the batter. Blueberries are filled with immune-boosting nutrients and antioxidants.

Best food choice(s) today:

....

....

....

EXERCISE RECORD

Walking or other aerobic activity: .... *minutes*

Resistance training: Upper body ....
                              Lower body ....
                                        Core ....

STRESS RECORD

Today my stress level is: Yellow .... *Orange* .... *Red* .... *Flashing red* ....

SUN DIARY

Today I got .... *minutes of sun exposure.*

THIS IS WHAT I DID TODAY TO IMPROVE . . .

My sleep:

....
....
....

My stress level:

....
....
....

My mood:

....
....
....

My environment:

....
....
....

 TIP OF THE DAY If you get about 10 to 15 minutes of sun exposure 2 or 3 days a week during your walking routine, you'll reap multiple benefits. For starters, sun exposure triggers the skin's production of active vitamin D, which protects against infection and many chronic diseases. What's more, sunlight is essential for setting the biological clock that regulates your 24-hour circadian rhythms, including your sleep/awake cycle.

Week 2 Review

Date ....

I'M MOST PROUD OF MEETING THE FOLLOWING GOALS:

Diet:

....

....

....

Exercise:

....

....

....

Stress reduction:

....

....

....

Sleep improvement:

....

....

....

Mood improvement:

....

....

....

Sun exposure:

....

....

....

Environmental improvement:

....

....

....

Areas I need to improve:

....

....

....

Get Set for Week 3

Date ....

Maximum Immunity Success Strategies

EXERCISE

Walking/aerobic: beginner, 25 minutes a day; veteran, 50 minutes or more a day
Resistance training: 10 minutes most days of the week, possibly doing a 20-minute routine one day so you can take off the next day without losing exercise time

SLEEP

Last week, you evaluated your bedtime rituals. Now examine the lifestyle habits that may be preventing you from getting your rightful amount of shut-eye. Are you drinking caffeinated beverages after 2:00 p.m. or alcoholic beverages within 3 hours of bedtime? Are you exercising in the evening? If so, consider pushing back these activities to an earlier time of day. Also, avoid working late on business or household finances.

STRESS

From the list that you created last week, try to eliminate at least one of the activities you identified as a time waster. When evaluating essential activities—such as work— consider ways to make more efficient use of your time. Nobody ever got to the end of their lives regretting that they didn't put in more unpaid overtime at the office.

MOOD

Take a closer look at your list from last week, in which you identified things that give you pleasure. Now go for it! Schedule—yes, schedule, because otherwise it might not happen—at least one activity per day that gets you to your happy place. This is one appointment you do not want to miss. Even anticipating a pleasurable event is enough to improve your mood and boost your immunity. Actually experiencing it is just icing on the cake.

ENVIRONMENT

During weeks 1 and 2, you took steps to germ-proof your personal space and your kitchen. But what should you do when a family member contracts a contagious disease? Protect yourself by separating towels, dishes, utensils, and toothbrushes; sleeping apart from the sick person; and disinfecting commonly shared surfaces such as kitchen counters, telephones, and computer keyboards.

Challenges I anticipate this week:

....

....

....

Strategies I can use to overcome them:

....

....

....

....

My goals for this week:

....

....

....

....

Your Maximum Immunity Workout

GET LOOSE

All you need for this stretch—which loosens the muscles at the backs of your legs, your inner thighs, and your lower back—is a chair. Stand about 2 feet in front of it with your feet as far apart as you can comfortably manage. Keeping your legs straight without locking your knees, turn your toes slightly inward and contract your leg muscles. With your back straight and your head aligned with your spine, bend forward from your hips and place your hands on the seat of the chair. Hold for 20 to 30 seconds, then return to the starting position. As your flexibility increases, you might try bending your elbows during the stretch so that your forearms rest on the chair.

GET FIT

A pedometer is an inexpensive device that snaps onto your belt or waistband and automatically counts every step you take. To help improve your cardiovascular fitness, you can use a pedometer in one of two ways.

■ Wear it during daily walks and write down the number of steps you take. Each day, try to go a bit farther, so you're tallying more steps. By keeping a log, you can measure your progress from day to day and week to week.

■ Wear it for an entire day. Remember, every step counts, whether it's part of a formal walking program or your daily routine. At first, aim for 10,000 steps a day, which is the government-recommended minimum for basic fitness. Your ultimate goal is to reach 20,000 steps per day. The more steps you take, the more immune-enhancing benefits you reap.

UPPER BODY: TRICEPS EXTENSION

Sit toward the front of a sturdy chair, with your back straight and your feet flat on the floor. Hold a dumbbell in your right hand and raise it straight above your right shoulder. Bend your right elbow and slowly lower the weight toward your right shoulder as far as you can comfortably manage. Be sure to keep your upper right arm rigid and the elbow close to your ear, pointed toward the ceiling. You might want to support your elbow with your left hand. This is the starting position.

Raise your right forearm straight above your head, just short of locking your elbow. Lower the dumbbell to the starting position and repeat. Work up to 2 sets of 8 to 12 repetitions per arm.

CORE: THE DIAMOND CRUNCH

Lie on your back on an exercise mat or another padded surface. Bend your knees, then drop them to the sides so that the soles of your feet are pressed together. Extend your arms above you at 45-degree angles to the floor and clasp your hands. "Hollow" your abdomen by pulling your navel toward your spine. Lift your head and shoulders off the mat by reaching as far forward as you can comfortably manage. Hold the position for several seconds, return to the starting position, and repeat without resting. Work toward 2 sets of 8 to 12 repetitions.

LOWER BODY: LUNGE

Holding a pair of dumbbells, stand with your feet hip-width apart and your arms at your sides. Take a large step forward with your left foot, keeping your back and torso perpendicular to the floor. Bend your left knee at a 90-degree angle without extending it beyond your toes. Bend your right knee at an angle a little wider than 90 degrees while lifting your right heel off the floor. Hold for a second, then return to the starting position by bringing your right leg forward. Repeat the exercise on your right side, starting with a large step forward with your right foot. Work up to 2 sets of 8 to 12 repetitions per side. *Note:* If you've never attempted lunges before, practice correct form before adding weights. If you have knee problems, check with your doctor before performing this exercise.

Week 3/Day 1

BREAKFAST

Mixed Berry Yogurt Parfait: 1½ cups fat-free vanilla yogurt layered with ½ cup low-fat granola, ½ cup blueberries, ½ cup raspberries, and ½ cup sliced strawberries

LUNCH

Roast Beef Sandwich: 2 slices hearty whole grain bread, 3 ounces deli roast beef, 6 spinach leaves, 2 slices tomato, and 2 teaspoons light mayonnaise

Sunflower and Three-Pepper Salad: 2 cups mixed romaine and spring greens; ⅔ cup chopped red, yellow, and orange bell peppers; 2 tablespoons chopped green onion; and 2 tablespoons sunflower seeds with 2 tablespoons light honey-mustard salad dressing

SNACK

1 chocolate chip cookie

1 cup 1% milk

DINNER

Pecan Mustard–Crusted Catfish: 4 ounces catfish fillet coated with 1 teaspoon Dijon mustard and 2 tablespoons finely chopped pecans before cooking

1 cup cooked brown rice seasoned with 1 teaspoon light margarine, a sprinkle of ground cinnamon, and ½ teaspoon orange zest

1 cup cooked Brussels sprouts with 2 teaspoons light margarine

1 cup papaya chunks

1,811 calories; 19% protein (86 g); 53% carbohydrate (249 g); 26% fat (52 g); 6% saturated fat (13 g); 135 mg cholesterol; 34 g dietary fiber; 9,880 IU vitamin A; 458 mg vitamin C; 14.4 mg vitamin E; 172 IU vitamin D; 4.1 mg vitamin B_6; 968 mcg folate; 12 mcg vitamin B_{12}; 2,443 mg sodium; 3,717 mg potassium; 1,153 mg calcium; 13 mg iron; 14.5 mg zinc

FOOD FACTS

■ All berries—raspberries, strawberries, blackberries, and blueberries—are packed with immune-boosting nutrients and antioxidants. Keep bags of frozen unsweetened berries on hand in case fresh aren't available.

■ Brown rice contains more fiber, vitamins, and minerals than white rice. You're no long limited to just the long-cooking type, either. Boxes and packages of quick-cooking and instant brown rice are readily available.

Best food choice(s) today:

....

....

....

EXERCISE RECORD

Walking or other aerobic activity: .... *minutes*

Resistance training: Upper body ....
.... *Lower body* ....
.... *Core* ....

STRESS RECORD

Today my stress level is: Yellow .... *Orange* .... *Red* .... *Flashing red* ....

SUN DIARY

Today I got .... *minutes of sun exposure.*

THIS IS WHAT I DID TODAY TO IMPROVE . . .

My sleep:

....

....

....

My stress level:

....

....

....

My mood:

....

....

....

My environment:

....

....

....

TIP OF THE DAY In the grade-B horror-movie classic *Mr. Sardonicus*, the doomed title character's face is frozen into a ghastly, grimacing smile. Believe it or not, that may be what lifted his mood enough for him to commit another hour and a half of mayhem. Research shows that the act of smiling—which involves 40 different facial muscles—triggers the brain to release mood-enhancing endorphins, which give you an instant lift and also enhance your immune function. What's cool is that it doesn't matter if your smile is real or fake. So the next time you're feeling down, pretend you're Mr. Sardonicus and give the mirror a big toothy grin. If you crack yourself up, so much the better. Laughter is immune-enhancing, too.

Week 3/Day 2

BREAKFAST

2 slices whole grain cinnamon-swirl bread topped with 2 tablespoons unsalted almond butter and ¼ cup chopped dried figs

1 cup 1% milk

LUNCH

Crabmeat Melt: 1 whole wheat English muffin, split in half and topped with crabmeat salad (3 ounces drained canned crabmeat mixed with 1 tablespoon light mayonnaise and 1 tablespoon finely diced onion) and 2 slices (1 ounce each) reduced-fat Cheddar cheese

¾ cup fresh cauliflower florets and 5 baby carrots with 2 tablespoons light ranch dressing for dipping

1 cup pomegranate juice

SNACK

4 whole wheat crackers topped with 2 tablespoons roasted garlic hummus

DINNER

Greek Salad with Chicken: 1½ cups spinach leaves, 1½ cups chopped romaine, 3 ounces grilled chicken strips cooked with ½ teaspoon dried thyme, ¼ cup crumbled feta cheese, 6 pitted kalamata olives, 3 table-spoons chopped red onions, 6 grape tomatoes, and ¼ cup chopped cucumber

3 tablespoons light olive oil vinaigrette

1 cup cantaloupe chunks

1,805 calories; 21% protein (95 g); 44% carbohydrate (199 g); 35% fat (70 g); 9.5% saturated fat (19 g); 232 mg cholesterol; 23 g dietary fiber; 19,990 IU vitamin A; 142 mg vitamin C; 16.8 mg vitamin E; 127 IU vitamin D; 1.8 mg vitamin B_6; 492 mcg folate; 3.2 mcg vitamin B_{12}; 3,208 mg sodium; 3,690 mg potassium; 1,631 mg calcium; 14 mg iron; 13 mg zinc

FOOD FACTS

■ Crabmeat contains protein, omega-3 fatty acids, and the essential antioxidant vitamin E. Enjoy fresh, frozen, or canned varieties.

■ Full-fat salad dressings ring up calories and fat grams quickly, so use light, reduced-fat versions instead. Fat-free isn't necessary, especially since fat helps absorb fat-soluble vitamins A, D, E, and K.

■ Hummus is a nutrient-dense spread made from chickpeas, also known as garbanzo beans. Look for plain or flavored hummus in the refrigerated case of your supermarket.

Best food choice(s) today:

....

....

....

EXERCISE RECORD

Walking or other aerobic activity: .... *minutes*

Resistance training: Upper body ....
Lower body ....
Core ....

STRESS RECORD

Today my stress level is: Yellow .... *Orange* .... *Red* .... *Flashing red* ....

SUN DIARY

Today I got .... *minutes of sun exposure.*

THIS IS WHAT I DID TODAY TO IMPROVE . . .

My sleep:

....

....

....

My stress level:

....

....

....

My mood:

....

....

....

My environment:

....

....

....

TIP OF THE DAY Fortify yourself against the stresses of the coming day by taking a spa-quality morning shower. Lather up with an aromatic bath gel or soap; gently scrub with a thick, soft sponge or loofah; and dry off with an extra-thick towel.

Week 3/Day 3

BREAKFAST

Sausage and Egg Burrito: 1 whole wheat tortilla filled with 1 scrambled egg, 2 tablespoons soy sausage-style crumbles, ¼ cup shredded reduced-fat Mexican-blend cheese, 2 teaspoons cilantro, and 2 tablespoons salsa

1 cup cranberry juice

LUNCH

2 cups split pea and ham soup

Crunchy Coleslaw: 1 cup shredded coleslaw mix with 1 tablespoon chopped dates, 1 tablespoon chopped walnuts, and 2 tablespoons low-fat coleslaw dressing

1 tangelo or tangerine

1 cup 1% milk

SNACK

1 Honeycrisp apple with 1 tablespoon peanut butter

DINNER

1 serving (10 ounces) lasagna (from a healthy brand of frozen entrée)

1 cup zucchini cooked with 1 teaspoon light margarine and a sprinkle of Italian seasoning

1 slice Italian bread, toasted, with 2 teaspoons light margarine and ⅛ teaspoon minced garlic

1 cup 1% milk

1,837 calories; 19% protein (87 g); 55% carbohydrate (253 g); 26% fat (53 g); 7% saturated fat (15 g); 285 mg cholesterol; 33 g dietary fiber; 6,396 IU vitamin A; 255 mg vitamin C; 5 mg vitamin E; 208 IU vitamin D; 1.6 mg vitamin B_6; 477 mcg folate; 4.5 mcg vitamin B_{12}; 2,837 mg sodium; 3,501 mg potassium; 1,386 mg calcium; 13 mg iron; 10.5 mg zinc

■ Eggs are perfectly fine on practically any eating plan. One average egg contains only 75 calories, 5 grams of fat, and 6 grams of protein—plus valuable vitamins and minerals. Look for the new eggs fortified with omega-3 fatty acids.

■ You can enjoy frozen entrées if you choose the healthier versions containing fewer calories and less fat and sodium. Enhance their nutritional value by adding a side vegetable, fruit, and/or a whole grain dinner roll.

Best food choice(s) today:

....

....

....

EXERCISE RECORD

Walking or other aerobic activity: .... *minutes*

Resistance training: Upper body ....
                       Lower body ....
                             Core ....

STRESS RECORD

Today my stress level is: Yellow .... *Orange* .... *Red* .... *Flashing red* ....

SUN DIARY

Today I got .... *minutes of sun exposure.*

THIS IS WHAT I DID TODAY TO IMPROVE . . .

My sleep:

....

....

....

My stress level:

....

....

....

My mood:

....

....

....

My environment:

....

....

....

TIP OF THE DAY To get the optimal immune-enhancing benefits of sunshine, try to expose 25 percent of your body to a moderate amount of sunlight 2 or 3 days a week. (Twenty-five percent is your hands, arms, and face or just your arms and legs.) If you live at a subtropical latitude—which includes a dozen of the southernmost states, as well as major cities such as Atlanta, Dallas, and Los Angeles—your skin can make vitamin D from sunshine year-round. If you live farther north, you may want to consider taking a vitamin D supplement during the winter months (between November and February). Currently, the government recommends a daily dosage of 200 IU for adults age 49 and younger, 400 IU for those 50 to 70, and 600 IU for those over 70. If you're taking a multivitamin, that should cover your vitamin D needs. Check the label to be sure.

Week 3/Day 4

BREAKFAST

Ginger Peach Smoothie: 1½ cups peach kefir, 1 cup fresh or frozen unsweetened peach slices, ¼ teaspoon minced refrigerated ginger, and ½ teaspoon almond extract

1 medium blueberry muffin (3 inches)

LUNCH

3 ounces tilapia cooked with salt-free onion-herb seasoning

1 cup cooked whole wheat rotini sprinkled with 1 tablespoon grated Parmesan cheese

1 cup cooked broccoli florets

1 purple plum

SNACK

1-ounce piece dark chocolate

½ cup low-fat chocolate milk

DINNER

1 cup tomato soup made with 1% milk

Grilled Cheese Sandwich: 1½ ounces sliced reduced-fat Cheddar cheese between 2 slices whole wheat bread coated with 1 tablespoon light margarine for grilling

Fruit and Spinach Salad: 1½ cups fresh spinach leaves, 1 chopped kiwifruit, ½ cup chopped strawberries, and 1 tablespoon pomegranate seeds with 2 tablespoons light raspberry vinaigrette

1,790 calories; 18% protein (81 g); 57% carbohydrate (255 g); 25% fat (49 g); 10% saturated fat (20 g); 138 mg cholesterol; 25 g dietary fiber; 8,898 IU vitamin A; 306 mg vitamin C; 7.5 mg vitamin E; 55 IU vitamin D; 1.1 mg vitamin B_6; 290 mcg folate; 5.2 mcg vitamin B_{12}; 2,739 mg sodium; 3,608 mg potassium; 1,439 mg calcium; 11 mg iron; 8 mg zinc

FOOD FACTS

■ Watch portion sizes on purchased muffins. Better yet, make your own with part whole wheat flour and extra immune-boosting blueberries.

■ Occasionally savor a small piece of dark chocolate, which contains more heart-healthy antioxidants than milk chocolate.

■ Chocolate milk contains the same amount of protein and calcium as regular milk. Stick with the low-fat version to keep fat and cholesterol in check.

Best food choice(s) today:

....

....

....

EXERCISE RECORD

Walking or other aerobic activity: .... *minutes*

Resistance training: Upper body ....
Lower body ....
Core ....

STRESS RECORD

Today my stress level is: Yellow .... *Orange* .... *Red* .... *Flashing red* ....

SUN DIARY

Today I got .... *minutes of sun exposure.*

THIS IS WHAT I DID TODAY TO IMPROVE...

My sleep:

....

....

....

My stress level:

....

....

....

My mood:

....

....

....

My environment:

....

....

....

TIP OF THE DAY When co-workers ask what you did over the weekend, are you as likely as not to say "I don't remember"? If so, it could be because you pid-dled away Saturday and Sunday performing tasks that you thought you "should" do, shelving activities that you really wanted to do. To reclaim your weekends, designate just 3 hours of each Saturday for "homework"—and set an alarm clock to signal your quitting time. Devote the rest of the weekend to whatever gives you pleasure.

Week 3/Day 5

BREAKFAST

1½ cups cooked oatmeal (made with 1% milk) topped with ¼ cup dried cranberries, 1 teaspoon ground cinnamon, and 2 tablespoons sliced almonds

1 cup orange juice

LUNCH

Fiesta Stuffed Baked Potato: 1 large baked potato topped with ½ cup black beans, ⅓ cup sweet-corn kernels, ⅓ cup shredded reduced-fat Mexican-blend cheese, and 2 tablespoons salsa

1 cup pineapple chunks

1 slice whole grain cinnamon-swirl bread, toasted and topped with 1 teaspoon light margarine

¾ cup fat-free lemon yogurt

DINNER

3 ounces grilled or broiled boneless pork loin chop

1 cup sauerkraut seasoned with 1 teaspoon light margarine and ¼ teaspoon caraway seed

1 cup cooked green beans seasoned with ¼ teaspoon minced garlic

1 cup fresh blueberries mixed with 1 tablespoon reduced-fat sour cream

1,793 calories; 18% protein (81 g); 62% carbohydrate (280 g); 20% fat (40 g); 7% saturated fat (14 g); 118 mg cholesterol; 37 g dietary fiber; 2,960 IU vitamin A; 248 mg vitamin C; 6 mg vitamin E; 128 IU vitamin D; 2.2 mg vitamin B_6; 353 mcg folate; 2.8 mcg vitamin B_{12}; 2,791 mg sodium; 4,318 mg potassium; 1,227 mg calcium; 16 mg iron; 11 mg zinc

FOOD FACTS

■ Sauerkraut is basically cooked, seasoned cabbage—and cabbage is one of those cruciferous vegetables (in the same family as broccoli and cauliflower) with powerful disease-fighting nutrients.

■ Mixing reduced-fat sour cream into fresh berries—like the blueberries for today's dinner—is like coating them in decadent cream but with less fat and calories.

Best food choice(s) today:

....

....

....

EXERCISE RECORD

Walking or other aerobic activity: .... *minutes*

Resistance training: Upper body ....
Lower body ....
Core ....

STRESS RECORD

Today my stress level is: Yellow .... *Orange* .... *Red* .... *Flashing red* ....

SUN DIARY

Today I got .... *minutes of sun exposure.*

THIS IS WHAT I DID TODAY TO IMPROVE ...

My sleep:

....

....

....

My stress level:

....

....

....

My mood:

....

....

....

My environment:

....

....

....

 TIP OF THE DAY If you aren't already doing so, and you feel up to the task, consider mowing your own lawn instead of hiring someone else to do it. You won't just save on the cost of a lawn service—using a power push mower, which has a gearing mechanism that helps propel the mower forward, burns 364 calories per hour. With a regular push mower, you can burn an astounding 486 calories per hour. As long as you take the proper precautions—wearing long pants, protective eyewear, and earplugs—a good 30- to 60-minute session of lawn mowing could easily fulfill your daily "requirement" of moderate aerobic activity.

Week 3/Day 6

BREAKFAST

Lox and Cream Cheese on Bagel: 1 multigrain bagel, split, toasted and topped with 2 tablespoons light cream cheese, 2 ounces thin smoked salmon, 4 slices tomato, 2 slices red onion, and 1 tablespoon capers and sprinkled with fresh lemon juice

¾ cup red or pink grapefruit juice

LUNCH

Ham and Swiss on Rye: 2 slices rye bread, 3 ounces lean deli honey ham, 1-ounce slice Swiss cheese, 6 spinach leaves, and 1 teaspoon zesty mustard

½ cup canned maple-and-brown-sugar baked beans

½ cup seedless green grapes

1 cup 1% milk

SNACK

1 fortune cookie

½ cup 1% milk

DINNER

Cashew Chicken with Rice: 2 ounces cooked chicken strips, ½ cup snow pea pods, ¾ cup cooked broccoli florets, ¼ cup sliced mushrooms, ½ cup bok choy, 2 tablespoons green onions, and 3 tablespoons cashews stir-fried with 3 tablespoons stir-fry sauce and 1 teaspoon oil

1½ cups cooked brown rice

1 cup mango chunks

1,834 calories; 21% protein (98 g); 58% carbohydrate (268 g); 19% fat (40.5 g); 8% saturated fat (16 g); 173 mg cholesterol; 24 g dietary fiber; 6,309 IU vitamin A; 215 mg vitamin C; 8 mg vitamin E; 205 IU vitamin D; 2.3 mg vitamin B_6; 385 mcg folate; 5.5 mcg vitamin B_{12}; 4,363 mg sodium; 3,585 mg potassium; 1,088 mg calcium; 16 mg iron; 13 mg zinc

FOOD FACTS

■ All nuts and seeds are calorie dense, but just a small amount can go a long way, nutrition-wise. Nuts and seeds are rich in vitamin E and other valuable nutrients. As a bonus, their fat is heart-healthy.

■ Lox is very thinly sliced smoked salmon, which makes it a good source of healthy protein and omega-3 fatty acids. Find it in the refrigerated seafood case of your supermarket.

■ Baked beans . . . pork 'n' beans . . . whatever you call them, they're jam-packed with fiber and immune-boosting nutrients. The extra calories from sweeteners are far outweighed by the protein, vitamins, and minerals.

Best food choice(s) today:

....

....

....

EXERCISE RECORD

Walking or other aerobic activity: .... *minutes*

Resistance training: Upper body ....
      Lower body ....
        Core ....

STRESS RECORD

Today my stress level is: Yellow .... *Orange* .... *Red* .... *Flashing red* ....

SUN DIARY

Today I got .... *minutes of sun exposure.*

THIS IS WHAT I DID TODAY TO IMPROVE . . .

My sleep:

....

....

....

My stress level:

....

....

....

My mood:

....

....

....

My environment:

....

....

....

TIP OF THE DAY
Keeping a regular journal—or even an irregular one—can significantly boost your immunity. Researchers at the University of Texas at Austin tracked one group of medical students who wrote about meaningful emotional issues for 20 minutes a day, 3 to 5 days week, and another group who simply wrote about everyday events. Each group was instructed either to mull over the events they wrote about or to just let go and move on. The students who took time to ponder their lives were more likely than those who didn't to produce higher levels of infection-fighting immune cells. Try to set aside at least 20 minutes 3 or 4 days a week to summarize and assess the important events in your life.

Week 3/Day 7

BREAKFAST

1½ cups mini frosted shredded-wheat squares with 1 cup 1% milk

1 banana

LUNCH

Citrus Salad with Shrimp: 3 cups mixed greens, 3 ounces cooked shrimp, ¾ cup red grapefruit sections, ½ cup mandarin oranges, ¼ cup julienned jicama, and ¼ cup chopped avocado with 3 tablespoons light poppy-seed or raspberry vinaigrette

4 whole wheat crackers

1 cup 1% milk

SNACK

¼ cup mixed nuts

DINNER

3 ounces grilled sirloin steak cooked with salt-free steak seasoning

1 cup cooked baby red potatoes seasoned with 2 teaspoons light margarine and 1 teaspoon chopped parsley

1 cup spinach sautéed with 1½ teaspoons olive oil and ¼ teaspoon minced garlic

1 whole wheat dinner roll

1,819 calories; 19% protein (89 g); 51% carbohydrate (232 g); 30% fat (60 g); 6% saturated fat (12.5 g); 240 mg cholesterol; 33 g dietary fiber; 13,655 IU vitamin A; 180 mg vitamin C; 15 mg vitamin E; 254 IU vitamin D; 3.4 mg vitamin B_6; 544 mcg folate; 7.3 mcg vitamin B_{12}; 1,398 mg sodium; 4,362 mg potassium; 935 mg calcium; 36 mg iron; 16 mg zinc

FOOD FACTS

■ Jicama is a crunchy, nutrient-rich vegetable that's a staple of Hispanic cooking. Use it on salads or simply as a fresh vegetable for dipping.

■ Precut grapefruit sections are available in cans or jars, packed in water or light syrup. Though all are rich in nutrients, the red/pink grapefruit contains more beta-carotene.

Best food choice(s) today:

....

....

....

EXERCISE RECORD

Walking or other aerobic activity: .... *minutes*

Resistance training: Upper body ....
Lower body ....
Core ....

STRESS RECORD

Today my stress level is: Yellow .... *Orange* .... *Red* .... *Flashing red* ....

SUN DIARY

Today I got .... *minutes of sun exposure.*

THIS IS WHAT I DID TODAY TO IMPROVE . . .

My sleep:

....

....

....

My stress level:

....

....

....

My mood:

....

....

....

My environment:

....

....

....

TIP OF THE DAY Consider substituting natural products for the cosmetics, fragrances, and toiletries you use each day. Most brands contain dozens of chemicals, some of which may cause serious harm. One example is dibutyl phthalate, a chemical that has been linked to birth defects in animals. According to one study, dibutyl phthalate is an ingredient in 37 nail products as well as other personal-care products.

For proprietary reasons, manufacturers are not required to divulge what's in their perfumes and colognes. So there's no way of knowing if a particular scent contains the essence of flowers—or the essence of carcinogens.

Week 3 Review

Date ....

I'M MOST PROUD OF MEETING THE FOLLOWING GOALS:

Diet:

....
....
....

Exercise:

....
....
....

Stress reduction:

....
....
....

Sleep improvement:

....
....
....

Mood improvement:

....
....
....

Sun exposure:

....
....
....

Environmental improvement:

....
....
....

Areas I need to improve:

....
....
....

Get Set for Week 4

Date ....

Maximum Immunity Success Strategies

EXERCISE

Walking/aerobic: beginner, 30 minutes a day; veteran, 50 minutes or more a day
Resistance training: 10 minutes most days of the week, adding more weight or repetitions (for moves that don't require dumbbells) if exercises have become easy

SLEEP

Revisit your sleep diary one more time. In addition to bedtime rituals and sleep-robbing lifestyle habits, are other factors preventing you from getting a decent night's shut-eye? The problem may be poor sleep hygiene—an uncomfortable mattress or pillow, for example, or a too-warm, too-bright, or too-noisy bedroom. Consider what you can do to make your bedroom more conducive to sleep.

STRESS

Continue using your time budget to organize, prioritize, and optimize this precious resource. In the long run, this is the most essential strategy that you can employ to de-stress your life. If you need a quick fix, splurge on a visit to a day spa—where you'll receive facials, massages, and other forms of pampering—or a once- or twice-weekly session with a massage therapist. Also consider adding tai chi or yoga to your daily routine. All of these interventions can make you feel great, not least because they reduce levels of cortisol, the hormone most strongly associated with stress and immune suppression.

MOOD

Continue scheduling activities that help you reach your "happy" place—and take it to the next level. Make a "fantasy" to-do list of those things that you've always dreamed of doing but have never quite managed to accomplish. It doesn't matter if your fantasies are relatively straightforward (such as taking a Mediterranean cruise or rafting through the Grand Canyon) or more complicated (such as building your dream home or starting a new career). The point is to recognize your dream, then create a step-by-step plan for achieving it; that alone can have a fantastic effect on your mood and your immunity.

ENVIRONMENT

Up to this point, you've considered how to germ-proof yourself and your kitchen and protect yourself from family members who bring home the latest bug. Now take a good hard look at your home environment. Have you already prohibited indoor smoking? You're off to a great start. Now try to rid your home of toxic products—especially those labeled "Danger" or "Poison" but also those labeled "Warning" or "Caution." Any substance identified as carcinogenic is hazardous to your immunity.

If you haven't done so, consider testing your home for radon. The test is cheap, and remediation efforts could help eliminate the toxin that's the second leading cause of lung cancer.

Challenges I anticipate this week:

....

....

....

....

Strategies I can use to overcome them:

....

....

....

....

My goals for this week:

....

....

....

....

Your Maximum Immunity Workout

GET LOOSE

While no single stretch can loosen all of the muscles in your body, the modified Triangle Pose comes close. It limbers up not only the muscles in your arms and chest but also those in your torso, hips, and legs.

Stand facing the seat of a chair. Position your left foot beneath the chair and turn your left toes slightly to the left. Step back about 3 feet with your right foot and turn your right toes slightly to the right. Keep your legs straight and contract your leg muscles as though you were hugging them to your bones. Now lengthen your spine and extend your arms out to the sides at shoulder level, your palms facing down.

Keeping your back tall, gently push your hips to the right as you lean left. Bend at your left hip and place your left hand on the chair seat. Look up as you stretch your right hand toward the ceiling. Now pull your shoulder up and back to keep your torso facing forward. Hold for 20 to 30 seconds, then return to the starting position. Relax a few seconds before repeating the stretch to the opposite side.

GET FIT

If you think mall-walking is just for the senior set, think again. Many of America's malls have organized walking clubs, and members don't just cruise the corridors to window-shop. Here's a program that incorporates brisk walking and light calisthenics to give you an all-in-one cardiovascular and resistance-training workout. You can perform it in a mall or outdoors in a park—anywhere there's a nice flat walking surface, benches, and stairs. *Note:* Although the program takes an hour and includes moderate to vigorous activity, feel free to adjust it to match your fitness, endurance, and comfort levels.

Start with 2 minutes of easy walking, followed by 2 minutes of moderate walking, then 6 minutes of brisk walking. If you're an experienced, fit walker, continue with another 20 minutes of fast walking. If not, try for another 20 minutes of brisk walking.

For the next 5 minutes, perform these two exercises.

Walking lunge. Step forward about 3 feet with your left foot, allowing your arms to swing naturally. Bend your left knee until your left thigh is almost parallel to the floor and your right knee is nearing the floor. Keep your left knee over your ankle and tighten your abdominal muscles. Bring your right foot forward and stand tall. Repeat the exercise by stepping forward with your right foot. Continue for 3 minutes.

Bench pushup. Place your hands shoulder-width apart on the back of an (unoccupied) bench or on a railing. Step back with your feet so that your body is on a diagonal. Bend your elbows and lower your chest toward the bench. Hold for 1 second, then straighten your arms and repeat. Continue for 2 minutes.

For the next 15 minutes, resume a brisk (or fast) walk. Follow with 6 minutes total of the following three exercises.

Squat walk-up. Stand facing a staircase and place your right foot on the second step. Bend your knees and sit back into a squat. Alternating your feet, climb the stairs two at a time while maintaining as deep a squat as possible. Continue for 2 minutes.

Stair hops. Stand facing a staircase with your feet together. Hop up onto the first step, landing with both of your knees bent. Carefully step backward one foot at a time. Repeat the exercise—only this time, step backward with the other foot first. Continue for 2 minutes.

Triceps dips. Sit on the edge of a bench with your hands next to your hips. Grasping the edge of the bench, slide your butt off the bench and walk your feet forward so that your knees are over your ankles. Lower your butt toward the ground while bending your elbows up to 90 degrees and keeping them pointing backward. Hold for one count, then straighten your arms and repeat. Continue for 2 minutes.

Finish your workout with another 6 minutes of brisk walking, followed by 3 minutes of easy walking to help you cool down.

GET STRONG

UPPER BODY: GET SUPER SHOULDERS WITH T-RAISES

Holding a pair of 3- to 5-pound dumbbells, stand with your feet hip-width apart and your arms at your sides, palms facing your thighs. Slowly raise your arms in front of you to shoulder height, then slowly lower. Work up to 2 sets of 8 to 12 repetitions.

Return to the same starting position as above, with your feet hip-width apart and arms at your sides. Keeping your arms straight, slowly raise the dumbbells out to the sides until your body forms a T. Slowly lower to the starting position. Work up to 2 sets of 8 to 12 repetitions.

CORE: ELBOW-TO-KNEE SITUP

Lie on your back on an exercise mat or another padded surface. Keep your knees bent and your feet flat on the floor. Place your hands behind your head, then lift your head and feet a few inches off the floor while pointing your elbows toward your knees. Contract your abdominal muscles until your elbows meet your knees, taking care not to pull on your head or neck with your hands. At this point, your body weight should be resting on the so-called sitz bones of your pelvis. Hold for a second, then return to the starting position. Work up to 2 sets of 8 to 12 repetitions.

LOWER BODY: PLANK LIFT

Lie facedown on an exercise mat or another padded surface. Bend your elbows and position your hands beside your ears. Raise your body so that you're supporting your weight on your forearms and toes. Keep your head, neck, and back in a straight line. Contract your abdominal muscles so your stomach doesn't sag toward the floor, and tuck your pelvis so your butt doesn't rise up.

Now raise your right leg 6 to 12 inches off the floor while squeezing the muscles in your buttocks. Hold for 3 to 5 seconds, then lower your right leg and repeat with your left leg. Work up to 2 sets of 8 to 12 repetitions.

Week 4/Day 1

BREAKFAST

Cheddar Scrambled Eggs: 2 extra-large eggs scrambled with milk, stirring in ½ cup shredded reduced-fat extra-sharp Cheddar cheese

1 soy sausage-style patty

2 slices whole wheat bread, toasted and topped with 2 teaspoons light margarine and 1 tablespoon sugar-free blackberry preserves

1 cup orange juice

LUNCH

Apple Turkey Pocket: 1 whole wheat pita filled with 3 ounces lean smoked deli turkey, ½-ounce slice provolone cheese, 6 spinach leaves, ½ thinly sliced apple, and 2 teaspoons mayonnaise-mustard spread

1 cup fresh sugar snap peas

½ apple (remainder from pita)

1 cup 1% milk

SNACK

Cherry Almond Smoothie: 1½ cups fat-free vanilla yogurt, ¾ cup cherries (fresh, frozen, or canned and drained), and 1 teaspoon almond extract

DINNER

Key Lime Tuna: 3 ounces grilled or broiled tuna steak seasoned with 2 teaspoons honey, ½ teaspoon soy sauce, 1 teaspoon lime juice, and ½ teaspoon lime zest

1 cup cooked whole wheat couscous

1 cup cooked broccoli florets seasoned with salt-free lemon-pepper seasoning and 1 teaspoon light margarine

1 cup honeydew melon and cantaloupe chunks

1,783 calories; 26% protein (116 g); 53% carbohydrate (239 g); 21% fat (41 g); 7% saturated fat (14 g); 548 mg cholesterol; 27 g dietary fiber; 6,073 IU vitamin A; 285 mg vitamin C; 5.4 mg vitamin E; 283 IU vitamin D; 2.3 mg vitamin B_6; 357 mcg folate; 6 mcg vitamin B_{12}; 2,483 mg sodium; 3,713 mg potassium; 1,175 mg calcium; 14 mg iron; 8 mg zinc

FOOD FACTS

■ One of the fastest-cooking whole grain side dishes is whole wheat couscous. You can find couscous—a Moroccan pasta—in the rice aisle. To prepare it, just boil water, add the couscous, and fluff.

■ For extra immune-boosting nutrients, choose the newer varieties of orange juice that have been fortified with vitamins A, C, D, and E, along with calcium and zinc.

Best food choice(s) today:

....

....

....

EXERCISE RECORD

Walking or other aerobic activity: .... *minutes*

Resistance training: Upper body ....
Lower body ....
Core ....

STRESS RECORD

Today my stress level is: Yellow .... *Orange* .... *Red* .... *Flashing red* ....

SUN DIARY

Today I got .... *minutes of sun exposure.*

THIS IS WHAT I DID TODAY TO IMPROVE . . .

My sleep:

....

....

....

My stress level:

....

....

....

My mood:

....

....

....

My environment:

....

....

....

 Now that you're well into your walking program, you may need some incentives to keep going. Mix up your routine with a walk in the woods or a hike along a mountain trail. Sign up for a 5-K walk that raises money for one of your favorite causes. Branch out into walking-related activities such as orienteering, bird-watching, or a *volksmarch* club, which sponsors noncompetitive 6-mile hikes with refreshments along the way. The clubs originated in Europe and grew to thousands of affiliates worldwide, all sponsored by the International Volkssport Federation.

Week 4/Day 2

BREAKFAST

1½ cups fat-free orange crème–flavored yogurt mixed with 2 tablespoons crunchy barley-nuggets cereal and 1 tablespoon wheat germ

1 cup blackberries

LUNCH

Thai Pork Lettuce Wraps: 3 ounces pork tenderloin cooked with Chinese 5-spice powder and sprinkled with 1 teaspoon sesame seeds, ⅓ cup bean sprouts, ⅓ cup grated or shredded carrots, ¼ cup chopped cilantro, and ¼ cup cooked rice noodles, divided between 2 very large or 4 small leaves butter or romaine lettuce, folded and served with ¼ cup Thai sweet chili or peanut satay sauce for dipping

1 cup steamed edamame (green sweet soybeans in the pod), salted

1 Asian pear

SNACK

2 small chocolate chip cookies

DINNER:

3 whole grain blueberry pancakes (made from packaged mix, using fat-free milk and egg) with 1 tablespoon light margarine and 2 tablespoons sugar-free pancake syrup

1 cup blueberries (⅔ cup for pancake batter and ⅓ cup for topping)

2 slices cooked turkey bacon

1 cup 1% milk

1 cup pineapple juice

1,792 calories; 21% protein (93 g); 53% carbohydrate (240 g); 26% fat (52 g); 7% saturated fat (14.5 g); 140 mg cholesterol; 34 g dietary fiber; 9,529 IU vitamin A; 105 mg vitamin C; 7.5 mg vitamin E; 202 IU vitamin D; 1.7 mg vitamin B$_6$; 442 mcg folate; 4 mcg vitamin B$_{12}$; 3,486 mg sodium; 3,734 mg potassium; 1,387 mg calcium; 21 mg iron; 14 mg zinc

FOOD FACTS

■ Mimic some of your favorite restaurant dishes at home, like the Thai Pork Lettuce Wraps in today's menu. They can be made with chicken, pork, or beef. Lettuce wraps are a great way to enjoy vegetables.

■ Edamame in the pod is fun to eat. Simply steam, salt, and squeeze the green soybeans into your mouth.

■ Asian pears are a cross between an apple and a pear. They're rich in fiber and valuable nutrients. Eat as is, or slice and add to salads or sandwiches.

Best food choice(s) today:

....

....

....

EXERCISE RECORD

Walking or other aerobic activity: .... *minutes*

Resistance training: Upper body ....
                    Lower body ....
                         Core ....

STRESS RECORD

Today my stress level is: Yellow .... *Orange* .... *Red* .... *Flashing red* ....

SUN DIARY

Today I got .... *minutes of sun exposure.*

THIS IS WHAT I DID TODAY TO IMPROVE . . .

My sleep:

....

....

....

My stress level:

....

....

....

My mood:

....

....

....

My environment:

....

....

....

 TIP OF THE DAY If you've made the switch from soda to black, green, or oolong tea, you'll get the same immune-enhancing benefits from both the regular and decaf versions. But don't flavor your tea with whole or fat-free milk, soy milk, or nondairy creamer. Recent research shows that these products cancel out the teas' antioxidant activity while adding unnecessary calories. Instead, try flavoring your tea with a cinnamon stick. Cinnamon contains methylhydroxy chalcone polymer, a substance that may reduce insulin resistance and diabetes risks. In one study, it increased cells' ability to process blood sugar by nearly twentyfold.

Week 4/Day 3

BREAKFAST

Cinnamon French Toast: 2 slices whole grain cinnamon-swirl bread dipped in mixture of 1 egg, 2 tablespoons 1% milk, and ½ teaspoon ground cinnamon, cooked and topped with 1 cup mashed or pureed peaches

2-ounce slice Canadian bacon

1 cup red grapefruit juice

LUNCH

Strawberry Almond Spinach Salad: 3 cups spinach leaves, ¾ cup sliced strawberries, 1 sliced kiwifruit, 2 tablespoons pomegranate seeds, 3 tablespoons honey-roasted almond slices, and 1 sliced hard-cooked egg with 3 tablespoons light red French dressing

1 whole wheat dinner roll with 2 teaspoons light margarine

1 cup 1% milk

SNACK

½ cup mango chunks

DINNER

Super Sloppy Joes: 1 whole wheat hamburger bun topped with mixture of 3 ounces ground turkey breast, 1 tablespoon minced onion, and ⅓ cup canned Sloppy Joe sauce

Carrot Slaw: ½ cup grated carrots, ¾ cup shredded cabbage, 1 tablespoon raisins, and 2 tablespoons low-fat coleslaw dressing

1 cup 1% milk

1,848 calories; 18% protein (83 g); 52% carbohydrate (240 g); 30% fat (62 g); 7% saturated fat (15 g); 561 mg cholesterol; 27 g dietary fiber; 22,408 IU vitamin A; 283 mg vitamin C; 19.4 mg vitamin E; 361 IU vitamin D; 1.7 mg vitamin B_6; 445 mcg folate; 4.6 mcg vitamin B_{12}; 3,191 mg sodium; 3,861 mg potassium; 1,258 mg calcium; 13.5 mg iron; 10 mg zinc

FOOD FACTS

▧ Make healthier versions of your favorite comfort foods—Sloppy Joes, meat loaf, spaghetti sauce, shepherd's pie—by using ground turkey breast, ground lean pork tenderloin, or extra-lean (95 percent) ground beef.

▧ Mango is incredibly high in beta-carotene, an antioxidant. It offers other nutrients and fiber as well. Choose fresh or frozen or even packed in light syrup or juice in bottles or jars.

Best food choice(s) today:

....

....

....

EXERCISE RECORD

Walking or other aerobic activity: .... *minutes*

Resistance training: Upper body ....
Lower body ....
Core ....

STRESS RECORD

Today my stress level is: Yellow .... *Orange* .... *Red* .... *Flashing red* ....

SUN DIARY

Today I got .... *minutes of sun exposure.*

My sleep:

....

....

....

My stress level:

....

....

....

My mood:

....

....

....

My environment:

....

....

....

 TIP OF THE DAY Most everyday chores don't burn anywhere near the number of calories you'd burn with 30 to 60 minutes of moderate exercise—but some do. Try enlisting your family for a sweat-busting cleaning frenzy that gets the house spic and span in just 1 hour. Afterward, congratulate each other for a job well done—and for a burst of activity that probably burned over 300 calories per person. Other chores that burn lots of calories include general gardening (404 per hour); painting, papering, and plastering (281); and raking leaves (322).

Week 4/Day 4

BREAKFAST

1½ cups cooked oatmeal (made with 1% milk) mixed with 1 tablespoon chopped walnuts, ¼ cup dried cherries, and 1 tablespoon ground flaxseed

1 cup pomegranate juice

LUNCH

Ham Sandwich: 2 slices mixed grain bread, 3 ounces lean smoked deli ham, 1 romaine lettuce leaf, 3 sliced tomatoes, and 1 teaspoon spicy brown mustard

Easy Three Bean Salad: ½ cup each canned and drained kidney, garbanzo, and black beans mixed with 2 tablespoons olive oil vinaigrette

1 cup 1% milk

SNACK

1½ cups microwave caramel popcorn

DINNER

Salmon Caesar Salad: 3 cups chopped romaine lettuce, 3 ounces grilled salmon, ⅓ cup marinated artichoke hearts, 8 whole grain croutons, and 2 tablespoons shredded Parmesan cheese with 3 tablespoons light Caesar dressing

1 red Anjou pear

1,852 calories; 19% protein (90 g); 54% carbohydrate (254 g); 27% fat (55 g); 7% saturated fat (14 g); 103 mg cholesterol; 43 g dietary fiber; 12,460 IU vitamin A; 189 mg vitamin C; 10.5 mg vitamin E; 130 IU vitamin D; 1.9 mg vitamin B$_6$; 543 mcg folate; 5.9 mcg vitamin B$_{12}$; 3,985 mg sodium; 3,976 mg potassium; 1,084 mg calcium; 13.3 mg iron; 11 mg zinc

FOOD FACTS

■ Even on a healthy eating plan, most of us can afford to enjoy small treats, like today's microwave caramel popcorn. Watching portion sizes is critical, however, so chew slowly and savor every bite!

■ Instead of serving chips with sandwiches, make protein-packed, nutrient-dense bean salads by mixing any combination of your favorite canned beans and stirring in a little light salad dressing.

Best food choice(s) today:

....

....

....

EXERCISE RECORD

Walking or other aerobic activity: .... *minutes*

Resistance training: Upper body ....
Lower body ....
Core ....

STRESS RECORD

Today my stress level is: Yellow .... *Orange* .... *Red* .... *Flashing red* ....

SUN DIARY

Today I got .... *minutes of sun exposure.*

THIS IS WHAT I DID TODAY TO IMPROVE . . .

My sleep:

....

....

My stress level:

....

....

My mood:

....

....

My environment:

....

....

TIP OF THE DAY Dove Dark contains Cocoapro cocoa, a proprietary blend with twice as many antioxidants as most other brands of dark chocolate. It's so dense with flavanols that scientists often use it in studies. In one such study comparing Dove Dark with lower-flavanol dark chocolate, only Dove Dark elevated blood levels of antioxidants and "good" HDL cholesterol, while reducing oxidation of "bad" LDL cholesterol. Dove Dark also contains procyanidins that trigger the release of nitric oxide, which relaxes arteries and improves bloodflow. Dark chocolate is just one of the nutritious daily snacks allowed in the Immune Essentials Plan. The recommended "dosage" is 1 ounce.

Week 4/Day 5

BREAKFAST

1½ cups raisin bran with 1 cup 1% milk

1 cup apricot halves packed in light syrup or juice

LUNCH

Cheese and Avocado Quesadilla: 2 corn tortillas (6 inches each), ½ cup shredded reduced-fat Mexican-blend cheese, and ¼ cup chopped avocado

¾ cup refried beans topped with 1 teaspoon chopped cilantro and ¼ cup salsa

1 orange or tangerine

SNACK

1 cup strawberry-banana kefir

DINNER

Lemon Chicken: 3 ounces cooked chicken breast seasoned with 2 teaspoons lemon juice, ½ teaspoon lemon zest, and ¼ teaspoon minced garlic

1 large sweet potato, baked and topped with 1 tablespoon light margarine, 1 teaspoon brown sugar, and 1 tablespoon chopped pecans

1 cup cooked cauliflower and broccoli florets sprinkled with chopped parsley

1 whole wheat dinner roll

1,836 calories; 19% protein (89 g); 60% carbohydrate (283 g); 21% fat (43 g); 8% saturated fat (15.5 g); 141 mg cholesterol; 49 g dietary fiber; 46,500 IU vitamin A; 250 mg vitamin C; 9 mg vitamin E; 190 IU vitamin D; 3.2 mg vitamin B$_6$; 445 mcg folate; 5.6 mcg vitamin B$_{12}$; 2,783 mg sodium; 4,664 mg potassium; 1,542 mg calcium; 16.2 mg iron; 14 mg zinc

FOOD FACTS

■ Canned refried beans are good sources of protein and fiber, as well as vitamins and minerals. Look for varieties that contain little or no fat.

■ Technically, avocado is a fruit, but it's mostly fat. Fortunately, it's the right kind of fat for good health. Avocados also contain vitamin E and other important vitamins and minerals.

■ Eat sweet potatoes with their skin for extra fiber, vitamins, and minerals.

Best food choice(s) today:

....

....

....

EXERCISE RECORD

Walking or other aerobic activity: .... *minutes*

Resistance training: Upper body ....
                         Lower body ....
                             Core ....

STRESS RECORD

Today my stress level is: Yellow .... *Orange* .... *Red* .... *Flashing red* ....

SUN DIARY

Today I got .... *minutes of sun exposure.*

THIS IS WHAT I DID TODAY TO IMPROVE ...

My sleep:

....
....
....

My stress level:

....
....
....

My mood:

....
....
....

My environment:

....
....
....

TIP OF THE DAY Think twice about using echinacea to ward off colds and flu. It's no better than sugar pills, according to a gold-standard double-blind, placebo-controlled study that appeared in a 2005 issue of the *New England Journal of Medicine*. After 437 volunteers took either echinacea or a placebo for 7 days, researchers sprayed cold viruses into their noses. None of the three echinacea extracts reduced infection rates or relieved cold symptoms better than the placebo.

Week 4/Day 6

BREAKFAST

2 multigrain frozen waffles, toasted and topped with 1 cup mashed or chopped strawberries

1 cup 1% milk

LUNCH

Sensible Chef's Salad: 3 cups mixed romaine and spinach greens, 2 ounces chopped lean smoked turkey deli meat, 2 ounces chopped lean honey ham, 1 sliced hard-cooked egg, 7 grape tomatoes, ⅓ cup chopped cucumber, ¼ cup shredded carrot, and 2 tablespoons roasted sunflower seeds with 3 tablespoons light cucumber ranch dressing

6 whole wheat crackers

1 purple plum

SNACK

½ cup light mint chocolate chip ice cream drizzled with 1 tablespoon chocolate syrup

DINNER

1 cup vegetable soup

3 ounces grilled beef tenderloin

¾ cup sautéed mushrooms

Chive and Garlic Smashed Potatoes: 1 cooked medium baking potato mashed with 2 tablespoons 1% milk, 1 tablespoon light sour cream, a dash of salt, 1 tablespoon chopped chives, and ⅛ teaspoon minced garlic

1 cup nectarine or peach slices

1 cup 1% milk

1,818 calories; 20% protein (93 g); 51% carbohydrate (233 g); 29% fat (59 g); 8% saturated fat (17 g); 380 mg cholesterol; 28 g dietary fiber; 20,959 IU vitamin A; 190 mg vitamin C; 9.5 mg vitamin E; 385 IU vitamin D; 3 mg vitamin B₆; 503 mcg folate; 6.1 mcg vitamin B₁₂; 3,759 mg sodium; 5,336 mg potassium; 1,127 mg calcium; 16.4 mg iron; 13 mg zinc

FOOD FACTS

■ Many convenience foods are now made with whole grains, like the frozen waffles for today's breakfast.

■ Today's chef salad isn't fat-laden like typical versions. The cheese is omitted, and lean deli meat and an egg provide the protein. Nutrient-dense spinach leaves replace iceberg lettuce, and sunflower seeds—one of the best dietary sources of vitamin E—are added for extra antioxidants and crunch.

Best food choice(s) today:

....

....

....

EXERCISE RECORD

Walking or other aerobic activity: .... *minutes*

Resistance training: Upper body ....
Lower body ....
Core ....

STRESS RECORD

Today my stress level is: Yellow .... *Orange* .... *Red* .... *Flashing red* ....

SUN DIARY

Today I got .... *minutes of sun exposure.*

THIS IS WHAT I DID TODAY TO IMPROVE . . .

My sleep:

....

....

....

My stress level:

....

....

....

My mood:

....

....

....

My environment:

....

....

....

A regular nap may reduce your risk of heart disease. For a 2007 study published in the *Archives of Internal Medicine,* Greek researchers tracked 23,681 men and women for a little over 6 years. The people who napped for 30-plus minutes at least 3 days a week were 37 percent less likely to die from heart disease than nonnappers. The benefit appeared particularly strong in men who worked and less strong in men who didn't work or who were retired. The data weren't sufficient to determine if working women experienced the same effect.

Week 4/Day 7

BREAKFAST

2 cups toasted O-shaped cereal with 1 cup 1% milk

1 cup raspberries

½ cup orange juice

LUNCH

Sunflower-Apple-Date Rollup: 1 whole wheat flour tortilla spread with 2 tablespoons sunflower seed butter, ½ sliced apple, and 1 tablespoon chopped dates

½ cup 1% cottage cheese

½ cup pineapple chunks

SNACK

¾ cup butterscotch pudding made from instant mix with fat-free milk

DINNER

BBQ Pork: 3 ounces grilled or broiled boneless pork loin chop topped with 1 tablespoon barbecue sauce

1 large ear sweet corn on the cob with 1 tablespoon light margarine

1 cup cooked kale, mustard, or collard greens, seasoned with 2 teaspoons light margarine and 1 tablespoon finely diced ham

1 cup barbecue baked beans

2 cups watermelon

1,814 calories; 19% protein (86 g); 60% carbohydrate (273 g); 21 percent fat (45 g); 5% saturated fat (10 g); 110 mg cholesterol; 41 g dietary fiber; 22,843 IU vitamin A; 211 mg vitamin C; 14.5 mg vitamin E; 210 IU vitamin D; 2.7 mg vitamin B_6; 676 mcg folate; 5.6 mcg vitamin B_{12}; 3,427 mg sodium; 4,200 mg potassium; 1,185 mg calcium; 38 mg iron; 31 mg zinc

■ Sunflower seed butter, like cashew, almond, soy-nut, and peanut butters, is nutrient dense. But sunflower seed butter stands apart as being the highest in fiber, vitamin E, and zinc. It's a good alternative for people with peanut allergies.

■ Bored with raisins? Try dates. They're naturally sweet and rich in fiber, potassium, and magnesium, among numerous other vitamins and minerals. Chopped dates make a great addition to baked goods, cereals, yogurt, and salads, while whole dates are perfect for snacking and satisfying that sweet tooth.

■ Watermelon is among the best sources of cancer-fighting lycopene. In fact, it surpasses even tomato products! Enjoy watermelon year-round by purchasing fresh-cut chunks in your supermarket's produce section.

Best food choice(s) today:

....

....

....

EXERCISE RECORD

Walking or other aerobic activity: .... *minutes*

Resistance training: Upper body ....
Lower body ....
Core ....

STRESS RECORD

Today my stress level is: Yellow .... *Orange* .... *Red* .... *Flashing red* ....

SUN DIARY

Today I got .... *minutes of sun exposure.*

THIS IS WHAT I DID TODAY TO IMPROVE . . .

My sleep:

....

....

....

My stress level:

....

....

....

My mood:

....

....

....

My environment:

....

....

....

TIP OF THE DAY Rid your home of unnecessary paints, aerosol sprayers, cleansers, air fresheners, and similar products. They release potentially hazardous chemicals into the air not only when you're using them but also while in storage. Ever wondered why your garage smells so funny? It could be because the air is a stew of chemicals that include known carcinogens such as methylene chloride fumes from aerosol spray paints, paint strippers, and adhesive removers and benzene fumes from stored paint and fuel. At the very least, get such products out of your living quarters. Throw away your air fresheners, too. They only cover up bad odors with additional chemicals, some of which are carcinogenic. Use air filters instead.

Week 4 Review

Date ....

I'M MOST PROUD OF MEETING THE FOLLOWING GOALS:

Diet:

....

....

....

Exercise:

....

....

....

Stress reduction:

....

....

....

Sleep improvement:

....

....

....

Mood improvement:

....

....

....

Sun exposure:

....

....

....

Environmental improvement:

....

....

....

Areas I need to improve:

....

....

....

PART IV

Immune Extras: Smart Strategies to Boost Immunity

If You Are Overweight . . .

For the first half of her life, Nicki Anderson was constantly sick. "I always had a cold or the flu—whatever was going around, I got it," she says. "I was heavy, not exercising, and eating very poorly—a lot of fried foods. Frustrated, I started doing my own research. I found that in underserved countries where nutrition is poor, infections and diseases are rampant. That's when I made the connection between my unhealthy lifestyle and my weak immune system. I realized that I had to make a major change."

Nicki did make a major change—in her diet. She lost 50 pounds. "As soon as I started eating better and losing weight, I slept better, and I began exercising," she says. "Today, I hardly ever get sick. There was clearly a correlation between being overweight and eating fried foods and being chronically ill."

Instead of fast food, Nicki—now age 45—eats tons of fruits and vegetables, "and I step up my consumption of greens, blueberries, and other antioxidant-rich foods around flu season," she says. She also owns her own fitness studio, where she helps others lose weight and—more important—enhance their health.

By teaching people how to make better food choices and shed pounds, Nicki is indeed boosting their well-being—and their immune function. Extra pounds weigh heavily on the immune system, not to mention the cardiovascular system, digestive system, and pretty much every other part of the body. Being overweight or obese puts a person at higher risk for cancer, heart disease, diabetes, and autoimmune disease, to name just a few ills.

Immunity Takes a Pounding

Although the terms are used interchangeably, *overweight* and *obesity* are not one and the same. Overweight is defined as a body mass index (BMI)—a measure of body fat based on height and weight—of 25.0 to 29.9. A BMI of more than 29.9 is considered obese. (To calculate your BMI, go to www.nhlbisupport.com/bmi/.)

Carrying too many pounds taxes the immune system. One reason is that fat cells release hormones called adipokines, which cause inflammation and suppress the immune system. "It is a matter of degree—the heavier you are, the more adipokines you make, and the more pro-inflammatory you are," says Gerard Mullin, MD, director of complementary and alternative medicine and gastrointestinal nutrition services at Johns Hopkins Hospital in Baltimore. "Higher inflammation leads to a higher risk of autoimmune disease and some forms of cancer."

Further, "it is very clear that obesity, particularly central obesity [also known as visceral fat], leads to oxidative stress because of the improper digestion and metabolism of fats," says Sam J. Sugar, MD, board-certified internist and staff physician for the Seaside Medical Group at the Pritikin Longevity Center and Spa in Aventura, Florida. During oxidative stress, free radicals—highly reactive molecules with unpaired electrons—attack the structure of DNA and impair the function of the B cells (white blood cells that help fight infection by producing antibodies) and T cells (which attack and kill invaders).

The direct effects of visceral fat are obvious. People with fat around their middles are at higher risk for cardiovascular disease, diabetes, allergies, and even cancer. "Instead of just being storage vehicles, fat cells are actually quite active metabolically," says Jana Klauer, MD, author of *How the Rich Stay Thin* and a New York City–based physician who specializes in the biology of fat reduction. Visceral fat cells produce small molecules that can't seem to sit still. These restless—and harmful— molecules travel to surrounding cells in the abdomen. "So with visceral obesity, there is an increase in cancers of the digestive system, pancreas, liver, gallbladder, colon, and small and large intestine," says Dr. Klauer. The molecules also jump into the blood and take a ride to distant sites, elevating the risk of prostate and breast cancers as well.

It's no secret that people who are overweight or obese are less likely to exercise than those who are thin, which may have something to do with why they gained weight in the first place. Because exercise stimulates the immune system, those who are less active or inactive miss out on a crucial immune-boosting benefit. Beyond giving short shrift to exercise, we, as a nation, have forgotten the benefits of eating well. Good nutrition has been pushed aside in the name of fad diets and calorie counting. We eat all the wrong things for all the wrong reasons. As a result, more than 60 percent of American adults (and more than 30 percent of the country's children and adolescents) are overweight or obese. This epidemic has taken a heavy toll on our immune systems.

Slim Down, Sneeze Less

The solution is obvious: We need to lose weight. "The lack of responsiveness in B and T immune cells that accompanies overweight resolves with weight loss, so taking off any extra pounds is imperative," Dr. Klauer says. If you are overweight or obese, here are some measures to help reduce the load and relieve your immune system of some of the burden.

Firm up with fish oil. "The omega-3 fatty acids in fish oil can help people who are overweight in a few ways," says Gretchen Vannice, MS, RD, research coordinator at Nordic Naturals in Watsonville, California. These beneficial fats reduce the inflammation associated with obesity, and they seem to support vigorous metabolism by maintaining healthy cell membranes. For people following a relatively low-fat diet, fish oil contributes to satiety—a sense of fullness and satisfaction after eating.

"There have been some studies out of Australia showing that people who took fish oil in addition to exercising three times a week for 45 minutes lost a higher proportion of body fat than people who didn't take fish oil," says Vannice. Another interesting finding involves the relationship between omega-3 fatty acids and obesity in children—a rapidly growing problem in the United States. "A Swedish study revealed that 4-year-olds who were obese had lower levels of omega-3 fatty acids than 4-year-olds of a normal weight," says Vannice. "Even more surprising: The obese kids ate less than the normal-weight kids, but they ate a higher proportion of sugar and fat."

What about mercury in fish? Despite past concerns about mercury levels, researchers at the Harvard School of Public Health say that the health benefits of fish outweigh the risks. In fact, their study reported that overall mortality was 17 percent lower among people who ate fish twice a week, compared with people who ate little or no seafood. Clearly, a good way to get the beneficial omega-3 fatty acids eicosapentaenoic acid (EPA) and docosahexaenoic acid (DHA) is from fatty fish such as salmon, herring, and mackerel. Aim for two to three servings per week.

If you don't enjoy fish, you can take an omega-3 fish-oil supplement—as long as you choose a brand that has been tested for mercury and lead. Look for a product that says something on the label like "free from heavy metals, dioxins, and PCBs" or "purified to ensure the absence of heavy metals, PCBs, and dioxins." Take a total of 1 gram of EPA and DHA in supplements per day. Fish oil can cause blood thinning, so be sure to talk to your health care professional before you begin supplementation.

Consume some krill oil. Another source of beneficial fats is the oil extracted from shrimplike crustaceans called krill. "In addition to being high in omega-3 fatty acids, krill oil is very high in phospholipids, which are great for cell membranes [and, therefore, metabolism]," says Keith DeOrio, MD, DHom, founder of the DeOrio Wellness Medical Center in Santa Monica, California. Krill oil is available in capsule form. Follow the dosage directions on the label.

Fill up on fiber. "Fiber is an important element of the diet that many of us in the US miss out on," says Dr. Klauer. "Our average consumption of fiber is 15 grams a day, but we need 25 to 30 grams a day for optimum health." She recommends getting fiber from fruits and vegetables instead of the typical whole grains. "I am not saying that grains aren't valuable—they certainly are," she says. "But they don't give you the antioxidants that fruits and vegetables do. Plus, per 100 calories, fresh fruit typically contains twice as much fiber as whole grains. Nonstarchy vegetables contain about eight times as much!

"For people with diverticulitis [common in people who are overweight], berries are wonderful because they don't leave behind little seeds," adds Dr. Klauer. Throw some blueberries, strawberries, or blackberries on your cereal in the morning; better yet, eat them by themselves. "Pretty much all berries are high in fiber, but blueberries are the top berry as far as I am concerned because they are rich in resveratrol, which has been shown to have antiaging properties," she says. "They're packed with vitamins and antioxidants, too."

For lunch, have a big mixed green salad with lots of colorful fruits and vegetables for extra phytochemicals. "Leafy greens provide not only healthful fiber but also omega-3 fatty acids, which are excellent for your body," says Dr. Klauer.

Avoid trans fats. "After seeing the dramatic change in my health after I gave up fried foods, I say you might as well smoke a cigarette if you are going to eat fried food," says Nicki. She's right. Like cigarettes, trans fats do all sorts of bad things to your body. They not only cause you to gain weight faster than you can say "crispy french fries," they also take a toll on your immune system and may even cause cancer.

Trans fats are made by adding hydrogen to vegetable oil, a process called hydrogenation. "Trans fats are great for the food industry because they last a very long time, but they are terrible for us because our bodies are not primed to process them," says Dr. Sugar. "When you eat foods cooked with trans fats, your body undergoes a lot of oxidative stress and stores fat cells quickly. This leads to even more oxidative stress."

In addition, trans fats appear to interfere with a cell membrane's ability to respond to insulin molecules. This creates a blood sugar imbalance that stimulates cravings for sugar and other junk foods containing trans fats, sparking the cycle to start all over again.

Trans fats are so dangerous, in fact, that they are now considered a public health hazard. Many cities have banned or are considering banning them from use in restaurants. "I strongly recommend that you avoid trans fats," says Dr. Sugar—but to do this, you need to know where they're lurking. Pretty much any food cooked in a deep fryer is prepared with the help of trans fats. On food labels, they hide behind names such as *partially hydrogenated vegetable oil, palm oil,* and *coconut oil.* "There can be plenty of trans fats in something that is labeled as containing zero," Dr. Sugar points out. "The federal government says that as long as a food contains less than 0.5 gram of trans fats per serving, it can be labeled as zero, so it's important to always check for these suspect oils in the ingredients list."

Flush away the pounds. Most people don't drink enough water. "I have patients who can't remember the last time they drank water—Gatorade, coffee, juice, and soda they can remember, but not water," says Janet Suvak, MD, a general practitioner specializing in preventive health care with offices in Newport Beach and Beverly Hills, California. "But drinking water is important. Even dehydration of a couple of percentage points affects all of your metabolic processes, including your immune system." Dehydration also makes you feel sluggish, so you will be less apt to exercise. To boost your metabolism, your mood, and your immune system, drink eight 8-ounce glasses of water per day. To get maximum pound-melting power from your water, add lemon, which helps prevent sugar cravings.

Guzzle green tea. Green tea contains anti-inflammatory antioxidants and polyphenols. It also helps boost metabolism, so it's great for both weight control and immune function, Dr. Mullin says. Replace your morning mug of coffee with a cup of green tea, drink it with lunch, and pair it with a piece of fruit for an after-dinner treat. When it comes to green tea, you can't have too much of a good thing.

Toss down some oolong tea. Oolong tea has been touted for its ability to restore the skin's youthful appearance. As a bonus, it boosts the immune system and promotes weight loss. "I started drinking oolong tea for the beauty benefits, but it has made me much more energetic and healthy—no colds so far this winter," notes Amanda Lazaro, a public relations specialist in Boston. "Plus, in the few months that I've been drinking two tea bags of oolong tea a day, I have lost weight." In a Japanese study, oolong tea was shown to help overweight mice shed pounds, and it appears to help humans do the same.

Put your body in motion. Exercise has invariably been proven to help regulate the immune system. It's also one of the best things you can do to keep your weight under control. If you are currently inactive, any physical movement you add to your life will be beneficial. "Walking is a great one to start with," says Mary Jo DiMilia, MD, assistant professor of medicine and pediatrics at Mount Sinai School of Medicine in New York City.

If you are severely overweight and haven't exercised in a long time, first get medical clearance from your doctor. Then start very slowly, walking just a few minutes or blocks at a time. "Before you know it, you will be walking for 15 to 20 minutes at a stretch," Dr. DiMilia says. For optimum health and immunity, gradually build up to 30 to 60 minutes of brisk walking (or another aerobic activity) most days of the week.

To help make your exercise routine stick, Dr. Klauer recommends doing it first thing in the morning. "People who work out in the morning are 40 percent more likely to maintain it than those who postpone their workouts until later in the day," she observes.

Balance your life with yoga. "One of my patients told me that yoga makes the difference between living life in color and living it in black-and-white," says Hema Sundaram, MD, a dermatologist in Washington, DC, and a devoted yoga practitioner. "It has a wonderful balancing effect, physically and psychologically, which helps regulate eating. You develop an understanding for and appreciation of the power of your body, so you are less likely to want to damage it by overeating or eating the wrong foods."

Practicing yoga on a regular basis has been scientifically shown to control weight. One observational study, conducted at the Fred Hutchinson Cancer Research Center in Seattle, tracked the effects of yoga on weight change over the course of 10 years. Compared with nonpractitioners, normal-weight participants who practiced yoga regularly for 4 or more years gained 3 fewer pounds through the study. Overweight participants who practiced yoga gained 18½ fewer pounds. For weight control and overall mental and physical health, Dr. Sundaram recommends thrice-weekly yoga sessions in tandem with a regular aerobic exercise routine.

Buddy up. Whether it's the friend with whom you drive to yoga class or the sibling who strengthens your willpower in the presence of cheesecake, a weight-loss buddy can do wonders for ensuring your success. "Having someone whom you will let down if you don't show up to exercise is really good for motivation," Dr. Sundaram notes. "And being able to bounce your thoughts and ideas off of somebody else as you lose weight is great for stress reduction."

Your buddy doesn't need to be someone with the same goals as you. "Maybe you need to lose 20 pounds and your buddy needs to lose 5," Dr. DiMilia says. "That's okay, as long as it's someone who will encourage you."

Junk your junk food. Junk food is terrible for both your immunity and your waistline. If you have processed foods chock-full of trans fats and other "junk" calling your name from your kitchen cabinets, by all means get rid of it, Dr. DiMilia says. "If you can't bring yourself to do that, wrap the food boxes and bags with scrap paper and tons of rubber bands, so you have to spend a lot of time getting to it before you can dig in," she suggests. "Hopefully, by the time you've unwrapped the food, you will have changed your mind about eating it or called your buddy for support."

Top food with turmeric. The herb turmeric promotes proper metabolism in the body and aids the digestion of protein. Even better: One of the compounds in turmeric, curcumin, has been shown to help prevent some of the DNA damage that can lead to cancer. Add a little turmeric to your more flavorful recipes for a weight loss/immune-boosting combo.

Crunch on crackers. "It's funny to me when diet plans tell you to snack on carrots and celery instead of potato chips . . . not quite the same thing," Dr. DiMilia says. To satisfy your craving for something crunchy and salty, she recommends seven-grain Kashi crackers. "They are low in sodium and calories and high in fiber," she notes. "You can have 15 crackers for 100 calories—and they are delicious."

Be patient. Weight loss—and the immune enhancement that accompanies it—takes time. "Patients come to me discouraged after losing only 1 to 2 pounds in a week, but they shouldn't be, because that is exactly the correct rate of weight loss," Dr. DiMilia says. To illustrate her point, she shows her patients a plastic model of 1 pound of fat. It's actually quite big, and it's not light. "I tell people to be happy about every ounce they lose," she says. "It gives your immune system, your heart, and your entire body such a boost."

If You're a Chronic Dieter . . .

For a moment, let's imagine that we've been invited out to lunch by a co-worker. We'll call her Janet. On the surface, Janet is very health-conscious. She carefully peruses the menu before choosing a spring-mix salad with fat-free balsamic vinaigrette (on the side, of course). She waves off the bread basket—"Gotta watch those carbs," she explains—and skips soda in favor of unsweetened tea. When the dessert tray arrives at the table, Janet doesn't give it a second glance. Though the server tries to tempt her, she politely refuses. "No thanks," she says. "I'm dieting."

It isn't the first time that Janet has been dieting. Although she expresses confidence that she finally has found a plan she can live with, she privately fears it won't be her last. From the time she reached puberty, Janet battled her weight with all kinds of diets—low-calorie, low-fat, low-carb, no-carb. Every one of them has worked . . . for a little while, at least. But she struggles to stick with a plan for the long term. Inevitably, pounds begin to creep back on.

All of us know someone like Janet. We may even recognize a bit of her in ourselves. Janet is a chronic dieter—and though she may not realize it, her erratic eating habits are affecting her immune function and her health.

The Ups and Downs of Dieting

Chronic dieting, also called weight cycling or yo-yo dieting, is a vicious cycle in which someone intentionally loses weight, only to unintentionally regain it. The cycle may repeat over and over, sometimes resulting in no bottom-line change in weight one way or the other. In this country, many of us—often women, but men, too—have this on-again/off-again, feast-or-famine attitude toward weight loss.

The diet industry bears some of the blame for chronic dieting. Every new diet plan is touted as being *the* one that works, explains Stuart Trager, MD, an orthopedic surgeon at Pennsylvania Hospital in Philadelphia and founder of Elite Health and Wellness, a program that provides comprehensive medical evaluations and treatment protocols to improve nutrition and cardiovascular fitness and decrease lifestyle risk factors. "Well, guess what? If you can follow them, they all work," he says. But they're too hard for most people to adhere to long-term, and it's the "long-term" part of a diet that is key to weight-loss success.

"The concept of dieting is a false security," says Sam J. Sugar, MD, a board-certified internist and staff physician for the Seaside Medical Group at the Pritikin Longevity Center and Spa in Aventura, Florida. "It means little or nothing for your long-term health to lose some weight temporarily."

In fact, the cycle may be more harmful than never losing weight in the first place. The problem is, with all these leaps on and off the diet bandwagons, our bodies start to get tired. We may not make an immediate connection between our last few head colds and the diet plans we were on—or off—at the time, but our eating habits probably weakened our immune systems.

A landmark study published in the *Journal of the American Dietetic Association* found that frequent intentional weight loss is associated with lower levels of natural killer (NK) cells, important immune cells that attack cancers and viruses. Researchers recruited 114 healthy but overweight and sedentary postmenopausal women and examined both their weight-loss patterns over the previous 20 years and their present immune function. The findings revealed nothing good about chronic dieting. Levels of NK cells were 6 percent lower among the women who reported ever intentionally losing more than 10 pounds, compared with the women who never dieted. If that isn't eye-opening enough, the researchers also found a correlation between the frequency of weight-loss attempts and the number of NK cells, suggesting that with each diet, immune function diminishes even more.

Beyond the direct effects of weight cycling on the immune system, poor nutrition is a concern. When people are malnourished, their immune systems suffer. New research suggests that it isn't only inadequate nutrition that affects immunity; it's also the overall calorie restriction and extreme weight loss that may be part of chronic dieting.

Some recent studies have supported calorie-restricted diets for general good health and longevity, as long as they contain enough essential nutrients. But a study conducted in the department of bioscience and biotechnology at Drexel University in

Philadelphia tells a different story. Researchers determined that mice on calorie-restricted diets without malnutrition were more likely to die after exposure to the flu virus than mice of the same age that ate a normal diet.

This finding suggests that low body weight may be associated with altered immunity, says Barry Ritz, MS, lead researcher on the study. "We know that weight, like many things in human health, is best described by a J-shaped curve," Ritz explains. "In other words, someone has to be at his or her ideal weight—not too heavy and not too thin—to be at his or her healthiest. Fighting infection and maintaining a healthy immune system may simply require energy that is not available if one's body weight is too low."

Get Off the Diet Roller Coaster

In a society in which 66 percent of women and 43 percent of men report having dieted, yet 64 percent of the population is overweight, what is the answer? Well, we certainly know what it *isn't,* and that is fad diets. "All you have to do is look at the life span of fad diets to see that they don't work," Dr. Sugar says. And the reason they don't work is that they are a temporary fix. "To achieve lasting weight loss, you have to change your whole life," he says. By adopting the modest lifestyle changes that follow, you can leave behind chronic dieting and head down the right path toward permanent weight control. You'll boost your immune system in the process.

Get moving. The problem with many of the fad diets out there is that they ignore one of the most important ingredients in the weight-loss recipe: exercise. "Daily physical activity is a basic element of good health," says Jana Klauer, MD, author of *How the Rich Stay Thin* and a New York City–based physician who specializes in the biology of fat reduction. "Without physical exercise, you will look and feel older than your chronological age. It is a well-documented scientific fact."

To lose weight or maintain your weight once you reach your goal, you should exercise for 45 to 60 minutes at least 6 days a week. If this sounds like too much, considering your busy schedule, look at it this way: "The president of the United States finds time to exercise, and somehow I think his schedule might be pretty full," Dr. Klauer says. "The health benefits of daily exercise are enormous, and the time spent exercising can actually extend your life. So you get a good rate of return on the investment you make, in terms of your time."

If you haven't been exercising, you shouldn't jump right in to the full 45 minutes, however. In fact, be sure to get clearance from your physician before you begin any fitness routine. Then start with whatever time interval you can handle—even 5 minutes will do—and gradually build up your time and intensity as you feel comfortable.

Be proactive with probiotics. The restricted diet associated with most weight-loss programs may directly affect the bacteria in your intestines and, thus, your immune function. "Chronic dieters sometimes end up altering their gut bacteria because they're eating limited types of foods," says Patricia David, MD, MSPH, president of the Healthy U wellness program in Columbus, Ohio. "So they diminish the number of nutrients their bodies are able to tolerate and digest, and their immunity decreases."

That's where probiotics—microorganisms that can alter intestinal flora and improve overall health—come in. "By balancing our intestinal bacteria, probiotics help stimulate our immune systems to be more 'alert,'" explains José Saavedra, MD, associate professor in the department of pediatrics, division of gastroenterology and nutrition, at the Johns Hopkins School of Medicine and School of Public Health and medical and scientific director of Nestlé Nutrition. "They also help to modulate the immune response, so it adequately protects the host [as from viruses] and prevents it from overreacting [as in allergies]."

A growing number of products claim to contain probiotics. But only certain ones supply the specific types of beneficial bacteria—certain strains of *Lactobacilli* and *Bifidobacteria*—that have been shown to support immune health. To ensure that you are getting the most effective bacteria for immunity, look for strains such as these on product labels.

- *L. casei*
- *L. reuterii*
- *L. rhamnosus GG*
- *B. breve*
- *B. lactis*

Among the products that contain these bacteria are yogurts such as Activia and Danimals and drinks such as DanActive. When it comes to consuming probiotic products, the more the better, Dr. Saavedra says. "It's almost impossible to overdose on bacteria present in yogurt," he notes. "When you eat a cup of yogurt, you may eat 10 million to a billion bacteria. That's nothing compared to the many trillions you already have in your intestines."

Fortify with fish oil. The beneficial fats in fish oil help counteract the inflammation that contributes to health problems related to weight cycling—like metabolic syndrome, which is a combination of insulin resistance and cardiovascular disease, says Keith DeOrio, MD, DHom, founder of the DeOrio Wellness Medical Center in Santa Monica, California. Omega-6 fatty acids promote inflammation in the body, while omega-3 fatty acids counteract it. "The healthy ratio between omega-6s and omega-3s is 4 to 1, but in this country, most people are between 10 to 1 and 20 to 1," Dr. DeOrio says.

A wonderful way to get omega-3 fatty acids is to eat two to three servings of fatty fish such as salmon, herring, or mackerel per week. Fish-oil supplements supply omega-3s as well. Just be sure to look for a brand that has been tested for both mercury and lead. The product label should say something like "free from heavy metals, dioxins, and PCBs" or "purified to ensure the absence of heavy metals, PCBs, and dioxins."

If you opt to take supplements, aim for a total of 1 gram of the omega-3 fatty acids eicosapentaenoic acid (EPA) and docosahexaenoic acid (DHA) per day, advises Gretchen Vannice, MS, RD, research coordinator at Nordic Naturals in Watsonville, California. Fish oil can cause blood thinning, so be sure to talk to your doctor before you start taking it.

Pump up your protein. "When people watch their calories too closely, they often limit protein," Dr. Klauer says. "Without sufficient protein, the body is unable to build and repair—and this will reduce immunity."

"You need about 1 gram of protein per kilogram of body weight, and a little more than that if you are physically active," she explains. "So a 120-pound female requires 60 to 70 grams [a little over 2 ounces] of protein per day, while a 170-pound man needs 80 to 90 grams [about 3 ounces]." Dr. Klauer's favorite source of protein is egg whites. "Because the yolk can be separated from the white, the fat content can easily be avoided," she says. Other good sources include fish and low-fat dairy products, followed by poultry and lean meat.

Make mineral water your cocktail of choice. Mineral water not only supports hydration by adding to your goal of 64 ounces of water a day—which is important for weight management—it also gives you a calcium boost, which will do wonders for your waistline and your overall health. "There are so many benefits from calcium that it really is a miracle mineral," Dr. Klauer says. "It lowers blood pressure, reduces the risk of cardiovascular disease and colon cancer, helps maintain skeletal mass, and keeps us slim." Perrier mineral water contains approximately 60 milligrams of calcium per liter (33.8 ounces), while San Pellegrino contains 120 milligrams, and Sanfaustino supplies a whopping 400 milligrams.

Just say no to addictive foods. Sure, you love chocolate—it tastes good! But if you can look back on your weight-cycling patterns and recall reaching for extra chocolate on days you were feeling blue or in the midst of a weekend where you decided to put your diet on hold, it may be more than the taste that feeds you. Chocolate contains not only sugar and caffeine, which are clearly addictive, but also theobromine, a very strong stimulant that releases the feel-good hormone serotonin in your brain, Dr. Sugar says.

If you tend to use chocolate—or any other food, for that matter—as a crutch, get rid of it. "Not having an addictive food around is the first step in not being able to eat it," Dr. Sugar notes. "For some people, foods are literally narcotics, and they need to be avoided." Other foods with particularly strong addictive powers include cheese, ice cream, and fast food.

Strengthen immunity with selenium. "There have been some incredibly interesting studies done by Melinda Beck, PhD, a professor in the departments of pediatrics and nutrition at the University of North Carolina at Chapel Hill School of Medicine, on the relationship between the mineral selenium and immunity," Ritz says. "The studies have shown that a selenium deficiency not only results in immune decline, it also creates an environment in which viruses get stronger and more dangerous. In other words, poor selenium nutrition [which may result from chronic dieting] forces viruses to strengthen in order to survive."

To make sure your selenium levels are up to par, choose selenium-rich foods such as Brazil nuts (1 ounce contains 544 micrograms, or 788 percent of the Daily Value, or DV), tuna (3 ounces supplies 63 micrograms, 95 percent of the DV), and lean beef (3.5 ounces serves up 35 micrograms, 50 percent of the DV).

If You Smoke . . .

One of the first television advertisements for cigarettes in the early 1950s featured a strangely oversize cigarette pack with gorgeous Rockette-like legs dancing aimlessly on a curtained stage. As the pack danced, the announcer promised a cigarette taste "made by tobacco men, not medicine men."

More than 50 years later, it's clear that cigarettes most definitely were *not* made by medicine men and that the frightening disconnect between cigarettes and good health is nothing to brag about. Since they were introduced to the public in the late 19th century, commercial cigarettes have contributed to hundreds of thousands of preventable deaths. Each year, an estimated 438,000 people die from smoking-related illness. Smokers are at increased risk for heart disease; chronic lung disease; autoimmune disease; and cancers of the lung, esophagus, bladder, kidney, and pancreas— just to name a few.

Nonsmokers exposed to cigarette smoke at work or at home—for example, those who work in restaurants or bars with smoking sections or who live with people who smoke—also are in danger. Each year, an estimated 3,000 lung-cancer deaths result from secondhand smoke, and 300,000 children who live with smokers suffer from respiratory tract infections.

One reason that cigarette smoke is such a health hazard is that it directly suppresses the immune system. "There is very good medical research showing that smoking actually impairs T cells [white blood cells that destroy virus-infected cells and other abnormal cells] and other components of the immune system," says Hema Sundaram, MD, a dermatologist in Washington, DC, and author of *Face Value*.

In a study published in the journal *Nicotine and Tobacco Research,* one group of adolescent rats was given 6 milligrams of nicotine (which produced blood levels of nicotine similar to those of smokers), a second group was given 2 milligrams (which produced blood levels lower than those of smokers), and a third group got a placebo. After just 1 week, T-cell levels were the lowest in the group receiving the most nicotine, followed by the group receiving 2 milligrams. Perhaps most interestingly, T-cell levels quickly returned to normal in both groups once the rats were taken off the nicotine, only to drop again when they reached young adulthood—even in the group receiving the lower dose. These results suggest that nicotine has both short- and long-term effects on immune function.

Another reason smoking is so tough on the body is that it causes oxidative stress, or an accumulation of free radicals (unstable oxygen molecules that are missing an electron). Oxidative stress is the same process that causes an apple or a banana that has been exposed to oxygen to turn brown. "Every time you take a puff of a cigarette, you get 10,000 molecules of free radicals," says Gerard E. Mullin, MD, MS, CNSP, director of complementary and alternative medicine and gastrointestinal nutrition services at Johns Hopkins Hospital in Baltimore.

Free radicals attack cell membranes (including the membranes surrounding immune cells) and damage DNA, which causes you to age faster and become more susceptible to cancer, Dr. Mullin explains. In other words, a similar process to the "rusting" of the apple or banana happens inside your body with every exposure to nicotine.

Smoking launches an assault on the physical barriers of your immune system as well. "Smoking causes cilia in the airways to shrink," says Chris D. Meletis, ND, executive director of the Institute for Healthy Aging in Portland, Oregon. "Imagine your fingers as normal healthy cilia, and then picture them as stumps cut off at the joint." These stumpy cilia are not nearly as effective at protecting the body from infection.

Boost Immunity by Butting Out

Unfortunately, regardless of the hazards associated with smoking—and let's face it, even those with a pack-a-day habit know about them—nearly 21 percent of the US population, or 45.1 million people, smoke. "Some smokers are scary. They will tell me right to my face, 'I am not quitting—that is ridiculous,'" says Mary Jo DiMilia, MD, assistant professor of medicine and pediatrics at Mount Sinai School of Medicine in New York City.

Why the strong resistance? For many people, smoking eases anxiety and balances emotions. Add to that the associations between cigarettes and eating, sex, and other routine behaviors—plus the highly addictive nicotine—and quitting can become very difficult.

But despite all the rationalizations for not giving up smoking, the dangers far outweigh any benefits. If you are a smoker, the very best thing that you can do for your immune system and for your overall health is obvious: You've got to quit.

"When someone gives up smoking, there are immediate improvements in the immune system," Dr. Sundaram says. "Quitting cold turkey is really hard, so don't be afraid to consult your doctor for advice. There are so many different methods, and everyone responds differently to them." The following measures also can help you stop smoking for good—and boost your immune system in the process.

Find support in fish oil. Fish oil does a number of things to counteract the negative effects of cigarettes. "The omega-3 fatty acids in fish oil reduce the oxidative stress caused by smoking and help protect cell walls," says Gretchen Vannice, MS, RD, research coordinator at Nordic Naturals in Watsonville, California. "Beyond that, fish oil helps calm your nerves, which is important when you are trying to quit." If you currently smoke, Vannice recommends taking a minimum of 1 gram of the omega-3 fatty acids eicosapentaenoic acid (EPA) and docosahexaenoic acid (DHA) in fish-oil supplements per day. If you are trying to quit, increase your DHA by taking 1 teaspoon of cod liver oil daily. "It will help ease the anxiety," she says. Fish oil can cause blood thinning, so be sure to talk to your physician before you start taking it.

Aim for one or two Emergen-Cs per day. Cigarettes contain 4,000 chemical compounds, 43 of which are proven cancer causers. "To counteract their effects, increase your intake of the antioxidant vitamin C," Dr. Meletis advises. "Research shows that smokers need more vitamin C than nonsmokers." A great way to get a quick 1,000-milligram dose is to pour an Emergen-C Immune Defense Formula packet into 4 to 6 ounces of water. The drink mix also delivers selenium, zinc, and vitamins A, B, and D—all of which offer additional immune-boosting benefits. He recommends two packets a day. Emergen-C Immune Defense Formula is available in most health food stores as well as online.

Get your fill of fruits and vegetables. Another great way to get your antioxidants is to eat at least five—ideally, 10—servings of fruits and vegetables per day. If you build up your antioxidant defenses, you can counteract some of the free radical damage caused by cigarettes, Dr. Mullin says. Produce rich in antioxidants includes blueberries, raspberries, citrus fruits, grapes, plums, onions, and leafy green vegetables.

The king of antioxidant-rich fruits appears to be the goji berry, a wild berry from the Himalayas. "Goji berries seem to have the highest concentration of antioxidants of any fruit," says Patricia David, MD, MSPH, a preventive medicine specialist and president of the Healthy U wellness program in Columbus, Ohio. "In the Himalayas, goji berries were dropping into the rivers and streams, and the people drinking that water were living to an extremely old age. The theory is that it had something to do with the high content of goji berries in the water." Goji berries aren't available in most local grocery stores, but you can order them online. Throw a few in a glass of water to mimic the delivery in the Himalayas, or munch a few each day to get their antioxidant effects.

Neutralize smoking's negative effects with NAC. In people with respiratory issues, N-acetylcysteine (NAC) helps break down mucus. In addition, it's a potent antioxidant. This combination of benefits makes NAC, which is available over the counter, an ideal remedy for smokers, Dr. Melitis says. It works by increasing levels of glutathione, an antioxidant substance found in animal tissues that assists in energy production and proper immune function. Take one 600-milligram capsule once or twice daily. "After you take NAC, blood levels peak in about 45 minutes, and it stays active for about 5 hours," he says.

Flush away the effects. Smoking irritates the mucous membranes, leaving them dry, cracked, and more susceptible to inflammation and invasion by viruses and bacteria, Dr. Meletis says. The best way to combat the irritation? Drink at least eight 8-ounce glasses of water per day, he advises.

Try a repulsive antidote. When a patient is struggling to quit smoking, Dr. DiMilia recommends the following: "Fill an empty mayonnaise or mustard jar one-quarter of the way with water. Collect a week's worth of ashes in the jar and place it on a windowsill or in another spot where it has some sun exposure for a few days. Then open the jar and smell it. It is the most horrific, noxious stimulant. Some people need that kind of turnoff to quit."

Wrap up your bad habit. "If you can, get rid of all your cigarettes so you can't easily smoke," Dr. DiMilia advises. "If you are not ready to go that far, wrap up your remaining cigarette packs in newspaper or scrap paper and surround them with tons of rubber bands. Then when you have the urge for a cigarette, you will have to unwrap . . . and keep unwrapping. Hopefully, by the time you get to the cigarettes, you will say to yourself, 'Is it really worth the trouble? I don't need to smoke this badly.'"

Visualize how smoking harms you. "Smoking affects almost all of your organ systems," Dr. DiMilia says. "To turn patients off on smoking, I tell them to envision the damage that smoking is doing to their organs, one by one, and to think about all of the diseases that they could get as a result of their habit." For example, smoking affects your heart, so you could end up with a heart attack or stroke. It takes a toll on your lungs (obviously), your intestines, even your skin. Thinking seriously about the physical cost of smoking can be a real deterrent for some people.

If You Are Under Extreme Stress . . .

It seems to be the American way: Many of us feel as though we have 25 hours' worth of responsibilities to squeeze into a 24-hour day. Often that doesn't even include the time necessary to take proper care of ourselves (and our immune systems) by eating nutritiously, exercising regularly, and sleeping adequately.

All that stress can deplete the immune system, just like a cell phone running on a low battery. It just takes one stressful conversation with a boss, a frustrating meeting with colleagues, or a fight with a spouse for the immune "battery" to run out of juice. That's when we get sick.

"On college campuses across the country, infirmaries consistently are the most full during final exams," notes Shawn Talbott, PhD, a nutritional biochemist in Salt Lake City and author of *The Cortisol Connection Diet.* "Students aren't sleeping, they're under stress, and they're up all night drinking Coke and eating Doritos—a recipe for getting sick."

From the standpoint of personal motivation, a little stress is a good thing. It's what pushes us to jump out of the path of an oncoming car, get started on a project for work, or shop for holiday gifts *before* Christmas Eve. When you encounter a stressful situation, your brain tells your adrenal glands to release the stress hormone cortisol, which shifts your body into a fight-or-flight mode. Your blood pressure rises, your heart beats faster, your pupils dilate—and you are ready to react. When the stress passes, your body returns to its normal state.

Stress can have a positive, stimulating effect on immune function, too, as cortisol readies the immune system to launch an attack against any invaders. "But *chronic* stress suppresses the immune system," Dr. Talbott says. Over time, cortisol limits your body's ability to produce antibodies, molecules in blood that fight disease. Chronic stress also lowers your white blood cell count, further weakening your immune response.

In addition, as cortisol increases, levels of secretory immunoglobulin A (IgA)—a substance that acts as a protective coating for the mucous membranes in your eyes, mouth, nose, and respiratory tract—decline. "Secretory IgA is like Scotchgard for your membranes," explains Chris D. Meletis, ND, executive director of the Institute for Healthy Aging in Portland, Oregon. When you lose some of this protective coating, your membranes become more vulnerable to the microbes that come their way.

If that weren't bad enough, chronic stress can cause your immune system to work so hard that it turns against the very body it's trying to protect. Your immune cells are constantly ready for battle, but they don't encounter enough pathogens to meet their increased forces. As a result, your overstimulated immune system may mistakenly kill your own tissues, possibly leading to an autoimmune disease such as lupus or rheumatoid arthritis.

Switch Off the Stress Response

The toll of chronic stress on immune health has been proven in studies. "When mice are put under stress for a few minutes, all of their immune cells—including natural killer [NK] cells, CD4, CD8, general macrophages—start working harder," Dr. Talbott says. "If that stress continues for hours, there is a 60 to 80 percent drop in immune cell function and overall immune system activity."

So how can we escape the vicious cycle of chronic stress? "One thing I don't like to tell people is to get rid of the stress in their lives, because in our current society, that's close to impossible to do," Dr. Talbott says. On the other hand, you can take steps to better cope with stress and protect your immune system from its harmful effects. For example:

De-stress with theanine. This amino acid is as close to a magic bullet for stress relief as you can get. "People who take theanine come back to me the next day to say, 'Wow, that was magical stuff,'" Dr. Talbott says. "They can feel the calming effect that quickly." Theanine occurs naturally in green tea leaves. It might be one of the reasons you can drink a cup of green tea and feel calm, despite the caffeine. "Theanine makes you feel energized but relaxed," he explains. "It can take the edge off of a stressful day or meeting almost immediately. I personally swear by it."

These days, most supplement shops and health food stores carry theanine products. Dr. Talbott recommends starting out with 50 to 100 milligrams of theanine a day and increasing to 200 milligrams, if necessary. "Going above 200 milligrams per day isn't dangerous, but it is unlikely to provide additional benefits," he says.

Fight stress with fish oil. There is a direct relationship between stress and inflammation, says Gretchen Vannice, MS, RD, research coordinator at Nordic Naturals in Watsonville, California. As your stress level increases, inflammation increases, too. To combat that effect, take fish oil—"a natural anti-inflammatory," she says. Fish oil also can offset the ill effects of stress on your heart by lowering triglycerides and reducing the risk of heart attack. "For people under stress, I recommend 1,000 to 1,500 milligrams of fish oil per day," Vannice says.

Wake up your immune system with beta-glucan. Beta-glucan is a yeast extract that contains sugar polysaccharides in its cell membranes. "When you eat this yeast extract, your immune system looks at the sugar polysaccharide–enriched cell membrane and says, 'Huh, that looks like a virus cell wall or a bacterial cell wall. I am going to be more vigilant now because something may be coming,'" Dr. Talbott says. In response to beta-glucan, your immune system wakes up its NK cells and tumor fighters, preparing them to attack any invader that your stressed-out body may let slip through the cracks. He recommends a specific beta-glucan product called WGP, made by Biothera. Follow the dosage directions on the label.

Relax with tai chi. Tai chi—a slow, graceful discipline with flowing movements based on the martial art of kung fu—is wonderful for relieving mental stress, says Ron Knaus, DO, a psychiatrist in Largo, Florida, and author of *A B Chi*. "Tai chi has become an exercise for the prevention of health conditions as well as for the promotion of mental strength and ability," he says. "Studies show that it improves relaxation a great deal."

You can learn a basic form of tai chi in 30 days and practice it for the rest of your life. Dr. Knaus recommends finding a tai chi class with a skilled but laid-back instructor. "You want someone who is just happy that you are moving—not someone who will be compulsive about the positioning of your elbow," he says. If you have trouble finding an instructor who motivates you, you could try a tai chi video or DVD. "You can do the short form of tai chi once or twice a day for only 10 minutes at a time and reap the benefits," Dr. Knaus says.

Mellow out with meditation. "To combat the effects of stress on the immune system, I advise people to meditate daily," says Mary Jo DiMilia, MD, assistant professor of medicine and pediatrics at Mount Sinai School of Medicine in New York City. Start with a very easy meditation in a quiet room or with some kind of soothing background music. "I use a CD called *Angels of Healing*, but you can use whatever music puts you into a relaxed state," she says. Sit on the floor in a comfortable position, and practice deep belly breathing. Close your eyes and slowly inhale and exhale, relaxing your whole body to a count of 10. Breathe very deeply, so you can feel your stomach expand. If you can, devote at least 5 minutes a day to meditation. It will help relieve your stress, Dr. DiMilia says.

Give yourself a pep talk. A lot of the stress in our lives comes from the pressure we put on ourselves. "People tend to go beyond their capacity, especially at times like the holidays," says D. V. Pasupuleti, MD, clinical professor of medicine at Michigan State University in East Lansing and author of *Change Your Mind.* "We spend beyond our limits—in money, time, and energy—for fear of being judged."

To take the edge off your stress, Dr. Pasupuleti recommends spending a few minutes alone each day to put things into perspective. "Look at yourself in the mirror and say, 'You look good. You are doing great. Compared to all of the bad things going on in the world, you're doing very well,'" he says. Positive thinking stimulates certain areas of the brain to release chemicals such as endorphins, serotonin, and dopamine, which instantly make you feel better.

Lend your diet a hand. It's been shown that people who demonstrate a higher level of dietary restraint—those who see a chocolate chip cookie and start stressing because they know it will go right to their hips—have a higher level of stress overall, according to Dr. Talbott: "The greater your fear of a chocolate chip cookie, the more cortisol you will secrete when you see one."

To stop worrying about the cookie and other potentially fattening foods, make room for them in your diet with what Dr. Talbott calls the Helping Hand technique. "What we do with Helping Hand is remove the diet stress from people's lives with a simple, easy-to-follow meal plan that teaches portion control," he says. It works like this: First, spread your fingers and thumb as far apart as you can. The size of your spread palm, including your digits, represents the amount of fruits and vegetables that you should eat with each meal. Next, make a fist. Its size equals the volume of pasta, oatmeal, bread, or other concentrated carbohydrates. Now unclench your fist. The size of just your palm is equal to a portion of meat, chicken, fish, or other protein. Finally, make an okay sign. The size of the circle formed by your thumb and index finger indicates the amount of butter, olive oil, full-fat salad dressing, or other fat or oil you can have.

Using this system, you can fit whatever you are hungry for into your daily diet, so you don't worry about a cookie or piece of cake. "You can have that treat as long as it fits within the Helping Hand criteria," Dr. Talbott says. "We see cortisol levels go down 20 percent in people with this dietary change alone." Because chronically elevated cortisol has been proven to suppress the immune system, lowering your cortisol level by removing some of the dietary stress in your life will give you an extra immune boost.

If You Are Blue . . .

Anyone who has ever experienced depression—either personally or through the eyes of a friend or loved one—knows its weight. Instead of rose-colored, the world appears dark and foreboding. Everyday tasks, from getting dressed in the morning to concentrating long enough to drive down the street, demand overwhelming effort. "To someone who is depressed, the air feels like Jell-O. Everything is bad," says Janet Suvak, MD, a general practitioner specializing in preventive health care with offices in Newport Beach and Beverly Hills, California.

Dismissed in generations past as a "weakness" or even a "choice," depression is recognized today as a real condition affecting millions of Americans. Although its exact cause remains unknown, scientists believe an imbalance of neurotransmitters in the brain—including dopamine, serotonin, and norepinephrine—is at least partially to blame. Beyond brain chemistry, lifestyle factors such as weight gain, poor diet, and lack of sleep also appear to play roles in triggering the condition.

It's important to distinguish between major and mild depression, or what might be called the blues. Occasional feelings of sadness can be normal, appropriate, and even necessary, especially during life setbacks or losses, such as a divorce or a job layoff. People may become unhappy or blue for short periods of time without really knowing why. This, too, is normal. But if such feelings persist for 2 weeks or longer or begin to interfere with your daily routine, you may be experiencing a major depressive disorder.

People with major depression may feel sad, hopeless, helpless, or constantly agitated. They may approach activities they once loved with an attitude of indifference or apathy. Other characteristic symptoms of major depression include anxiety, irritability, fatigue, insomnia, weight gain or loss, digestive trouble, and physical pain.

Whether it's a persistent episode of major depression or a temporary case of the blues, it takes a toll on the mind and body—specifically, on the immune system. Studies have shown that even people with mild depression have impaired immunity, compared with those who are mentally fit. "The connection between mind and body is incredibly strong—it's impossible to separate the two," notes Chris D. Meletis, ND, executive director of the Institute for Healthy Aging in Portland, Oregon. "So as we go mentally, we go physically."

A study published in the *Archives of General Psychiatry* supports this point. In the study, older people with clinical depression had higher levels of interleukin-6 (IL-6), a chemical marker of inflammation in the body, than older people with good mental health. Chronically high levels of IL-6 are known to increase the risk of illnesses such as heart disease, osteoporosis, diabetes, and certain types of cancer.

Other research has shown that people with depression have lower levels of natural killer (NK) and T cells, two important types of white blood cells that attack and kill invaders. In addition, adults with depression are more likely to develop shingles, a condition that occurs when suppressed immune function allows the chickenpox virus—which has been lying dormant in certain nerve cells—to reactivate.

Beat the Blues, Boost Immunity

The good news is that, in most cases, depression is treatable. Sometimes it may require prescription antidepressants, which can help the person to function—and possibly improve immunity as a bonus. In one study, people with depression who were not taking antidepressant medication showed weakened immunity, while those on medication had healthy immune function. This suggests that antidepressants may be protective in terms of physical as well as mental health.

Antidepressants don't work for everyone, however. "Recent research shows that some people taking antidepressants continue to be depressed," says D. V. Pasupuleti, MD, clinical professor of medicine at Michigan State University in East Lansing and author of *Change Your Mind*. "Why? Because if you do not tackle the factors that are activating the mechanism for depression—such as poor eating habits or lack of sleep—it is like putting a bandage on a dam," he says.

If you experience any symptoms of major depression, it's critical for you to see your doctor, who can make a proper diagnosis and recommend an appropriate course of treatment. The following self-care measures can help enhance your mood and boost your immunity in the process.

Douse depression with DHEA. "One chemical factor associated with depression is the balance between the hormones dehydroepiandrosterone [DHEA] and cortisol," says Gerard Mullin, MD, director of complementary and alternative medicine and gastrointestinal nutrition services at Johns Hopkins Hospital in Baltimore. Through a natural circadian rhythm over 24 hours, your body makes melatonin at night to help you sleep and secretes cortisol in the morning to get you going. Usually, DHEA helps maintain the balance between cortisol and melatonin—but in some people, it fails to do its job. "People with low DHEA—and, therefore, high cortisol—are more likely to be depressed," Dr. Mullin says. In addition, research has shown that higher DHEA levels are associated with better immune function.

To find out if low DHEA is to blame for your dampened spirits, Dr. Mullin recommends testing your hormone levels with a hormone profile kit such as the one from BioHealth Diagnostics in San Diego (www.biodia.com). "The profile uses a salivary test to check your hormone levels every 6 hours over a 24-hour period," he explains. "If your results reveal an abnormality that's correctable with DHEA, you can try taking an over-the-counter DHEA supplement. A reasonable starting dose is 25 milligrams a day."

Improve your outlook with omega-3s. "I cannot say enough about omega-3 fatty acids," says Mary Jo DiMilia, MD, assistant professor of medicine and pediatrics at Mount Sinai School of Medicine in New York City. "They not only have wonderful effects on the cardiovascular system, they also help prevent mood disorders and depression."

The ideal ratio of omega-6 to omega-3 fatty acids is 4 to 1, but most of us get between 10 and 20 to 1. "We're way undernourished in omega-3s," explains Gretchen Vannice, MS, RD, research coordinator at Nordic Naturals in Watsonville, California. "And if you look at epidemiological research, you'll see that as dietary intake of omega-3 fatty acids has decreased over the last 200 years, the rate of depression has increased."

Studies suggest that the best sources of the beneficial omega-3 fatty acids eicosapentaenoic acid (EPA) and docosahexaenoic acid (DHA) are fatty fish such as salmon, herring, and mackerel. If you're concerned about mercury content, a team of scientists from Harvard School of Public Health says that the health benefits of eating fish far outweigh the risks. Most people (with the exception of pregnant women and children) should be eating two to three servings of fatty fish per week.

That said, if you just aren't a fan of fish, you may choose to get your omega-3 fatty acids from fish-oil supplements instead. Dr. DiMilia recommends reading supplement labels to find a product that has been tested for mercury and lead. Aim for a total of 1 gram of EPA and DHA per day. Fish oil can cause blood thinning, so be sure to talk with your doctor before beginning supplementation.

Bolster your B vitamins. If you are a woman experiencing symptoms of depression, it could be a sign that you're running low on B vitamins. "Research has shown that women on hormone replacement therapy [either birth control pills or hormone replacement for menopause] have lower levels of B vitamins, particularly B_6," Dr. Meletis says. Vitamin B_6 helps make serotonin, a neurotransmitter that affects mood, so low levels can lead indirectly to depression. "For women who report feeling depressed while taking hormone replacement therapy, I recommend 50 milligrams of a B-complex vitamin once or twice a day," he says.

Say good-bye to the blues with St. John's wort. The herb St. John's wort (*Hypericum perforatum*) has been used for centuries to treat mental disorders. "Some studies have shown that St. John's wort is as effective for mild depression as prescription antidepressant medications," Dr. DiMilia says. Look for an herbal extract that's standardized to 0.3 percent hypericin, and take 300 milligrams three times daily for a total of 900 milligrams per day. Do not take St. John's wort if you already are on antidepressants, because of the potential for a negative additive effect.

Lift your mood with 5-HTP. The neurotransmitter 5-hydroxy-tryptophan (5-HTP) helps regulate serotonin levels in the brain. Taken in supplement form, it can help combat depression in some people. The recommended dose is 50 to 200 milligrams per day, according to Dr. Meletis. "Start at the lower dose and work your way up as needed," he says. If you already are taking antidepressants or another medication for depression, he advises against adding 5-HTP to your treatment regimen because of a potential negative interaction.

Be sure to drink enough water. Many people aren't getting the eight 8-ounce glasses of H_2O their bodies need each day. "Even slight dehydration will make you feel cranky," Dr. Suvak says. So keep a water bottle in your car, at your desk, next to your bed. Sip whenever you can to reach your goal of 64 ounces a day.

Talk to yourself nicely. "Depression often manifests as a lack of self-esteem and a fear of being judged," Dr. Pasupuleti says. "We spend so much time trying to please others when we really should be pleasing ourselves." To overcome these feelings, engage in positive self-talk each morning. "Before you even get out of bed, say, 'I have the freedom of choice, and today I choose to be happy. Today I choose to stop worrying about what others think,'" he says. "Don't wait for someone else to say, 'You look nice' or 'You're doing great.' Instead, say these things to yourself. Daily positive thoughts like these stimulate certain areas of the brain to release chemicals such as serotonin and dopamine, which will instantly make you feel better—both mentally and physically."

Stimulate your mind with yoga. Research has shown that yoga can help counteract depression. It can be so effective, in fact, that it enables some people to reduce their dosage of antidepressants or stop taking the drugs altogether. In one study conducted at UCLA, half of the participants (28 young adults with mild depression) took an hour-long yoga class once a week for 5 weeks. At the conclusion of the study, those practicing yoga reported lower levels of depression and anxiety, compared with a second group of nonpractitioners.

What is it about yoga that makes it such potent therapy for the blues? For one, it prompts your body to release mood-elevating endorphins. It also helps turn off your external surroundings, so you can focus inward and think positive thoughts, Dr. Pasupuleti says. Try practicing yoga three or four times a week—either by joining a class or learning from a DVD.

Get sunny. In the early 1980s, a Japanese study revealed that people living in cold, gloomy climates were more prone to depression during the winter season than in the summer or spring. This phenomenon, now known as seasonal affective disorder (SAD), affects between 10 and 20 percent of Americans. If you're one of them, a 10- to 15-minute stroll outside in the sun can do wonders for your mood. As a bonus, sun exposure enables your body to manufacture vitamin D, which can help lift your spirits, Dr. Suvak says.

Swap a light dessert for a light walk. In Oriental medicine, walking improves the flow of chi, which represents the movement of the lymph system, says Dan Kenner, ND, OMD, a naturopathic physician and licensed oriental medicine doctor in Forestville, California, and author of *Building Immunity Naturally*. "Oriental medicine literature shows that movement of the lymph system is important both for immunity and for the prevention of mood disorders like depression," he explains. Lymph doesn't have a heart to pump it as blood does, so one way to get it moving is with physical exercise. "I recommend a daily walk after meals because chi flow and the digestive system are closely related," Dr. Kenner says. "For chi flow, it isn't necessarily the length or intensity of your walk that matters. It is just the fact that you get out there and move."

Fake it till you make it. "Some people with depression have to pretend they are happy in order to actually feel that way again," Dr. Suvak says. "Concentrate on completing small tasks that make you feel a little better and give you a sense of accomplishment at the same time—for example, preparing and eating a healthful meal." Dr. Suvak suggests doing one small thing for a little while before adding another. "Start with something like the healthful meal and do it for 3 days," she says.

"If you make it for 3 days, try to do it for 3 weeks. After 3 weeks, the activity starts to become a habit. Then add another activity, such as a 15-minute walk, and so on. These little steps will help lift you out of your depression and, in turn, boost your immune system."

Have a good laugh. When you're blue, nothing feels better than a hearty belly laugh. And there's good reason: Researchers have found that the positive emotions evoked by laughter not only make you feel happier, they also increase levels of certain immune cells. In a study conducted at Loma Linda University School of Medicine in California, 10 healthy men who laughed while watching a funny video for an hour showed significant increases in immune system activity. To add humor to your own life, rent a comedy, read a book by your favorite comedian, or spend more time with friends who tickle your funny bone.

If You Are Having Trouble Sleeping . . .

To strengthen our bodies, we make major investments in time, money, and energy. We lift weights, sweat through aerobics classes, and take herbal and nutritional supplements. But ironically, the activity that makes us the strongest involves the least effort of all. It's sleep.

"If you look at the word *restoration,* which means bringing people back to their original state, the first four letters are r-e-s-t—*rest*," says Chris D. Meletis, ND, executive director of the Institute for Healthy Aging in Portland, Oregon. "Whether you want to have a healthy immune system, reduce some of the stress in your life, or heal from surgery, you have to rest."

A good night's sleep does more than leave you feeling relaxed and refreshed in the morning, though that's certainly an important benefit. Just like proper diet and regular exercise, sleep is essential to good health. While you're asleep, your body replenishes its energy stores and tends to vital physiological and psychological housekeeping. When you don't get enough sleep, these chores don't get done, and your health suffers. There is evidence that just 2 to 3 days of total sleep deprivation can lead to serious problems with mental function and judgment. After 4 to 5 days, it can cause psychosis; after a week, it can be fatal.

Plenty of studies have shown that our bodies take care of important business specific to the immune system during sleep. "A number of research projects, some ongoing, point to the fact that immunity can be affected by disrupted sleep, because of either poor sleep habits or a sleep disorder," says Carol Ash, DO, medical director of the Sleep for Life Program at Somerset Medical Center in New Jersey.

One such study, conducted at Mount Sinai School of Medicine in New York City, revealed that people who got adequate sleep not only felt less tired during the day, they also had more natural killer (NK) cells—immune cells that kill foreign bodies and abnormal cells (such as cancer cells)—than people who didn't get enough sleep. This finding suggests that sleep deprivation impairs NK cells. In a separate study, men who were restricted to between 4 and 6 hours of sleep per night showed changes in their carbohydrate metabolism and hormone function similar to those in much older men, a sign that the lack of sleep was physically aging them.

In other research, sleep deprivation has been shown to affect cytokines, proteins secreted by white blood cells to regulate the duration and strength of an immune response. Specifically, sleep deprivation leads to a decline in the cytokine interleukin-2, while inhibiting the normal protective rise in interleukin-6 that occurs during a full night's sleep.

"Sleep deprivation also disrupts your body's rhythm of the stress hormone cortisol," says Hema Sundaram, MD, a dermatologist in Washington, DC, and author of *Face Value*. Your body's cortisol levels are highest in the morning and then drop throughout the day, reaching their lowest point at midnight. When you are sleep-deprived, you may get a cortisol surge at the wrong time—at night, for example—because your body is out of balance. This surge can leave you awake and anxious, unable to go to sleep. And because sleep deprivation is stressful to both body and mind, you react by pumping out even *more* cortisol, which has suppressive effects on the immune system.

A Costly National Debt

Many things can disrupt our normal sleep patterns. Some are within our control, while others are not. With all of our responsibilities and obligations in the course of a day—from working long hours to preparing dinner to carting kids to sports practice—getting the necessary 8 or so hours of sleep can seem next to impossible. According to the National Sleep Foundation's 2005 Sleep in America poll, the average American sleeps 6.8 hours per night. That's 1.2 hours too little, for an average total yearly sleep debt of a whopping 438 hours.

Sometimes it is not the number of hours but the quality of sleep that's the problem. The Sleep in America poll found that up to 75 percent of Americans have at least one symptom of a sleep disorder. For instance, an estimated 54 percent of the population occasionally lies in bed for minutes to hours before falling asleep. "Problems falling asleep—a condition called insomnia—has a proven impact on the immune system," Dr. Ash says.

Another common disorder is sleep apnea, which causes an estimated 18 million Americans to stop breathing as often as 20 to 60 times an hour. As Dr. Meletis describes, "Imagine putting your hands firmly around your neck and choking yourself for 6 to 8 hours. Basically, that's what happens to people with sleep apnea." You don't get enough oxygen to your brain or your tissues, and your immune system sputters, he says. Beyond that, sleep apnea puts sufferers at risk for diabetes, cardiovascular disease, high blood pressure, and digestive problems. Other sleep disorders, including restless legs syndrome, snoring, narcolepsy, and sleep paralysis, also deplete immunity.

Wake Up Your Immune System by Putting Your Sheep to Rest

If you've been experiencing sleep disturbances—not falling asleep, not staying asleep, awakening well before the alarm sounds—you should talk with your doctor to rule out any underlying medical problem. "In many cases, insomnia is a symptom of a larger sleep disorder," Dr. Ash explains. "So as a first step, it needs to be evaluated."

Once you have some sense of why you're not sleeping well, you can take steps to correct the problem. You should try to get approximately 8 hours of shut-eye a night. "Some people need a little more, some need a little less, but 8 hours is a good goal," Dr. Meletis says. With this in mind, here are some things you can do on your own to improve the quantity and quality of your sleep.

Practice good sleep hygiene. "We all recognize the importance of good dental hygiene, but many people aren't familiar with the phrase 'sleep hygiene,'" Dr. Ash says. "These sleep hygiene rules are things that all of us should do to maintain good health." For example:

1. Maintain a regular sleep-wake schedule, even on weekends. "A good general rule is to fall asleep by 10:00 p.m. and get up around 6:00 a.m.," Dr. Meletis says.

2. Establish a regular, relaxing bedtime routine. Soak in a warm bath, listen to soothing music, read a good book—whatever relaxes you.

3. Create a sleep-conducive environment that is quiet, dark, cool, and comfortable. Lower the thermostat, draw the shades to block out streetlights and the morning sun, and do anything else that makes your surroundings more sleepworthy.

4. Invest in a comfortable mattress and pillow. A sunken 10-year-old mattress and pancake pillows can put a damper on a good night's sleep. Quality sleep furnishings are worth the expense.

5. Reserve your bedroom for sleep and sex. Sure, your bed makes a great place to wrap gifts, work on a scrapbook, or eat a sandwich—all while watching TV. But these and other activities belong elsewhere in your home.

6. Finish eating no less than 2 to 3 hours before bedtime. If your body is busy digesting food, it will be less likely to fall asleep.

7. Exercise regularly, but make sure that you complete your workout at least 2 to 3 hours before going to bed. As with eating, exercising too late at night can keep you awake.

Soothe with Seriphos. The nutritional supplement Seriphos contains serine phosphate derivatives, which help combat high cortisol levels so that you can sleep better. "Take a couple of Seriphos capsules before bedtime and one in the morning, if necessary, for a total daily dose of up to 1,000 milligrams," Dr. Meletis says. "As a nice side benefit, Seriphos improves mental clarity." You can find it in many supplement shops and health food stores, as well as online.

Ease jangled nerves with L-theanine. "L-theanine, an amino acid derived from green tea, is helpful for people who are a little worked up and need to relax to go to sleep," Dr. Meletis says. Taking 200 to 400 milligrams about half an hour before bedtime does a splendid job of reducing anxiety and inducing sleep, he says.

Just say no to caffeine. "Caffeine not only disrupts your sleep patterns, it also generates free radicals that stress your body's antioxidant defenses," Dr. Sundaram says. In her view, the best thing you can do for a good night's sleep is give up caffeine altogether. "But if you currently are drinking several cups of coffee a day, try to cut down to a cup a day—or better yet, switch to green tea," she advises. "Green tea contains some caffeine, so you will get your little boost. But it also is highly antioxidant, which means that it can help counteract the negative effects of the free radicals in caffeine on your immune system."

Ease your worries with flower essences. "When people have emotional upheavals in their lives, they often can't sleep," observes Melissa Wood, ND, a naturopathic physician based in San Antonio. "In these cases, I recommend flower essences." The original flower essences were developed by the English physician Dr. Edward Bach, who believed that diseases of the body occur because of emotional imbalances in the brain and soul. Once such emotional imbalances are corrected, he theorized, the body can heal on its own.

"The essences that work best for sleep problems are those directly related to emotions—White Chestnut and Aspen," Dr. Wood says. "White Chestnut is good for worrying thoughts or mental arguments that go round and round, while Aspen is effective for unknown anxiety and vague fears.

"Since the flower essences are homeopathic in nature, they are most effective when applied directly in the mouth or under the tongue," she adds. "Or they can be added to water and sipped throughout the day or right before bedtime." Flower essences are sold in health food stores such as Whole Foods, Sun Harvest, and Wild Oats, as well as in some grocery stores. They're also available online.

Calm yourself with chamomile tea. The herb chamomile is soothing in and of itself. Taking it in tea form makes you feel nice and warm inside, which also promotes truly restful sleep. "I wouldn't slurp down a 20-ouncer because you'll be up all night going to the bathroom, but sipping a nice 6-ounce cup of chamomile tea does the trick for most people," Dr. Meletis says. If you find that you're waking up to urinate even after a small cup, he suggests trying chamomile in capsule form—about 500 milligrams a half hour before retiring.

Abstain from alcohol. Though alcohol may help you fall asleep, its effects quickly backfire, disrupting sleep cycles for a few hours into the night. And because it has been shown to reduce the number of NK cells, booze serves up a double shot in terms of immune system suppression.

Wind down with valerian. A mild sedative, valerian root works well for many people with sleep problems. "Take about 500 milligrams about a half hour before bed," Dr. Meletis suggests.

Lull yourself to sleep. It isn't just the motion of a car or train that makes so many of us nod off; it's also the whirring of a motor or the soft *thump thump* of the tracks. That's why so many people sleep better with a white-noise machine in their bedrooms, says Nikol Margiotta, DN, a naprapathic physician in Chicago. (Naprapathy is a therapeutic discipline that uses the manipulation of connective tissue to promote healing.) A white-noise machine can provide the right kind of nonspecific noise to help you get to sleep and stay asleep, whether it's the sound of a babbling brook, a gentle breeze rustling through tree branches, or a soft motor that soothes you. Don't want to invest in a machine? "A fan works just as well for some people," Dr. Margiotta says.

Doze off with passionflower. The leaves and roots of the passionflower have a long history of use by Native Americans for treating insomnia. "You can drink passionflower as a tea, but I think that the capsule form is best," Dr. Meletis says. "Take 300 to 500 milligrams about a half hour before bedtime."

End the day on a high note. As we climb into bed at night, our minds often are far from ready to settle down. "If you are like most people, you think about things like what you need to do the next day and what you are going to wear, which keeps you awake," says D. V. Pasupuleti, MD, clinical professor of medicine at Michigan State University in East Lansing and author of *Change Your Mind.* "Instead, shift your mental focus to all of the positive things that happened to you during the day that's just ending. By doing this, you not only will relax your body, you also will sleep better and have more pleasant dreams. Plus, your brain will be rested and ready for the next day."

If You Work Swing Shift . . .

Sandy*, a psychiatric nurse, volunteered for a swing-shift schedule a few years ago to earn extra money. "For 2 weeks, I work from 7:00 a.m. to 3:00 p.m. Then I move to evenings for 2 weeks; I'm on duty from 3:00 p.m. to 11:00 p.m. After that, it's 11:00 p.m. to 7:00 a.m. for 2 weeks. And then the cycle starts all over again," says the 42-year-old mother of two.

Although the schedule has paid off financially, otherwise Sandy has suffered. Since moving to swing shift, she has gained 30 pounds, constantly feels tired, and has taken more sick days than ever before. She's beginning to wonder if the extra pay is worth the cost to her health.

Sandy is not imagining the downturn in her health that has accompanied the swing in her shift. Our bodies are programmed to be awake during the day and asleep at night . . . period. When we mess with this natural rhythm by working a schedule that begins at sundown—or worse, a schedule that starts sometimes at dawn and sometimes at dusk—our bodies and our immune systems suffer.

"In a perfect world, there would be no swing shift. But with our society demanding that we be on call 24 hours a day, 7 days a week, shift work is an issue that is not going away," says Carol Ash, DO, medical director of the Sleep for Life Program at Somerset Medical Center in New Jersey. "Any change to the normal sleep-wake schedule impacts physiology. And poor sleep, whether caused by a sleep disorder or by swing shift, has been shown in several studies to affect the immune system."

The impact of shift work on health becomes even more alarming when you look

*Not her real name

at the statistics. From an epidemiological perspective, shift workers die at a younger age than those who work a normal schedule of 9:00 a.m. to 5:00 p.m., says Chris D. Meletis, ND, executive director of the Institute for Healthy Aging in Portland, Oregon. "So for some people, it simply may not be worth the pay differential when they consider the years of their lives that they may be trading for," he says.

Why is a swing-shift schedule so detrimental to the immune system and overall health? It has to do with what's known as the circadian rhythm, the body's natural 24-hour cycle of activity. The circadian rhythm prompts your brain to produce melatonin at night, so you can sleep, and cortisol during the day, so you can stay awake. The brain's pineal gland, which is responsible for making melatonin, is regulated by sunlight. In the morning, the rising sun alerts the pineal gland that it's daytime. The gland responds by cutting back on melatonin production.

"In people who work swing shift, the circadian rhythm goes out of sync, and the pineal gland becomes damaged," says Keith DeOrio, MD, DHom, founder of the DeOrio Wellness Medical Center in Santa Monica, California. As a result, melatonin and cortisol are secreted at incorrect times and in incorrect amounts. Melatonin isn't just important for sleep. The hormone has antioxidant properties and helps maintain a healthy immune system. So when you aren't making the right amount of melatonin, your immune function—and the rest of your body—must deal with the consequences, Dr. DeOrio says.

Beyond the direct physical toll of swing shift, it tends to promote bad eating habits, which further impair immunity. "A lot of people who work swing shift have poor nutrition," says Patricia David, MD, MSPH, president of the Healthy U wellness program in Columbus, Ohio. They eat the wrong things at the wrong times and for the wrong reasons—for instance, Twinkies and coffee at midnight to stay awake.

How to Outsmart Swing Shift

With all of the above in mind, "if you can avoid shift work, avoid shift work," Dr. Meletis says. Unfortunately, many of us don't have a choice. If you're a shift worker, these tips can help your body and immune system better deal with the constant change in sleep-wake pattern.

Turn day into night. "If sunlight is shining into your bedroom, your pineal gland will create a melatonin level in sync with daytime, and you will have trouble falling asleep," Dr. Meletis says. If you must regularly sleep during the day, hang the thickest darkening shades you can find on your windows, and wear an eye mask to block light. "Completely black out your bedroom to make your own night," he says.

Create a comfortable sleeping environment. Whether your bedtime is at midnight or 8 o'clock in the morning, a comfortable sleeping environment is essential to sound sleep. Make sure your bedroom is not only dark but also quiet and your bed is clean, fluffy, and cozy.

Go right home. Although it's tempting to run a few errands or stop for a snack on your way home from work, please refrain, for your health's sake. "The time you spend traveling from work to home exposes you to sunlight, which tells your brain that it's time to wake up as opposed to time to go to sleep," Dr. Ash says. The less this happens, the better.

Supplement nighttime sleep with melatonin. To replace some of the melatonin that you may be shortchanged on as a result of your irregular sleep schedule, consider taking supplements, suggests Gerard Mullin, MD, director of complementary and alternative medicine and gastrointestinal nutrition services at Johns Hopkins Hospital in Baltimore. Supplemental melatonin has been recommended for a variety of conditions, but most often it's used as a sleep aid. The standard dose is one 3-milligram capsule 30 to 60 minutes before retiring.

Stabilize your system with good nutrition. Because people who work swing shift are at higher risk for poor nutrition and obesity, pay close attention to your diet—especially when and why you are eating certain foods, Dr. David says. Using food as a tool to stay awake is a sure bet for gaining weight. Instead, make a point of eating for good nutrition. Each day, aim for 3 to 4 ounces of whole grains, 2½ to 3 cups of vegetables, 1½ to 2 cups of fruit, 3 cups of low-fat dairy products, 5½ to 6½ ounces of lean meats and/or beans, and 5 to 7 teaspoons of oils (less than 7 percent of calories from saturated fats and no trans fats). For more specific information on nutritional goals, check out www.mypyramid.gov.

Fight the effects of disrupted sleep with fish oil. Another way to combat impaired nutrition: Take fish-oil supplements. "The omega-3 fatty acids eicosapentaenoic acid [EPA] and docosahexaenoic acid [DHA] in fish oil help maintain a healthy nervous system and reduce stress, both of which support sleep," says Gretchen Vannice, MS, RD, research coordinator at Nordic Naturals in Watsonville, California. She recommends taking fish-oil supplements that supply at least 650 milligrams of EPA and DHA, total, per day.

Become antisocial. Right after work, that is. Just like sunlight, socializing with friends or family will stimulate your brain so that it thinks it should be awake. When your shift is over, head straight home to your bedroom to catch some z's. "Ask your family members to limit interruptions, such as phone calls or noise, so you can get some good-quality sleep during the day," Dr. Ash says.

Stick to set sleep schedules. Your sleep schedule already is way out of whack. But the more regular you can keep this irregular schedule, the better, Dr. Meletis says, so try to establish a sleep-wake pattern for each shift. For example, always sleep from 8:00 a.m. to 4:00 p.m. on the days you work third shift, or from midnight to 8:00 a.m. when you work second shift. Aim for about 8 hours of sleep.

Wind down with Seriphos. To fight the confusion in your sleep-wake cycle, Dr. Meletis recommends Seriphos. This nutritional supplement contains serine phosphate derivatives, which help counteract high cortisol levels so you can sleep better. "Take two capsules before you go to sleep and one when you wake up, if necessary, for a total daily dose of up to 1,000 milligrams," Dr. Meletis says. As a bonus, Seriphos improves mental clarity, so you'll be more alert when you wake up, he adds.

Just say no to overtime. "Frequently with shift work, people will stay a few extra hours for more pay or because a co-worker is running late," Dr. Ash says. "But the more hours you stay awake, the worse the effects will be on your health, and the greater the likelihood you will be an impaired driver on the way home.

"People think they can adjust to shift work and staying up late, but that's a myth," she adds. "If you have gone without sleep, it is going to affect your alertness and your ability to stay awake. Sooner or later, sleep will take over. It is a basic physiological need."

If You Are 50 or Older . . .

Most of us know an older person who defies nature. While her friends are crocheting and playing bingo, she's out playing tennis. While his friends are lounging in their recliners watching reruns, he's out looking at sports cars.

"One person can be 50 and act 100, while another person can be 80 and fitter than anyone. There definitely is a difference between chronological and biological age," says Chris D. Meletis, ND, executive director of the Institute for Healthy Aging in Portland, Oregon. "They say that 50 is the new 30, so the question is, if someone is fit and healthy, can that person actually be in better shape than he or she was at 30? In some cases, in part because of the increased stability of careers and relationships that comes later in life, I think yes."

But lifestyle and personality aside, everyone ages. "As people approach or pass 50, their bodies can't quite keep up with physiological processes as they once did," says Janet Suvak, MD, a general practitioner specializing in preventive health care with offices in Newport Beach and Beverly Hills, California. DNA becomes more fragile and breaks down; metabolism slows, leading to weight gain and fatigue; and a person begins to look and feel . . . well, older.

The immune system is just as vulnerable to the effects of aging as the rest of the body is. As people get older, they don't respond as well to vaccinations (which may be why the flu shot doesn't work as well for them). In addition, their immune cells can't attack and kill invaders as forcefully as they once did, nor can they communicate with each other as clearly, says Barry Ritz, MS, a researcher at Drexel University in Philadelphia who specializes in the effects of aging on the immune system. "Aging correlates with an increase in infectious diseases, autoimmune diseases, and cancers—all of which have at least some connection to age-related immune decline," Ritz says. "However, research shows us that there is a tremendous amount of variability in the immune systems of the elderly."

Factors behind Immune Decline

So why is it that some 65-year-olds have the immune systems of twenty-somethings, while others experience a relative plunge in immunity? "One important factor is nutrition," Ritz says. "We know that the leading cause of immunosuppression worldwide is malnutrition, so there is a clear relationship between nutrition and immunity." As some people get older, they don't pay as close attention to their diets as they once did. Others have been eating a diet of chicken fried steak and potatoes for 50 years, and it's finally catching up with them.

Another factor is depression, which affects between 8 and 20 percent of older adults in the community and 37 percent in primary care settings. A study from the American Psychological Association (APA), published in the *Journal of Abnormal Psychology*, compared the immune systems of older adults who were depressed with the immune systems of those who were not depressed. The researchers found that people with mild chronic depression had poorer immune responses and that the *duration* of depression—not the severity—had a more crippling effect on immunity.

The weakened immunity common among older people also may be due to long-term exposure to infectious agents such as cytomegalovirus (CMV), a member of the herpes virus family. A report published in the journal *Immunity and Ageing* revealed that persistent activation by CMV may cause the immune system to grow tired over time. Most of us have been exposed to CMV by the time we reach 40. The theory is that this virus and similar long-term infections keep our immune cells constantly stimulated, which causes them to respond less forcefully in the presence of a real threat.

Reinforce Your Disease Defenses

Considering all of the immune-suppressing hurdles that we face later in life, those tennis-playing, sports car–buying older people should serve as an inspiration. They're proof that we do have some power to fight the effects of aging. The following measures can help outsmart immune system declines and safeguard your health well into old age.

Rev up immunity with vitamin C. Vitamin C helps stimulate the immune system just by virtue of being an antioxidant. The body uses vitamin C to manufacture interferon, an immune system protein that helps destroy viruses. Vitamin C also may enhance levels of a compound called glutathione, which has been shown to strengthen immune function. And to combat the increased inflammation and slowed wound healing that accompanies aging, "vitamin C helps hold together collagen bundles, which is important for surgery recovery and wound healing in general," says Jana Klauer, MD, author of *How the Rich Stay Thin* and a New York City–based physician who specializes in the biology of fat reduction.

You can take vitamin C in supplement form, but you get extra benefits with berries. "Strawberries contain more vitamin C than oranges do, plus they provide additional antioxidants," Dr. Klauer says. "And because they are not high in calories, you can eat a whole cup of berries a day. They are a wonderful addition to your diet." Other good sources of vitamin C include guava, papaya, kiwifruit, tomatoes, broccoli, spinach, and citrus fruits.

Energize your immunity with vitamin E. "Vitamin E, which works together with vitamin C, appears to rescue T-cell functioning in aging," Ritz says. "In a study done at Tufts University, 200 IU of supplemental vitamin E per day reduced the rate of the common cold among nursing home elderly." Some research has shown an increased risk of death with high doses (over 400 IU) of vitamin E supplements, but daily amounts of 200 IU or less are safe. Good food sources of vitamin E include nuts, leafy green vegetables, wheat germ, avocados, and whole grains.

Eat like Bugs. Bunny, that is. Vitamin A and the carotenoids (beta-carotene, lutein, and lycopene) have long been studied for their immune-boosting effects. There has been some controversy surrounding the safety of vitamin A supplements, so your best bet is to get this essential nutrient from foods. "For efficient immune system function, I tell people to eat a lot of vitamin A–rich foods such as carrots, sweet potatoes, pumpkin, and kale," says Patricia David, MD, MSPH, president of the Healthy U wellness program in Columbus, Ohio.

Maintain vitality with vitamin D. Another nutrient that plays a role in immune function is vitamin D. "Vitamin D receptors are found on a variety of immune cells, including T-cells, macrophages, and dendritic cells," Ritz says. Unfortunately, vitamin D deficiency is pandemic in this country, particularly among older people. And because vitamin D does so much else for the body—from maintaining bones, joints, teeth, and gums to supporting the brain and heart—getting enough is important.

Vitamin D is unique because we can't get enough from dietary sources alone. It's found in a limited number of foods (mainly dairy). However, the human body can make its own vitamin D when exposed to the sun, Ritz adds. Your best bet is to get 10 to 15 minutes of direct sunlight, without sunscreen, per day.

Drink from the fountain of youth. "As people get older, they go from grapes to raisins, in part because they are dehydrated," Dr. Meletis says. "Some refrain from drinking enough water because of leaky bladders, but it is very important for them to be getting 64 ounces of water per day."

For an extra antiaging benefit, add goji berries to your glass. "The goji berry grows wild in the Himalayas, and scientists discovered that people who drank from streams into which goji berries fell were healthy and living to a very old age," Dr. David explains. "The scientists think that it has something to do with the high antioxidant content of the berries." To get the age-defying benefits, Dr. David suggests putting a few of the berries into a glass of water before drinking. "The berries are not available in most grocery stores, but you can buy them online," she says.

Sprinkle with cinnamon. "Cinnamon enhances immune function, and it helps regulate blood sugar and insulin," says Mary Jo DiMilia, MD, assistant professor of medicine and pediatrics at Mount Sinai School of Medicine in New York City. Since the risk of diabetes rises with age, cinnamon can be especially beneficial for older people. The great thing about cinnamon is that you can sprinkle it on just about any food—fruit, cereal, yogurt, you name it.

Get a little help from your friends. An interesting finding from the APA study mentioned earlier is that lack of social support is a risk factor for depression and, therefore, for impaired immunity. "Research has shown that if a woman has a strong support network, she is healthier than if she doesn't, and that men who have wives or partners are healthier as well," Dr. Meletis says. So make a point of getting together regularly with family and friends, or join a book club, a walking club, or other social group that interests you. Do whatever you can to get out there and mix and mingle with people whom you enjoy.

Fish for better health. People in their fifties and older generally are at higher risk for heart disease, dementia, depression, and diabetes. The omega-3 fatty acids in fish oil help with all of these conditions, says Gretchen Vannice, MS, RD, research coordinator at Nordic Naturals in Watsonville, California. In fact, the omega-3 fatty acids eicosapentaenoic acid (EPA) and docosahexaenoic acid (DHA) are so beneficial for heart disease that the American Heart Association (AHA) recommends 1 gram total per day as a preventive. This amount appears to help protect against depression and diabetes as well. "If you have elevated triglycerides, however, the AHA recommends upping the dose to 2 to 4 grams of EPA and DHA per day," Vannice says.

"You can get EPA and DHA from fatty fish such as salmon, herring, or mackerel, though getting a whole gram per day from fish alone is pretty hard," she adds. So for older adults, a fish-oil supplement containing both EPA and DHA is a good bet. Look for a supplement product that has been tested for mercury and lead; it should say so on the label. Because fish oil can cause blood thinning, be sure to check with your doctor before beginning supplementation.

Keep your body in motion. In general, older people are less active than younger people, which means they are missing out on a key immune system stimulant. "Exercise has invariably been shown to regulate our immune systems," Dr. Meletis says. It's never too late to adopt an exercise program. If you currently are inactive, any movement you add to your life will be beneficial. (Be sure to check with your doctor before you start, though.) For optimum health and immunity, you should build up to 45 to 60 minutes of aerobic activity—like brisk walking—6 days a week.

Put yourself first. "A lot of adults end up becoming caregivers for their parents—sometimes in addition to their own children—and they stop taking care of themselves," Dr. Suvak says. Instead of taking time to go to the gym or cook a healthful meal, they do something for Mom or Dad. "It doesn't have to be an either/or," she says. "You need to get exercise and sunshine, and you need to laugh. All of these things tie back into your immune system. Ultimately, you will not be taking away from anybody by taking good care of yourself. In fact, you will feel better, so you will have *more* to give."

Activate immunity with AHCC. Active hexose correlated compound (AHCC) is a fermented mushroom product first developed in Japan and now available in the United States as a dietary supplement. AHCC has overall immune-boosting power, as well as a stimulating effect on certain white blood cells. In a recent study at Drexel, laboratory mice were given AHCC for 1 week before being infected with the flu virus. "Results showed that AHCC indeed appeared to boost natural killer cell activity, reduce the severity of the influenza infection, and enhance the mice's ability to clear the virus from their lungs," says Ritz, co-author of the study.

In addition, AHCC shows promise as a cancer treatment. "It is being used in over 700 clinics in Japan as an adjunct cancer therapy, and it was shown to increase the longevity of liver cancer patients in a 12-year study," says Dan Kenner, ND, OMD, a naturopathic physician and licensed oriental medicine doctor in Forestville, California, and author of *Building Immunity Naturally*.

Because of its immune-enhancing effects, Dr. Kenner recommends AHCC to older people as both a preventive and treatment for certain conditions such as bronchitis and pneumonia. "AHCC is what I call a superfood—it helps everyone across the board," he says. It's available in most health food stores (one brand name is ImmPower) and online at www.vitaminshoppe.com and www.iherb.com. Dr. Kenner recommends what he calls the cancer dose for immune restoration. "That's four 500-milligram capsules three times a day for 6 weeks, for recurrent infections or infections that don't resolve," he says. "For prevention and general immune enhancement, I recommend two capsules twice a day for adults."

If You Are Around Young Children . . .

During his 4th year of medical school, 30-year-old Steven Barnes* spent 2 months on a pediatrics rotation. "I knew I was being exposed to a lot of germs on a daily basis, but I remember one incident in particular," says Dr. Barnes, who has since graduated from medical school and is currently in residency. "A baby came in with a case of diarrhea and sneezed right on me. I thought, 'Uh-oh'—and then I spent the next day and a half with a terrible stomach virus."

Each day, medical students like Dr. Barnes, practicing physicians, nurses, daycare workers, and, of course, parents are exposed to millions of germs thanks to the most fertile petri dishes around: children. By virtue of being in the presence of young children, you are exposed to more viruses and bacteria than people who aren't. And if you are caring for kids of your own, you likely are sleep deprived and under stress to boot, so the strain on your immune system is multifold.

Plus, if a youngster passes on a respiratory infection or strep throat and you end up taking antibiotics, you alter your own gut bacteria and, ironically, become even more susceptible to getting sick. "The bacteria colonization in the gut is very much associated with immune function," says Patricia David, MD, MSPH, president of the Healthy U wellness program in Columbus, Ohio. "The good bacteria control the bad bacteria and, therefore, prevent you from getting ill." Unfortunately, antibiotics cannot distinguish between good and evil, so when you swallow tetracycline or penicillin, it kills the villain that made you sick, but it also kills the good guys that are on the lookout for new invaders.

*Not his real name

No Kidding Around—You Need Immune Protection

We love our children, so we're more than willing to risk the germ exposure that goes along with caring for them. But wouldn't it be great if we could strengthen our immune systems enough so that we wouldn't need to worry about picking up viruses and bacteria when we're cuddling with our kids? In some cases, it appears that we can.

"People think that just because they've been exposed to the flu or another bug, they're going to get the infection, but that isn't necessarily true," says Keith DeOrio, MD, DHom, founder of the DeOrio Wellness Medical Center in Santa Monica, California. "The key is to bolster your immune system integrity in preparation for the exposure." The following measures can help strengthen your immune system against the viruses and bacteria that are part and parcel of caring for a child.

Promote immune health with probiotics. To build up healthy gut bacteria after taking antibiotics—and to maintain a healthy intestinal environment in general—you can take probiotics. Probiotics help stimulate the immune system to be more alert for invading viruses and bacteria by balancing your intestinal bacteria, explains José Saavedra, MD, associate professor in the department of pediatrics at the Johns Hopkins School of Medicine and School of Public Health and medical and scientific director of Nestlé Nutrition.

Many products, ranging from pills to drinks, claim to contain probiotics. But only certain ones supply the specific types of bacteria—*Lactobacillus* and *Bifidobacterium*—that promote immune health. To be sure you are getting the most effective bacteria for immunity, make sure the product label mentions those two bacteria. Two yogurt brands that do: DanActive and Activia. As for the proper "dose" of probiotic yogurt, you simply cannot eat too much. For best results, aim for at least a serving a day, preferably more.

Encourage good bacteria with prebiotics. "To keep your immune system healthy and on alert, in addition to probiotics, you should regularly consume prebiotics—nondigestible food components that selectively stimulate the growth of good bacteria in the gastrointestinal tract," Dr. David says. Natural sources of prebiotics include greens (such as dandelion greens, spinach, and kale), artichokes, legumes (lentils, kidney beans, and chickpeas), members of the allium family (onions, leeks, and garlic), whole grains (oats, flax, and barley), and soy yogurt.

For extra immune vigor, eat vitamin C. "Some studies suggest that vitamin C helps boost immunity, but other research suggests that nutrients like vitamin C in and of themselves may not be beneficial," Dr. David says. "So I advise people to get their vitamin C from foods rather than from supplements." She recommends aiming for five or more servings of fruits and vegetables high in vitamin C per day. Among your choices are kiwifruit (depending on its size, it might be higher in vitamin C than an orange), guava, strawberries, spinach, grapefruit, oranges, tomatoes, and broccoli. "Juices made from these fruits and vegetables also are beneficial, as long as they're not from concentrate," Dr. David says. "Juices from concentrate have been processed, so the nutrients aren't as active."

Zap colds with zinc. "Zinc appears to diminish cold symptoms," Dr. David says. As with vitamin C, she recommends getting zinc from foods rather than from a pill. "Foods high in zinc include pumpkin seeds, seafood [particularly oysters and crab], beans, and eggs," she says.

Drink the right kind of water. Because hydration is vital to good immune health, you should be drinking at least eight 8-ounce glasses of water a day, says Chris D. Meletis, ND, executive director of the Institute for Healthy Aging in Portland, Oregon. He recommends nonfluorinated, nonchlorinated water because chlorine can interfere with beneficial gut bacteria. "If chlorine is strong enough to kill bacteria in a swimming pool, it is strong enough to kill the beneficial critters in your colon," Dr. Meletis says. "Good bacteria are like powder puffs—they are easily destroyed. The healthier your gut is from a *Lactobacillus* and *Bifidobacterium* standpoint, the healthier your immune system will be."

Give your immune system an edge with EpiCor. "One of my favorite supplements for immune function is EpiCor," Dr. Meletis says. EpiCor was discovered accidentally when a group of workers in a cattle-feed plant realized that their health insurance premiums had never gone up. In fact, some of them hadn't taken a sick day in 30 years. A research team looked into the abnormally resilient health of the group and found that the workers were being exposed to an airborne yeast derivative, later named EpiCor.

"EpiCor has been shown to increase natural killer [NK] cells, which attack and kill invaders, as well as secretory immunoglobulin A [sIgA], which I call the Scotch-gard of the immune system," Dr. Meletis says. "Plus, EpiCor is very high in natural antioxidants, which makes it even more immune-protective. I not only prescribe EpiCor to patients who have a lot of exposure to viruses and bacteria, such as those who are around young children, I also take it every day." He recommends a dosage of one 500-milligram capsule per day. You can find EpiCor in vitamin shops and health food stores, as well as online.

Wash your hands, from A to Z. Should you use antibacterial soap or shouldn't you? One study found that antibacterial soaps are no more effective than regular ones at preventing infection. More important is the amount of time you spend scrubbing up. "Practice the ABCs of hand washing—wash your hands for the length of time it takes you to slowly recite the entire alphabet," Dr. Meletis says. "This technique is great for kids, too."

If you have kids, wipe things down often. "Think about it: Your kids use the bathroom, wash their hands—sort of—and then touch the doorknob," Dr. Meletis says. "Or worse, they don't wash their hands, and then they touch the doorknob." Voilà—contamination. "To prevent spreading toilet contamination throughout the house, clean bathroom and other doorknobs and surfaces regularly with Lysol or other antibacterial wipes," he advises.

Don't share foods or containers with kids. If you have children of your own, it's tempting to share their juice boxes and ice cream cones, and it seems harmless to kiss them on the lips. But those cute little mouths have been on toys and blocks that other kids have chewed and pawed, Dr. Meletis says. So for the sake of your immune system and your weight (yes, the rest of an ice cream cone is fattening, even if it wasn't originally yours), be mindful of the kissing and sharing.

Carry antibacterial gel everywhere. "The antibacterial gel that evaporates without water is the best thing since sliced bread if you are around lots of young children," says Janet Suvak, MD, a general practitioner specializing in preventive health care with offices in Newport Beach and Beverly Hills, California. The "soap without water" antibacterials have been shown to get rid of more than 90 percent of bacteria on hands.

"Kids constantly put their hands on their faces and then transmit germs everywhere," Dr. Suvak says. "But if you teach them to use the antibacterial gel, you will stop some of that transmission." She recommends putting bottles of gel all over the house. "Kids love squirt bottles, and they will like the feeling of the gel because it's cool and it evaporates quickly," she says.

Keep your hands off your face. One of the easiest ways to spread germs is to touch them—and then touch your face, eyes, or mouth. "All of us touch our faces, and our hands go in our mouths much more than we realize," says Hema Sundaram, MD, a dermatologist in Washington, DC, and author of *Face Value*. "In a dermatological study, researchers coated people's hands with a fluorescent Vaseline-based ointment and asked them to avoid touching their faces. The participants swore up and down that they hadn't, but when researchers fluoresced them, they had touched *all over* their faces, including their mouths."

The lesson? Try to pay attention to when you're touching your face, and as soon as you realize that you are, remove your hands. Beyond that, use an antibacterial wipe or gel if you know that you will be in contact with germs or contamination, Dr. Sundaram says.

Arm your immune system with AHCC. Active hexose correlated compound (AHCC) is a fermented mushroom product from Japan that has been shown to improve the survival rate of some cancer patients, Dr. David says. AHCC works by stimulating certain white blood cells and by boosting immune function in general. In a study at Drexel University in Philadelphia, laboratory mice were treated with AHCC for 1 week before being infected with a flu virus. "Our results suggested that AHCC improved the activity of natural killer cells, reduced the severity of the influenza infection, and enhanced the mice's ability to clear the flu virus from their lungs," says researcher Barry Ritz, MS, a co-author of the study.

Because of the immune-boosting effects of AHCC, some conventional and naturopathic physicians—including Dan Kenner, ND, OMD, a naturopathic physician and licensed oriental medicine doctor in Forestville, California, and author of *Building Immunity Naturally*—recommend it as a general preventive and immune stimulant. AHCC helps everyone across the board, including people who are around young children, Dr. Kenner says. AHCC is available in most health food stores (one brand name is ImmPower) and online at www.vitaminshoppe.com and www.iherb.com. For general immune enhancement, Dr. Kenner recommends two capsules twice a day for adults.

Ask your doctor about antibiotic alternatives. These days, as antibiotic-resistant germs become more of a threat after years of antibiotic use, many people are searching for an alternative. "Luckily, some new drugs aim to spare the immune system, even while you are treating an infection," Dr. Sundaram says. One example is Oracea, a prescription treatment for rosacea. "The conventional way of treating rosacea was to give someone an oral antibiotic," she notes. "It did improve rosacea, but it also killed good bacteria, contributed to yeast overgrowth, and led to antibiotic-resistant bacteria." Oracea, on the other hand, is a very low dose of the antibiotic doxycycline that doesn't kill bacteria. "It is the first of a new genre of therapy that reduces inflammation without killing bacteria," Dr. Sundaram says. "It addresses the issue at hand without causing collateral damage to the immune system."

So the next time you see your doctor about a bacterial infection, for the sake of your immunity and everyone else's, ask about these new drugs.

If You Spend a Lot of Time Indoors . . .

When Gerard Mullin, MD, first moved to downtown Baltimore, he chose a brand-new apartment building. "But after a few weeks, I wasn't feeling well. I decided to have the air quality tested," says Dr. Mullin, director of complementary and alternative medicine and gastrointestinal nutrition services at Johns Hopkins Hospital. "I discovered that the building had high levels of formaldehyde, so I moved out. I found another building with older construction. Since then, I've had no problems."

What Dr. Mullin experienced in his first apartment was indoor air pollution, a common problem that is of particular concern to people who spend most of their lives under roofs and behind closed doors.

Believe it or not, indoor air pollution can be more severe than outdoor pollution. "In fact, indoor air pollution is up to five times worse," says Keith DeOrio, MD, DHom, founder of the DeOrio Wellness Medical Center in Santa Monica, California. Things that seem harmless—such as new carpeting, computers, microwaves, plug-in air fresheners, and even everyday household cleaners—can actually be quite harmful for your immune system and your general health.

Part of the problem is the positive ions that reside indoors. Ions are charged particles that form when energy acts on a molecule to eject one of its electrons. That ejected electron attaches itself to another molecule, which then becomes a negative ion. The ion that is left without its electron is the positive ion.

Positive ions can make people feel tired, depressed, and irritable. They also have been linked with sick building syndrome. "Negative ions, which exist in outside air, are helpful because they bind with toxins and immediately drop them to the ground,"

Dr. DeOrio says. "Positive ions, on the other hand, do the opposite—they keep chemicals hovering in midair, which is why they build up indoors."

Beyond the toxins and positive ions that stress your immune system when you spend time indoors, you miss out on fresh air and sunshine. Sun exposure allows your skin to manufacture vitamin D, a crucial vitamin for a healthy immune system. In addition, unless you work at a gym or a health club, you probably are more sedentary when you're inside. Lack of exercise further suppresses immune function.

Cultivate an Immune-Friendly Environment

Thanks to the Internet, video games, and home shopping networks, Americans spend more time than ever indoors. As a result, according to the American Lung Association, poor indoor air quality is one of the top five most urgent environmental risks to public health, a risk that an estimated 50 percent of the population is unaware of. As a member of the informed half, you can take steps to offset the immune-suppressing effects of an indoor lifestyle. Here's what to do.

In with the negative, out with the positive. When it comes to ions, negative is good. So to combat indoor air pollution, Dr. DeOrio recommends increasing the number of negative ions in the air. One way: Open a window to let in some fresh air—and negative ions along with it. Even in the winter, it's better to crack a window and turn up the heat a little higher. You also can buy an air-regeneration system like the one made by Alpine Technologies to release more negative ions into the air. Or you can place items in your environment that naturally release negative ions, such as rocks, plants, and salts, Dr. DeOrio says.

Catch rays to raise vitamin D. Vitamin D is tremendously important for boosting immunity. To make vitamin D, your body needs sunlight. "We tend to tell people that when they catch a cold, it's from the cold weather," says Dan Kenner, ND, OMD, a naturopathic physician and licensed oriental medicine doctor in Forestville, California, and author of *Building Immunity Naturally*. "But researchers at the University of Manchester in England have proposed that it is not the drop in temperature in winter that leads to colds but, rather, the decline in sunlight and, therefore, vitamin D." For maximum immunity, many physicians recommend 10 to 15 minutes of sun exposure, without sunscreen, per day. Some recommend even more. "I think that people should get as much sun as possible during the fall and winter seasons," Dr. Kenner says.

Have a sunnier disposition. Beyond its role in the manufacture of vitamin D, sunlight has a beneficial effect on mood and, therefore, immunity. "Even people who are homebound due to a disability or illness should try to get outside in the sun, if only for 5 minutes," says Mary Jo DiMilia, MD, assistant professor of medicine and pediatrics at Mount Sinai School of Medicine in New York City. "There is a strong connection between sunlight and a cheery mood."

Make yourself comfortable. If your job or lifestyle requires hours on end indoors, you might as well make your space as pleasant as possible. "Use full-spectrum lighting instead of fluorescent lightbulbs to mirror a more natural environment," suggests Chris D. Meletis, ND, executive director of the Institute for Healthy Aging in Portland, Oregon. "Set up an ergonomically healthy workspace, where you look straight across at a monitor rather than down at a laptop. The physiological stress and muscle tension that accompanies uncomfortable surroundings will slowly but surely wear on you."

Conduct meetings on the move. If your job permits, hold an occasional meeting outdoors by going for a walk instead of gathering around a conference table, Dr. Meletis suggests. "You're going to have at least 30 minutes anyway, so why not use the time to stroll around outside?" he asks. Cover your agenda while you get some exercise—and fresh air and sunshine to boot.

Get rid of smelly things. If you can smell a chemical, whether it's coming from a cleaning product or a plug-in air freshener, you are inhaling substances that are harmful to your body and your immunity, Dr. Meletis says. Don't use anything that throws a strong odor into the air. "If you are trying to eliminate a noxious odor, get rid of the source of it, and then open a window rather than attempting to mask it with chemical air fresheners or cleaners," he says.

Disinfect indoor air. "An aromatic diffuser can help disinfect the air, particularly when you use natural lavender or eucalyptus essential oils," Dr. Kenner says. "Viruses and bacteria usually travel in particles of moisture, and these oils help eliminate the particles and keep air clean." Aromatic diffusers are available in various sizes for different rooms. "The more expensive ones use ultrasound to disperse the liquid into a gas form, and the less expensive models use a candle," he says. He recommends running the diffuser for about 10 minutes to infuse the air in your bedroom or living room with the oil.

Be on the lookout for black mold. "Water damage can lead to indoor mold toxicity and *Stachybotrys,* the worst kind of black mold," Dr. DeOrio says. "It causes harm to the immune system and can affect the brain and other organs." Symptoms of mold toxicity include new allergies to chemicals and foods, fatigue, brain fog, bloating, restless sleep, blurred vision, headaches, muscles aches and pains, and hormonal disturbances. If you have any of those symptoms and your home is older and/or showing signs of mold growth—such as a musty odor, peeling paint, water stains, warped wood, or visible mold—consider getting a mold test. You can obtain a do-it-yourself test or hire an inspector. "If you discover that you have mold in your home, for the sake of your immune system, you need to get rid of it," Dr. DeOrio says.

Filter the air you breathe. To reduce the number of germs you breathe in, consider investing in an air-filtration system. "The fewer irritants floating around the room, the better," Dr. Meletis says. "Irritants will make your airways more inflamed and cause more mucus, and mucus is a breeding ground for viruses and bacteria." Home-improvement stores carry all kinds and sizes of air-filtration systems. "Some actually incinerate viruses in the room, while others just remove larger molecules that are hanging around," he says.

Utilize natural cleaning products. "A lot of the cleaning agents we use every day are not healthy," Dr. Mullin says. "I personally buy cleaning products that are toxin free." Look for natural cleaning products at your local organic market or in the organics section of your nearest supermarket. You also can mix your own using baking soda, lemon, vinegar, olive oil, and water. One part vinegar to 1 part water will clean and disinfect most areas of your home. One cup olive oil to ½ cup lemon juice makes a wonderful furniture polish. Deodorizing baking soda can be used in place of abrasive household cleaners to scrub sinks and stove tops. Small changes like these can do wonders for your immune system in the long run.

Energize yourself and your immunity with ashwagandha. The shrub ashwagandha, also known as Indian winter cherry, has a long history of use for stimulating immunity and energy, Dr. DiMilia says. To give your cooped-up self a boost, take one-half to one 500-milligram capsule (5:1 extract) a few times a week.

Brighten your working environment. It may sound simple, but a photo of your child or puppy on your desk or computer screen instantly cheers a drab cubicle. Happy thoughts and images during the workday reduce stress, which in turn helps improve immunity. "It's up to you to make your workspace uplifting and nurturing, as opposed to cold and sterile," Dr. Meletis says. "We all need that dangling carrot, something to look forward to at the end of the day."

If you are able, get out and mingle. Research has shown that people who have strong social networks are healthier than those who lack them, Dr. Meletis says. So regularly hang out with friends and family. Join a cooking class, a photography class, or another community group that interests you. Stimulating interactions with pleasant people will have a positive impact on your immune function.

Laugh a lot. "As they say for cancer patients, give 15 hugs and get 25 laughs per day," Dr. Meletis says. This same immune-enhancing prescription can apply to people who spend a lot of time indoors. Just because you are inside doesn't mean you can't have some fun. "Throwing some humor into conversations and seeing the glass as half full throughout the day really contributes to a nourishing environment," he says. In fact, some scientific evidence confirms the power of laughter. Researchers at Loma Linda University School of Medicine in California found that the positive emotions evoked by laughter actually increase levels of certain immune cells.

PART V

Immune Accelerators: Fight Back against Illness

Allergies

If TV ads for allergy medications are to be believed, life without nasal allergies means feeling like Maria from *The Sound of Music*—standing in a hilltop meadow, arms outstretched, twirling and singing, "The hills are alive . . . " For someone *with* nasal allergies, the hills are alive with allergens, and the sound of coughing and sneezing drowns out any music.

The symptoms of nasal allergies are all too familiar to most of us: sneezing; stuffy nose; coughing; postnasal drip; watery eyes; and itchy eyes, nose, and throat. Afflicted children may end up with allergic shiners (dark circles under their eyes, caused by increased bloodflow near the sinuses) and an allergic salute (a crease mark on the nose caused by too much upward rubbing). The misery certainly has lots of company: Thirty-five million Americans suffer from nasal allergies. Each year, seasonal allergies—nasal allergies that occur at certain times of year—are responsible for 4 million sick days and $3 billion in medical costs.

A different type of allergy, food allergy, affects 2 percent of adult Americans and 8 percent of kids younger than 3. Symptoms of food allergies include flushing, hives, rash, swelling, runny nose, coughing, wheezing, and anaphylaxis (symptoms of which include a decline in blood pressure, trouble breathing, and shock).

The Immunity Link

Have you ever heard of a situation in which a local fire department—lights flashing, sirens blaring—races to answer a call, only to discover someone tripped the alarm by burning popcorn in the microwave? An allergy attack is something like that. It's your body's immune system responding to a false alarm.

In the case of nasal allergies, the immune system mistakes a normally harmless substance—such as grass pollen, household dust, or mold—for a threat and launches an attack against it. As soon as the allergen lands on the lining inside your nose, it triggers a chain reaction that prompts immune cells called mast cells to release histamine and other chemicals. These powerful chemicals contract certain cells that line small blood vessels in the nose, allowing fluid to escape and causing nasal passages to swell. This sets the stage for nasal congestion, as well as other allergy symptoms—sneezing, itching, irritation, and excess mucus.

"The main player inducing an allergic response is an antibody called IgE [immunoglobulin E]," says Michele Columbo, MD, a specialist in allergy and immunology in private practice in Bryn Mawr, Pennsylvania. "People with allergies produce IgE antibodies against foods or inhalants. These antibodies in turn trigger a series of biologic reactions, the end result of which is allergy symptoms.

"Other substances such as cytokines also play a very significant role in inducing the allergy symptoms and perpetuating their occurrence," she adds.

You can develop allergies at any age, but exposure to allergens at times when your body's defenses are depleted, such as after a viral infection or during pregnancy, increases your risk.

To add insult to injury, people who have allergies often are sensitive to more than one substance. Among the most common allergens are pollens, dust mites, mold spores, latex rubber, insect venom, and certain medications. The top allergy-causing foods are shellfish, fish, and nuts.

Protect Yourself

Allergies do tend to occur before adulthood, so it may be too late for you to avoid them, but you can take steps to help protect your kids or grandkids.

Get a pet. Scientists have discovered that during the first year of children's lives, those who are raised in homes with two or more dogs or cats are 66 to 77 percent less likely to develop allergic diseases than kids without furry pets. The bacteria carried by the animals might inhibit the immune system's allergic response. Interestingly, this appears to protect kids not only from pet allergies but other allergies as well.

Put down the Swiffer. Exposure to dust and dirt at an early age may make kids less likely to develop allergies. These days, our environments are so clean and sterile that babies don't encounter things in the environment that normally would cue the immune response in a nonallergic direction.

If you're a new mom, breastfeed. Several studies have found that babies who are breastfed for 6 months or more are less likely to develop food or nasal allergies.

Hold off introducing some foods. Wait until your child's digestive system matures (after age 1) to introduce cow's milk, wheat, corn, citrus, and soy—and even longer (after age 2) before adding fish, shellfish, peanuts, and tree nuts (such as almonds, cashews, and pecans).

"Individuals can be genetically predisposed to developing allergies," Dr. Columbo notes. "However, a genetic predisposition is not by itself sufficient to cause allergic disease. What you need is a recurrent exposure to the substance that triggers allergy symptoms."

Heal Yourself

If you already have allergies, you needn't just live with them. The following measures can help alleviate symptoms—if not reduce your chances of an allergic response in the first place.

Just stay away. "Once a person has developed an allergy, the first, most important measure is to try to reduce or eliminate exposure to the offending agent," Dr. Columbo says. This is absolutely essential with food allergies, for which reactions can be serious and even fatal.

Try the herbal route. A new herbal supplement called Aller-7 may stop your sneezing. It seems to control mast cells, which contain allergy-inducing chemicals. Scientists in India gave 545 people with hay fever 1,320 milligrams a day (the recommended dosage) of Aller-7. Incredibly, more than 90 percent reported improvement in their symptoms. You can buy Aller-7 at www.drugstore.com or www.gnc.com.

Another herb, butterbur, has shown promise in providing relief from nasal allergies. One Swiss study found the herb to be just as effective as prescription allergy medication at halting congestion, runny nose, and coughing. The researchers came to this conclusion after giving 330 people with allergies 24 milligrams of butterbur extract, a dose of fexofenadine (Allegra), or a placebo every day for 2 weeks. Look for butterbur supplements that contain 7.5 milligrams of petasin, which is the herb's active ingredient.

A third herbal remedy, the blue-green algae spirulina, also may prove helpful against allergies. In a study conducted at the University of California, Davis, spirulina reduced by 32 percent levels of the immune proteins that can trigger allergy symptoms. One brand is Earthrise Spirulina IL-4. The dose is one pill, four times a day.

Clean house. Making small changes in your home environment can yield big results in getting rid of potential allergens. You might want to try the following:

- Dust and vacuum weekly.

- Get rid of wall-to-wall carpeting, which is an allergen trap.

- Try an antiallergen carpet cleaner to kill mites. You can find these cleaners in home-improvement centers.

- Sleep on hypoallergenic pillows and a synthetic mattress.

- Seal your pillows and mattress in covers designed to block allergens.

- Wash bedding once a week in hot water.

- Keep any pets out of your bedroom.

- Keep your bedroom especially clean, as it probably is the room where you spend most of your time.

- Ban smoking from your home.

- Get rid of roaches. Their excrement can trigger allergies (and also asthma).

- Open your windows periodically to improve ventilation and usher out indoor pollutants.

- Buy the best air cleaner you can afford.

- Shower after being outdoors to remove pollen from your skin and hair.

- Dry clothes and bedding indoors to keep them from collecting pollen.

- Replace high-allergen outdoor plants (such as juniper) with low-allergen plants (such as yew).

Stimulate your immune system. Homeopathy is based on the principle that minuscule doses of a substance that normally triggers symptoms can instead stimulate healing. One study conducted in Scotland found that allergy symptoms declined by 28 percent in people given homeopathic remedies, compared with 3 percent in people given a placebo. The study used a homeopathic nasal spray called Dolimed, which you can find online.

Head to the drugstore. According to one study, over-the-counter drugs may be more effective than prescription medications at controlling allergy symptoms. Researchers at the University of Chicago gave 58 people with hay fever either the prescription drug montelukast sodium (Singulair) or OTC pseudoephedrine hydrochloride (Sudafed 24 Hour) for 2 weeks. While both medications relieved sneezing and itchy eyes, Sudafed cleared stuffy noses more than twice as well.

Stick it to your allergies. Acupuncture is thought to stimulate the body's infection-fighting and painkilling chemicals. They, in turn, help to restore the body's energy flow, which can be disrupted by the allergic response. Visit the American Academy of Medical Acupuncture's Web site (www.medicalacupuncture.org) for a list of accredited therapists.

Read labels. Manufacturers are required by law to list potential allergens on their food labels. People with severe food allergies should wear medical alert bracelets and carry injectable epinephrine (it comes in a portable container that looks like a pen), which helps prevent a full-blown allergic reaction. When injected into the thigh and absorbed into the bloodstream, epinephrine works rapidly to contract blood vessels, preventing them from leaking fluid, and it relaxes airways, relieves gastrointestinal cramping, reduces swelling, and blocks itching and hives.

"If you have food allergies, paying attention to what you put on your skin is almost as important as what you put into your mouth," says Rallie McAllister, MD, MPH, a board-certified family physician and author of *Healthy Lunchbox: The Working Mom's Guide to Keeping You and Your Kids Trim*. "A new study at Children's Memorial Hospital in Chicago revealed that more than one-quarter of all children's skin-care products tested contained at least one common allergenic food, such as cow's milk, egg, soy, wheat, peanuts, or tree nuts. In some cases, the use of allergen-containing skin-care products can trigger the symptoms of an allergic reaction in susceptible people."

On the Horizon

Stay tuned for these possible breakthroughs in allergy treatment.

Chocolate-flavored medicine. Scientists from Imperial College London gave theobromine, a compound found in chocolate, to 10 volunteers, who then received capsaicin to induce coughing, a common allergy symptom. The theobromine proved to be nearly three times more effective than codeine-based cough medicine at calming the coughs. Could chocolate-flavored allergy medications be far behind?

Allergy gene identification. Heredity is a huge factor in determining who will develop allergies. For example, a child of two parents with allergies is 75 percent more likely to develop allergies than a child of parents without allergies. Likewise, the sibling of a child with a peanut allergy is 10 times more likely to be allergic than a child from an allergy-free family. Scientists are trying to identify and describe the genes that make people susceptible to allergies.

Low-allergen peanuts. USDA researchers found that when they added polyphenol oxidase—an enzyme in apples—to nuts, it restructured the proteins that cause allergic reactions. The change may prompt the body to recognize these proteins as nutrients, not invaders. If additional research is successful, this technology could yield new food-processing techniques that could lower the risk of allergic reactions to peanuts.

Perhaps even better, scientists at North Carolina Agricultural and Technical State University in Greensboro have discovered a fermentation process that could reduce the peanut's ability to trigger an allergic response. The process breaks down two major allergenic proteins into easily digested particles. The researchers hope to engineer a 100 percent allergen-free peanut.

TEST YOURSELF

Is It Allergies or a Cold?

It's hard to tell for sure, but if a runny nose, sneezing, and cough last longer than a week or two, it's most likely allergies.

Alzheimer's Disease

As we age, we expect our memories to falter now and then. "I'm having a senior moment," we joke. But the symptoms of Alzheimer's disease are more than just lapses in memory. And they certainly are no laughing matter. According to the Alzheimer's Association, the 10 most common signs of Alzheimer's are:

- Memory loss
- Difficulty performing familiar tasks
- Problems with language
- Disorientation to time and place
- Decreased judgment
- Problems with abstract thinking
- Misplacing things
- Changes in mood or behavior
- Changes in personality
- Loss of initiative

This list may be all too familiar to the loved ones of the estimated 4.5 million Americans with Alzheimer's disease. And that number is climbing rapidly. In fact, it has more than doubled since 1980 and, by 2050, could reach between 11.3 million and 16 million, as life expectancies continue to increase. Nationally, the cost of caring for people with Alzheimer's is at least $100 billion a year.

The Immunity Link

While the exact cause of Alzheimer's disease is unknown, one leading theory attributes it to the development of plaques or tangles in the brain, according to Rallie McAllister, MD, MPH, a board-certified family physician and author of *Healthy Lunchbox: The Working Mom's Guide to Keeping You and Your Kids Trim*. These structures, which interrupt the transmission of messages between nerve cells, occur with the accumulation of protein fragments called beta-amyloid plaques.

Because the brains of people with Alzheimer's show signs of chronic inflammation, another theory proposes that the immune system contributes to progression of the disease. Researchers suspect that a seizure, head trauma, or stroke causes the brain to release a chemical called glutamate. Too much of this chemical reduces the ability of certain brain cells to protect themselves from the immune system, leaving the brain vulnerable to diseases like Alzheimer's.

Protect Yourself

The good news is, you can take steps to reduce your risk of Alzheimer's disease. For example:

Drink to your health—prudently. By now, you probably have seen or read reports of how resveratrol, a compound in red wine, can lower levels of beta-amyloid peptides, a characteristic feature of Alzheimer's. But other research, published to less fanfare, also has pointed to the potential protective effects of moderate alcohol consumption. For example, in a study at the University of Wisconsin–Madison involving 500 people with family risk factors for Alzheimer's, those who averaged one or two drinks per week scored 6 percent higher on word-recall tests than those who abstained or averaged less than one drink a week. A separate study found that people who consumed up to seven drinks a week had 7 percent lower levels of a chemical linked to Alzheimer's risk than people who were heavy drinkers. Interestingly, abstainers had even higher levels of this chemical.

The key here is *moderation*. Too much alcohol can be toxic to the brain. If you don't drink, you shouldn't start just for your brain's benefit. If you do drink, be very careful not to overdo. Healthy drink limits are two a day for men and one for women. But put down that 32-ounce beer stein! A drink is defined as 12 ounces of beer, 5 ounces of wine, or 1½ ounces of liquor. Each contains 12 to 14 grams of alcohol.

Go fish. When researchers from the US Department of Health and Human Services analyzed almost 500 medical studies, they found that consuming high amounts of eicosapentaenoic acid (EPA) and docosahexaenoic acid (DHA) may help ward off

Alzheimer's disease and dementia. These are two of three types of omega-3 fatty acids, the beneficial fats found in significant amounts only in marine life—particularly cold-water fish, which need more fat for insulation in frigid seas.

The Alzheimer's Association asserts that "high intake of omega-3 fatty-acids may reduce the risk of dementia and cognitive decline." However, the organization doesn't offer specific recommendations for how much fish to eat. Because omega-3 fatty acids offer protection against heart disease as well, the American Heart Association recommends two to three 3- to 4-ounce servings of cold-water fish per week. The best sources of omega-3s include salmon, mackerel, sardines canned in oil, trout, mussels, sea bass, and white tuna canned in water.

Don't like fish? Fish-oil capsules seem to work just as well. Take 500 to 600 milligrams a day of EPA and DHA combined. Studies show that daily supplementation can reduce Alzheimer's risk by as much as 60 percent.

Find berried treasure. Berries are full of plant hormones called lignans, which may help prevent Alzheimer's disease. A study by Dutch researchers of 394 women found that those who consumed at least 1 milligram of lignans per day had 49 percent better memory scores. "When it comes to boosting your brainpower, the blueberry seems to be especially beneficial," Dr. McAllister says. "Natural substances in blueberries help block the action of damaging free radicals on brain tissue.

"According to researchers at Tufts University, eating a diet rich in blueberries may reverse much of the mental and cognitive decline that occurs with aging," she continues. "The researchers found that diets rich in blueberries significantly bolster levels of brain chemicals that influence learning and memory." Broccoli is another good source of lignans.

Lace up your running shoes. Exercise slows changes in the brain associated with the progression of Alzheimer's disease. How? Researchers at the University of California, Irvine, may have the answer. They discovered that active mice that spent time running on wheels developed fewer plaque-forming beta-amyloid protein fragments in their brains than sedentary "couch potato" mice. The researchers hope that more studies will show whether exercise has the same effect in humans.

But don't just go for a mindless jog day after day after day. Mix up your fitness routine. Researchers at Johns Hopkins University found that seniors who always did the same workout were 56 percent more likely to suffer from dementia than people who pursued four or more physical activities each week. Researchers suspect that the physical and mental challenge of changing workouts may engage more areas of the brain.

Slim down. Add Alzheimer's disease to the very long list of problems brought on by too many trips through the drive-thru. (Do you *still* want fries with that?) Excess weight may raise Alzheimer's risk by contributing to insulin resistance. Researchers at the University of Washington found that people with insulin resistance had 50 percent higher levels of brain and spinal cord inflammatory chemicals as well as beta-amyloid proteins. These two levels are believed to be building blocks of Alzheimer's disease.

In fact, researchers from Brown University in Providence, Rhode Island, think that Alzheimer's could be a third type of diabetes—after the insulin- and non-insulin-dependent types. When they examined the brains of people who had died, they found that insulin levels were five to six times lower in the brains of those who'd had Alzheimer's, compared with the brains of those who were healthy. Lower insulin levels are a sign of insulin resistance. If brain cells develop insulin resistance, the researchers say, it could explain the tangled fibers and plaques characteristic of Alzheimer's.

Heal Yourself

As researchers continue to work toward a cure for Alzheimer's disease, conventional medicine offers several medications that may delay the progression of symptoms. A few nondrug treatments may help as well.

Consider this herb. Ginkgo biloba is a staple of Chinese medicine. "Individual ginkgo trees have been known to survive as long as a thousand years," Dr. McAllister notes. "So it's not surprising that the Chinese believe that the herb promotes human longevity. Traditional Chinese healers employ ginkgo biloba extract in the treatment of most age-related disorders." The herb also has become popular in Europe, where it's used to ease the cognitive symptoms associated with a number of neurological conditions.

On the US side of the pond, a study conducted at the New York Institute for Medical Research found that some people with Alzheimer's showed modest improvements in cognition, activities of daily living such as eating and dressing, and social behavior when taking ginkgo biloba. However, more research is needed to confirm the possible benefits. A multicenter trial with about 3,000 participants is investigating whether ginkgo may help prevent or delay the onset of Alzheimer's. "Scientists aren't sure exactly how ginkgo biloba extract works," Dr. McAllister says. "But they do know that it promotes bloodflow and prevents damage to tissues, especially in the brain. Ginkgo compounds also may block chemicals that injure and destroy nerve cells.

"Like all herbs, ginkgo is a potentially powerful drug," she notes. "If you're thinking about taking it, be sure to talk it over with your doctor first. Your best bet is to buy a product labeled EGb 761, the preparation used in most clinical studies. It also is the formulation approved by Germany's Commission E, the organization recognized as the world's leading authority on herb and plant medicines."

Don't be a rolling stone. One moss might help fight Alzheimer's disease: huperzine A, a moss extract that has been used in traditional Chinese medicine for centuries. Interestingly, it has properties similar to those of tacrine (Cognex) and donepezil (Aricept), both FDA-approved Alzheimer's medications. These drugs are cholinesterase inhibitors; they prevent the breakdown of acetylcholine, a chemical messenger in the brain that is important for memory and other cognitive skills. Small studies have shown that huperzine A may be as effective as the drugs, but large-scale trials are needed to confirm the results.

In spring 2004, the National Institute on Aging launched the first US clinical trial of huperzine A as a treatment for Alzheimer's disease. The doses in the studies range from 60 to 200 micrograms of natural (not synthetic) huperzine A each day. As of this writing, the study is ongoing. For now, you should try huperzine only with your doctor's recommendation and monitoring.

Fight AD with E (and C). Doctors often prescribe vitamin E supplements to their Alzheimer's patients because the supplements may help brain cells defend themselves from attacks by free radicals. These renegade oxygen molecules can injure cell structures and genetic material. The damage, known as oxidative stress, may play a role in Alzheimer's. A study from Johns Hopkins found that among 4,700 people, those who took vitamin E along with vitamin C were 64 percent less likely to develop Alzheimer's. Interestingly, taking the supplements together reduced risk more than taking them separately.

Safe ranges are 150 to 200 IU for vitamin E and 250 to 500 milligrams for vitamin C. Most people can take vitamins C and E without side effects, but it's best to consult your doctor before beginning supplementation. This is especially true if you are taking blood thinners, since vitamin E can act as a blood thinner, too.

On the Horizon

Look to the future for these possible breakthroughs in Alzheimer's treatment.

Sage. How ironic! The herb sage is being studied as a possible therapy for Alzheimer's disease.

New drugs. Scientists are working to develop new drugs to protect against Alzheimer's by blocking or reducing levels of glutamate after a brain injury.

A vaccine. Researchers continue their search for a possible Alzheimer's vaccine.

Could You Have Early Alzheimer's Disease?

This simple test, developed by researchers in Great Britain, may identify early Alzheimer's disease. Grab a watch with a second hand and write down all of the animals that you can think of in 1 minute. The researchers found that healthy people could name 20 to 25, while those with Alzheimer's could name only 10 to 15. They also tended to choose simpler words, such as *dog*. So give yourself extra credit if you included *platypus* in your list.

Asthma

Asked to describe an asthma attack, one little girl put it this way: "I feel like a fish out of water." Coughing, wheezing, and shortness of breath are hallmarks of this breath-taking condition.

Approximately 11 million Americans—10 to 12 percent of the population—have asthma. And the number keeps growing. Since 1980, asthma cases have increased by 75 percent. Asthma is the most common reason for pediatric emergency room visits and hospital admissions and the leading cause of school absences. By some estimates, the economic costs of the condition exceed $12 billion a year.

The Immunity Link

Though the actual cause of asthma isn't known, studies have identified several factors that predispose a person to the condition. These include genetics, the growth and development of the lungs and immune system, various types of infection, and certain exposures in the environment. Some experts think that asthma is a sign of an overactive immune system. Research has shown that the immune systems of children and adults with asthma respond differently than those of people who are asthma free. Many people with asthma also have allergies, which means that their immune systems overreact to substances such as pollen, mold, and cat dander that generally don't cause problems. In some cases, the immune system may overreact to substances such as a virus or bacteria, which also could increase asthma risk.

When asthma begins in adulthood, 25 percent of the time it's because of exposure to an occupational toxin such as isocyanates, chemicals used in manufacturing to make, for example, paints and plastic. Experts believe these chemicals can cause the immune system to go into hyperactive mode. "In the development of asthma, there's something called the hygiene hypothesis," says Michael G. Marcus, MD, director of pediatric pulmonology and allergy/immunology at the Maimonides Medical Center in Brooklyn, New York. "Over the past 20 years, we generally have seen more and more allergic diseases such as asthma, eczema, and hay fever. All of these diseases seem to be on the rise in developed, Western countries. In Third World countries where hygiene and infections are more of a problem, we don't see allergy-related diseases quite as often.

"One of the things that we've learned is that there's a portion of our immune system—cells called T lymphocytes—that can travel one of two different roads," he explains. "If these cells are exposed to an infection, they will walk the road to help fight that infection. If these cells are not exposed to an infection, then in people with a genetic predisposition, they will walk the road to trigger an allergic response.

"The key is that these cells can do only one thing at a time," he says. "You can never have an elevation of your infection-fighting T lymphocytes at the same time that you have an elevation of your allergy-producing T lymphocytes. So the theory goes that because we live in an environment where we tend to have less infection [because we practice good hygiene and vaccinate] and use lots of antibiotics, we suppress the portion of the immune system that fights infection. This allows the allergy portion of the immune system to dominate, and we end up with more allergy-related diseases."

Protect Yourself

In about 75 percent of cases, asthma first appears in childhood, when developing lungs are more susceptible to it. If you're concerned that asthma may affect the children in your life, or think that you may be at risk, here's what you can do to help stave off the disease.

Breastfeed. "Breastfeeding's impact on asthma risk is controversial," says Dr. Marcus. "The studies go both ways. But breastfeeding at an early age decreases the severity of viral infection, so I do encourage it."

Stay well. "One thing that you can do to try to prevent asthma in your children is to minimize their risk of getting a viral infection in the first 6 months of life," Dr. Marcus says. "This is especially important in premature infants, who are at high risk for RSV [respiratory syncytial virus]. That's why all premature babies should be given the RSV vaccine." According to the Centers for Disease Control and Prevention, RSV is the most common cause of bronchiolitis and pneumonia among infants and children under 1 year of age.

Follow doctors' orders. "Make sure that your children take their medications appropriately," Dr. Marcus says. "For example, don't ask for antibiotics for every red throat. Work with your child's doctor to avoid antibiotics whenever possible."

Butt out. Keeping kids away from secondhand smoke is one of the best ways to reduce their asthma risk. "Exposure to cigarette smoke increases the risk of developing asthma five- to tenfold," Dr. Marcus notes. "In fact, if you're pregnant, or even trying to get pregnant, stop smoking now."

Breathe free. Long-term exposure to irritants such as indoor chemicals and air pollutants is a major risk factor for developing asthma. Keep your environment as nontoxic as possible.

Stay slim. Some research points to a possible link between obesity and asthma. In one study conducted at the University of New Hampshire in Durham, researchers found that levels of immunoglobulin E (IgE), a marker for asthma, were three times higher in obese women than in normal-weight women. Another study, this one from the Norwegian Institute of Public Health, found that as weight increases, so does asthma risk. The researchers examined data collected from 135,000 people over the course of 21 years. They found that for every 1 percent increase beyond a body mass index of 25, a person's chances of getting asthma go up by 10 percent. Some experts theorize that excess weight pressing on the lungs may trigger asthma.

Frequent the produce aisle. Antioxidants may cut asthma risk. A study at Cornell University in Ithaca, New York, found that kids with higher blood levels of the antioxidants vitamin C, beta-carotene, and selenium were 10 to 20 percent less likely to have asthma than kids with lower levels of these antioxidants. So fill your plate with strawberries, raspberries, and sweet bell peppers for vitamin C; cantaloupe, mangoes, and pink grapefruit for beta-carotene; and nuts and fish for selenium.

Pass the margarine. When German scientists examined the diets of more than 500 people, they found that men who ate 4 grams of margarine a day, on average, were 2½ times more likely to develop asthma than men who ate less of the spread. The scientists suspect that the culprit is a certain type of trans fat found in margarine. So make the switch to trans fat–free margarine, or use butter instead.

Heal Yourself

Once you develop asthma, it's critical to find ways to minimize attacks. Here are a few ideas to try, with your doctor's blessing.

Find a fishy solution. A study found that fish-oil supplements may keep asthma symptoms at bay. Researchers at Indiana University in Bloomington gave 16 people with exercise-induced asthma either fish-oil capsules or a placebo. The people who took the fish oil daily for 3 weeks showed a 64 percent improvement in lung function, and their use of emergency inhalers declined by 31 percent. The researchers concluded that the healthy fats in fish oil may reduce inflammation in the airways. The supplements used in the study contained 3.2 grams of eicosapentaenoic acid (EHA) and 2 grams of docohexaenoic acid (DHA), two of three types of omega-3 fatty acids. Other than supplements, these fats are found in significant amounts only in marine life—particularly cold-water fish, which need more fat for insulation in frigid seas.

Breathe better with herbs. A joint study between China and the United States found that a blend of three Chinese herbs—reishi mushroom, licorice, and sophora root—may ease moderate asthma symptoms as effectively as a prescription medicine. In the study, researchers gave more than 90 people with asthma either the herb blend or the steroid prednisone. After a month of daily treatment, both groups had less than half as much wheezing and shortness of breath. However, just 5 percent of those taking the herb blend experienced side effects, compared with 15 percent of those taking steroids. In addition, those taking the medication gained an average of 6 pounds and were three times more likely to report stomach discomfort.

Houseclean. People who don't dust (surely you're not one of *them*!) may be at increased risk for asthma, according to a study by researchers at the University of Iowa in Iowa City. The researchers first interviewed 831 families, then analyzed their homes (wearing white gloves, no doubt). Those living in dusty conditions were twice as likely to suffer from asthma symptoms as those living in clean conditions. The researchers suspect that endotoxins—chemicals that are released by the bacteria in dust and can irritate the lungs—are to blame.

According to the study, the highest concentrations of endotoxins occur in kitchen and living room dust. But that's no excuse to simply shut your dusty bedroom door. The study showed that the chances of having asthma symptoms were nearly three times greater in people exposed to high levels of endotoxins in the bedroom, where most of us spend 8 to 10 hours each night. For tips on how to minimize allergens in your home, see "Clean House" on page 293.

Time exercise right. After tracking almost 5,000 people with asthma for 5 years, researchers from Long Island Jewish Medical Center in New Hyde Park, New York, concluded that the lungs are 20 percent more powerful at 5:00 p.m. than at noon. Why? Lung function is governed by circadian rhythms, much like sleep, body temperature, and even pain tolerance.

Say ohm. Taking 20-minute hatha yoga classes three times a week for 6 weeks can significantly improve breathing capacity, according to researchers in Thailand. Poses such as Camel, Cat, and Tree help increase expansion of the chest wall.

Try biofeedback. With biofeedback training, subconscious or involuntary bodily processes (such as heartbeats or brain waves) become perceptible to the senses, so they can be regulated by conscious mental control. One study found that people with asthma who received biofeedback training experienced fewer symptoms, used less medication, and improved their lung function.

Get a shot. "A cold or the flu can play a significant role in aggravating the symptoms of a person with asthma," says Michele Columbo, MD, a specialist in allergy and immunology in private practice in Bryn Mawr, Pennsylvania. "While there are no very effective means to avoid a cold, all patients with asthma should receive the flu shot prior to flu season. In fact, the occurrence of flu in an asthmatic patient presents an increased risk of pneumonia."

On the Horizon

"We're learning that people with asthma respond very differently to medications, depending on their genetics," Dr. Marcus says. "We're beginning to identify different genes that will allow us to predict what medication a person will respond to best. Ten years from now, we may be able to take a blood sample from someone, send it to a genetics lab, and receive a report that the person should respond to medications A, B, and C but not D or E. That will give us the means to treat that patient in the best possible way. Right now, it's more trial and error."

TEST YOURSELF

Is It Asthma or a Cold?

Ask yourself the following questions.

1. Are you coughing, especially after exercise or at night?
2. Are you wheezing?
3. Do you have difficulty breathing?
4. Does your chest feel tight?
5. Do you *not* have a runny nose, congestion, sneezing, or fever?

   Answer more with yes than no? You're most likely dealing with asthma. More noes? It's probably a cold.

Cancer

Flip a coin. If you're a man, that coin tumbling in the air represents your chances of developing cancer. If you're a woman, your odds are slightly better. According to the American Cancer Society, one of two American men and one of every three American women will have some type of cancer at some point.

Although there are many different kinds of cancer, all of them begin the same—with cells in a part of the body growing out of control. Normal cells grow, divide, and die in a nice, orderly manner. Cancer cells also grow and divide, but they don't die. Instead, they outlive normal cells and, like reproducing rabbits run amok, continue to form new abnormal cells. The scary thing is that all of this can be happening inside your body, and you're blissfully unaware. Often cancer produces no symptoms. Among the early warning signs that can occur:

- Persistent cough or blood-tinged saliva
- A change in bowel habits
- Blood in the stool
- Unexplained anemia
- A lump in the breast or discharge from the breast
- A lump in the testicles
- Change in urination
- Blood in the urine
- Persistent hoarseness or swollen glands

- A change in a wart or mole
- Indigestion
- Trouble swallowing
- Unusual vaginal bleeding or discharge
- Persistent genital itching
- Unexplained weight loss
- Sores that won't heal
- Headaches
- Back pain
- Pelvic pain
- Bloating

It's important to talk with your doctor about any lingering symptom that doesn't clear on its own. Odds are that it isn't cancer—but if it is, early diagnosis and treatment offers the best possible chance of a cure. And if you're healthy? You still can make lifestyle changes to reduce your cancer risk.

The Immunity Link

"The immune system is responsible for protecting the body against that which is not the body; it's the issue of self versus nonself," says John Rothman, PhD, vice president of clinical development at Advaxis, a biotechnology company working to develop cancer vaccines. "When the immune system recognizes something nonself, it attacks it, kills it, and clears it from the body.

"The immune system evolved to deal with pathogens like bacteria and viruses," he continues. "Cancer is a tough case, however, because it starts out as self and ends up as nonself over a slow process that can fool the immune system. Cancer also has evolved in ways that enable it to hide from the immune system." There are three aspects to the cancer–immunity connection.

1. A strong immune system protects you against cancer. Tumors develop when the immune system breaks down or becomes overwhelmed. "We know that the immune system has tremendous power for preventing cancer," says Susan Silberstein, PhD, founder and executive director of the Center for Advancement in Cancer Education (www.BeatCancer.org). "Research shows that a healthy body can seek out and destroy 100 to 1,000 cancerous cells every day as part of its built-in surveillance mechanisms."

Tumors can only grow in laboratory animals that have been bred with malfunctioning immune systems. "Also, organ-transplant patients will reject their foreign tissue unless they're given the same immunosuppressive drugs that are given to cancer patients," Dr. Silberstein notes. "Because of this, they get cancer at a higher rate than the average population.

"When the United States bombed Japan, there was a lot of radiation fallout and a vast increase in cancer incidence," she continues. "But there were a lot of people right in the radiation area who never got sick. The question isn't why those who got cancer got it but why those who didn't get cancer didn't. The answer is: the integrity of their immune systems."

2. Immune cells, like other cells, can grow uncontrollably, resulting in cancer. Leukemias, for example, occur with the proliferation of white blood cells, or leukocytes. Likewise, the uncontrolled growth of antibody-producing plasma cells can lead to multiple myeloma. Cancers of the lymphoid organs, known as lymphomas, include Hodgkin's disease.

3. Long-term overactivation of the immune system may cause cancer. When the immune system goes into overdrive, it leads to the inflammation of tissues. This creates the conditions necessary to encourage the growth and spread of cancer.

Protect Yourself

Though some risk factors for cancer, such as age and family history, are beyond our control, others involve our lifestyle habits and choices. For example, study after study has shown that a healthful diet—eating fewer "bad fats" and more fruits, vegetables, legumes, and whole grains—can vastly reduce cancer risk. In fact, research indicates that if all of us ate more of the right foods and less of the wrong ones, the incidence of all cancers would drop by at least 30 percent.

Get moving. An extensive amount of research has shown that you not only feel better when you're physically active, you're also healthier. "It's been estimated that about one in every three people in Westernized countries is physically unfit and sufficiently sedentary to raise the risk of breast, colon, and prostate cancers," says Keith I. Block, MD, cofounder and medical and scientific director of the Block Center for Integrative Cancer Care in Evanston, Illinois. "This represents a large part of the cancer burden—one that could be greatly reduced if people took up a regular exercise program.

"I tell my patients that the anticancer benefits they derive from exercise depend on how much energy they wish to put into it," he continues. "Even if you burn as few as 500 calories a week in exercise—the equivalent to about an hour's worth of brisk walking, or less than 10 minutes a day—you'll lower your cancer and heart disease risks substantially, compared with people who are almost completely sedentary. On the other hand, if you burn 2,000 calories a week [about 4 hours of brisk walking], your risk drops far more."

Keep stress in check. "Battling what's eating you is also important in the prevention and treatment of cancer," Dr. Silberstein says. "The field of psychoneuroimmunology, now 30 years old, demonstrated that emotional stress is absolutely connected to susceptibility to all disease, and definitely to cancer. We know that stress affects nervous system function, hormone levels, and immunological response.

"You can't get away from stress. How you cope is the question," she observes. "As Sir William Osler, the father of modern medicine, said, it's less important what kind of disease the patient has than what kind of patient has the disease. There's been a great deal of research looking at coping strategies and risk for cancer, as well as personality types and risk for cancer. Some personality types were found to be a greater predictor of death from lung cancer than even smoking.

"The important thing isn't the stress that you experience, which you can't change, but your perception of that stress, which you can change," Dr. Silberstein concludes. (For tips and tools to help cope with stress, see page 255.)

Wash up. "It's becoming increasingly clear that certain cancers, such as cervical cancer, are associated with other forms of transmissible diseases, such as viruses," Dr. Rothman says. "The cleaner you are, the fewer transmissible diseases you will catch. You can't avoid all of these diseases simply by washing. However, if there is a link between certain cancers and ingested pathogens—which you could pick up from utensils, cups, and other surfaces and then transfer into your body when you touch your eyes, nose, and mouth with dirty hands—the cleaner you are, the lower your cancer risk will be."

Skip the saturated fat. "Most of immunity boils down to lifestyle factors—in particular, what you're eating and what's eating you," Dr. Silberstein says. "There are foods that can suppress immune function and foods that can enhance immune function." At the top of Dr. Silberstein's list of dietary changes to prevent and control cancer is the elimination of saturated fat. "We know that saturated fat from animal sources is associated with increased growth of cancer," she says.

Another concern revolves around growth hormones such as bovine growth hormone, which has been implicated in breast and prostate cancer. "Organic meats and dairy products are better [than nonorganic], but you can't eat or drink them with impunity," Dr. Silberstein notes. "Even if you buy organic dairy products, they contain insulin-like growth factors that instruct cancer cells to replicate."

Stifle that sweet tooth. "White sugar is dangerous in terms of promoting cancer," Dr. Silberstein says. "Sugar is cancer's favorite food. We call cancer tumors obligate glucose metabolizers because they are sugar feeders. Cancer cells will use up glucose [blood sugar] five to 10 times faster than healthy cells." What's more, eating sugar suppresses the immune response—and the more sugar you eat, the more your immune system falters. "If you eat 10 teaspoons of sugar a day—whether it's in your tea, breakfast cereal, dessert, or even ketchup—you're going to see a 50 percent decline in phagocytosis," she says. This is the process by which immune cells called phagocytes engulf and ingest bacteria and other foreign microorganisms.

It isn't just the amount of sugar you eat that matters; it's also the frequency with which you eat it. Research has shown that within an hour of eating a moderate amount of sugar, immune response declines by 38 percent. It drops even further, by 44 percent, after 2 hours. "The curve eventually comes back up to baseline, but only after 5 hours," Dr. Silberstein says. "By then, you're probably ready for another sugar fix."

Color your plate. Carotenoids—the pigments that naturally occur in plants, such as the beta-carotene that gives carrots and cantaloupe their orange color—are very high on the list of foods and beverages with antitumor activity. "A lot of people focus on beta-carotene, but there are more than 600 carotenoids," Dr. Silberstein says. These substances have two main benefits. The first is their antioxidant properties, which enable them to neutralize free radicals. The second is their ability to support immune function.

"Hundreds if not thousands of studies have shown how carotenoids inhibit cancer and boost immune function," she says. "They stimulate the T-helper cells that turn on the immune response, and they help the body produce its own interferon." (Interferons are proteins released in response to challenges by foreign agents, such as viruses, bacteria, parasites, and tumors.) For example, a study by the National Cancer Institute found that people with the highest intakes of carotenoids were up to six times less likely to develop skin cancer than those with the lowest intakes.

Experts recommend getting carotenoids from foods rather than supplements, as foods contain other compounds that may be interacting with the carotenoids to enhance their protective effects. Good sources include carrots, pumpkin, sweet potato, mango, and kale.

Read the tea leaves. Tea is one of the most popular beverages in the world, ranking second only to water, according to Rallie McAllister, MD, MPH, a board-certified family physician and author of *Healthy Lunchbox: The Working Mom's Guide to Keeping You and Your Kids Trim.* "Traditionally, Americans have been more likely to go for a slug of coffee than a spot of tea, but times are changing," she says. "And with good reason. In the past decade, dozens of studies have demonstrated the healing powers of the tasty brew." In some of those studies, tea has proven its ability to prevent certain kinds of cancer. For example, women who drank 2 cups of tea a day were 46 percent less likely to develop ovarian cancer. Each additional cup of tea per day was associated with an additional 18 percent decline in risk.

Tea helps maintain the immune system through its abundant antioxidant supply. "The polyphenols in teas serve as powerful antioxidants," Dr. McAllister says. "In the body, these agents help neutralize unstable molecules called free radicals, high-energy renegades that contribute to the development of a number of deadly diseases, including cancer. As antioxidants go, those in tea seem to be far more potent than the ones in most fruits and vegetables. They're also about 100 times more effective than vitamin C and nearly 25 times more effective than vitamin E."

Green tea (*Camilla sinensis*) in particular is very stimulating to the immune system. "It contains polyphenols, catechins, and EGCG (epigallocatechin-3-gallate)—all antioxidant compounds," Dr. Silberstein says. "White and black teas also contain antioxidants, but in nowhere near the amounts in green tea."

There's a catch, however. "In order to get the health benefits of green tea, you have to drink lots of it," Dr. McAllister says. "In preliminary studies, scientists have found that people who gulp 4 to 10 cups of green tea every day seem to have a lower overall risk of cancer."

That said, if you can get even a modest immune boost by sipping green tea, why not give it a try? If you don't like the taste of green tea, steep it with an herbal type that you do like, or add a little stevia to it. (Stevia is an herbal sweetener that's been in use in South America for hundreds of years. The leaves can be 30 times sweeter than sugar.)

Brew up some more antioxidants. Tea may be a great source of antioxidants, but another beverage tops it as the number one source of antioxidants in the standard American diet. It's coffee.

Researchers at the University of Scranton in Pennsylvania found that no other food or beverage in the US diet comes close to coffee in contributing to our total antioxidant intake. Truth be told, of all the fruits and beverages in the study, even dates have more antioxidants than coffee, per serving. Then again, people drink a whole lot more coffee than they eat dates. And that may not be a bad thing at all.

"Although scientists once believed that coffee might increase the risk for a variety of cancers, it has since been disproved," Dr. McAllister says. "As it turns out, regular consumption of the brewed beverage appears to offer a measure of cancer protection." One study, from Japan, found that people who drank coffee daily or almost daily were about half as likely to develop a certain type of liver cancer, compared with people who never drank coffee. Most interestingly, the risk of cancer declined with an increase in the amount of coffee consumed each day.

Coffee may have another protective effect as well. Researchers determined that drinking 2 or more cups of decaf coffee appears to lower the incidence of rectal cancer by a whopping 52 percent. The researchers theorize that coffee's benefit comes from its ability to speed transit time and increase bowel movements. (They don't know why decaf is more protective than regular coffee, however; after all, both decaf and regular brews supply the same amount of antioxidants.)

Of course, as with other dietary strategies, moderation is key. One study found that people who drank 2 or more cups of java a day had higher levels of the inflammatory markers linked to heart disease. You should talk with your doctor about your coffee consumption if you have blood pressure problems because the caffeine in regular coffee can increase heart rate. It also can interfere with sleep, of course.

Go fishing. Fish has a well-earned reputation as a cancer fighter. In one Harvard University study involving nearly 48,000 men, those who ate fish more than three times a week were 40 percent less likely to develop advanced prostate cancer than those who ate fish only twice a month.

Among the beneficial nutrients in fish are omega-3 fatty acids. "There are three main types of unsaturated fats: omega-3s, omega-6s, and omega-9s," Dr. Silberstein explains. "What's important is the ratio between them. Omega-3s stimulate the immune system, in effect turning it on. Too many omega-6s suppress the immune system, in effect turning it off. Omega-9s are essentially neutral.

"What you want is an immune system that isn't turned off all the time nor on all the time," she continues, "so your ratio of omega-6s to omega-3s should be 1 to 1. However, in the typical American diet, it's about 25 to 1. That's 25 to 1 *against* your immune system."

Don't like fish? Try flaxseed. "Another food that has specific anticancer properties is flaxseed," Dr. Silberstein says. "Like fish, flaxseed is a good source of omega-3 fatty acids. It also contains lignans. Because it's high in fiber, it decreases intestinal transit time, which reduces the risk of colon cancer. Flaxseed also influences prostaglandin E, which is a type of chemical that can slow down your immune system and allow tumor cells to metastasize. Flaxseed can inhibit tumor growth by influencing prostaglandin chemistry and keeping it from doing its dirty work." One study of 25 men with prostate cancer found that a low-fat diet supplemented with ground flaxseed reduced serum testosterone, slowed the growth rate of cancer cells, and increased the death rate of cancer cells.

Dr. Silberstein recommends taking 2 heaping tablespoons of freshly ground gold flaxseed per day. "Start with 1 teaspoon and work your way up, so your gut can get used to the extra fiber," she says. "You can stir the flaxseed into smoothies or applesauce, roll it on a banana, sprinkle it on cooked grain or cereal, or serve it on salad or steamed vegetables."

On the Horizon

"We are really on the cusp of significant immunological advances against cancer," Dr. Rothman says. "The learning curve was a lot steeper than we thought 30 years ago. We are learning how to work with the immune system by using a lot of different modalities together—to stimulate some areas of the immune system and inhibit others, and to stimulate the immune system in ways that get it to recognize cancers as being nonself needing attack and allowing that attack to occur in a therapeutic way. We're not all the way there yet, but over the next decade, possibly as close as 5 years, you're going to start hearing more about very effective immune therapies for cancer." For more information on therapeutic cancer vaccines, see page 16.

Colds and Flu

Achoo! Cross your fingers that the woman standing behind you in the supermarket checkout line covered her nose and mouth when she sneezed. Infectious particles from a sneeze can spray at speeds of up to 200 miles an hour, land at a distance of 3 feet, and survive there for more than 24 hours. No wonder colds spread so easily.

According to some estimates, we Americans suffer a collective one billion colds a year. Adults average two to four a year—though the number drops to less than one a year among those over age 60. Children average six to 10. That means that every second, someone somewhere in the United States is catching a cold. (There goes another person, and another, and another. . . .) The economic tally is substantial, with colds costing 50 million sick days and $5 billion in remedies.

The news about influenza isn't much better. Every year, 5 to 20 percent of Americans come down with the flu. It's responsible for about 36,000 deaths annually.

The Immunity Link

Simply put, your immune system helps protect you from colds and flu by fending off viruses before they gain a foothold. If by chance you do get sick, your immune defenses will continue to fight until the cold or flu bug is out of your system. "The immune system is critical in preventing both viral and bacterial infections, as well as in supporting recovery from infections," agrees Michael G. Marcus, MD, director of pediatric pulmonology and allergy/immunology at the Maimonides Medical Center in Brooklyn, New York. "Different sections of the immune system respond at different times in the process. Some sections stop bacteria and viruses from entering the body or at least limit their ability to do so. Other sections actually fight the infection once it starts."

"Surprisingly, most of the symptoms associated with colds are caused not by cold viruses themselves but, rather, by the reaction of your body's immune system," adds Rallie McAllister, MD, MPH, a board-certified family physician and author of *Healthy Lunchbox: The Working Mom's Guide to Keeping You and Your Kids Trim*. "The copious mucus secretions that make you cough, sniffle, snort, and blow are a big part of the problem.

"In as little as an hour after a cold virus has infected the lining of your nose and throat, the invaded cells begin to release chemicals called prostaglandins," she explains. "These chemicals attract white blood cells to the site of infection to battle the meddling microbes. As the disease-fighting white blood cells report for duty, they begin to pile up by the millions in your nose, throat, and chest, producing the massive flow of mucus that contributes to stuffiness and congestion."

Protect Yourself

Before you decide to lay in supplies and hole up at home for the next cold and flu season, read on. There's much you can do to keep cold and flu bugs at bay.

Clean up. According to Dr. Marcus, the most important self-care strategy for avoiding colds and flu is to keep viruses from gaining entry into your body in the first place. This means practicing good oral hygiene (including brushing your teeth regularly), washing your hands frequently, and avoiding contact with people who are sick.

As for washing your hands, you may be wondering whether you should be using an antibacterial soap, especially during cold and flu season. Actually, at least one study has shown that ordinary soap eliminates germs just as well. What's more important than which type of soap you use is how long you scrub. The Centers for Disease Control and Prevention recommends washing your hands in warm water for about 10 to 15 seconds. Incidentally, only 58 percent of people wash their hands after sneezing or coughing. That's enough reason for you to be extra-diligent about it.

Replace your toothbrush. The American Dental Association recommends changing your toothbrush every 4 months. This is especially true for electric brushes, which harbor more germs than manual brushes.

Eat yogurt. When researchers compared 94 workers who took a daily dose of the probiotic *Lactobacillus reuteri* with 87 workers who took a placebo, they found that the probiotic group reported 56 percent fewer colds. The researchers suspect that the beneficial bacteria may have helped stimulate the immune system. Currently, the only brand of yogurt available in the United States with this strain of bacteria is Stonyfield Farm. As an alternative, you can take a daily dose of 100 million live bacteria in supplement form. Look for the supplements in the refrigerated section of health food stores.

C some protection. Increasing your intake of certain vitamins and minerals may help prevent colds and flu, Dr. Marcus says. Vitamin C, for example, can be helpful if it's taken at the first sign of symptoms. "An extra 1,000 milligrams a day probably is sufficient," he says. "Don't take more than 2,000 milligrams a day."

In addition, don't continue taking vitamin C after your cold is gone. "Chronic use doesn't help as much as a short-term extra burst," Dr. Marcus explains. "If you take vitamin C all of the time, your body adapts to it and eliminates any extra to bring levels back to normal."

Try an herbal boost. In one study, only 10 percent of people who took 400 milligrams of the herb American ginseng every day from November to February got two or more colds, compared with 23 percent of people who took a placebo. In addition, those in the herb group reported milder symptoms.

But buyer beware. "Lots of natural products say that they prevent colds and flu, but the problem is that many of them aren't standardized," Dr. Marcus explains. "So you don't know how much of the active ingredient you actually are getting in each pill."

One product, Cold-fX, *is* standardized, and studies have shown that it has some benefit. "Cold-fX contains polysaccharides from the herb ginseng, which has been shown to enhance the immune system," Dr. Marcus says. "It seems to both prevent colds and shorten their severity if you take it at the first sign of infection."

Move your body. Another way to boost immune function is to get active. "We're not sure why exercise enhances the immune system," Dr. Marcus says. "In part, it improves cardiovascular conditioning, so your heart and lungs work more effectively. Your heart and lungs are responsible for delivering immune cells to the site of an infection. With better conditioning, the cells get to where they need to be faster, and they work better."

Through 10 years of studies, researchers at Appalachian State University in Boone, North Carolina, monitored the effects of exercise on the immune system by comparing the illness rates of couch potatoes with those of people who were physically active. Participants who went for a brisk 45-minute walk every day ended up taking half as many sick days as the nonexercisers. "Taking a 20- to 30-minute walk 3 or 4 days a week is a good target for your immune system to work optimally," Dr. Marcus says. Don't overdo it, though, as too much exercise actually can undermine immune function. "Ultramarathoners and even marathoners tend to have problems with their immune systems because they over-exercise," Dr. Marcus says.

Slim down. A bonus of all that exercise is that it can help achieve and maintain a healthy weight. "Obesity makes the immune system less effective," Dr. Marcus says. When researchers from Tufts University in Boston asked a group of slightly overweight people to cut 100 to 200 calories from their daily intakes, the participants lost weight as expected. In addition, their immune systems showed improved response to disease-causing microorganisms.

Be a social butterfly. Spending too much time alone can weaken your immune system. We're talking not about a few glum weeks after, say, you take a new job but, rather, about persistent loneliness lasting more than 4 months.

Researchers at Carnegie Mellon University in Pittsburgh studied the social interactions of 83 people and compared them with blood samples taken before and after flu shots. They found that people who were isolated had 21 percent weaker immune responses than people who were more social. The researchers surmised that the stress of social isolation may cause physiologic changes that interfere with immune function.

Cheer up. Studies dating back 20 years show that people who are suffering from depression have impaired immune responses. Those same studies show that if people deal with their depression, their immune systems begin to work effectively again. "Mental health clearly has an impact on how well we're able to fight infection," Dr. Marcus says. He encourages people to maintain a positive outlook on life and seek treatment for persistent depressive symptoms. (For more on the connection between depression and immune function, see page 258.)

Stay warm. Chalk up another one for Mom: Being cold actually may make you more susceptible to cold viruses. Welsh scientists had half of their 180 volunteers put their feet in cold water for 20 minutes. Within a month, 29 percent of the chilled participants caught colds, compared with just 9 percent of those who got to stay warm and dry. In theory, getting chilled may hamper immune function.

Try a new tissue. If you're especially worried about getting sick—let's say your spouse or office mate has come down with a cold—hand the person a box of antiviral tissues, which contain a special layer that traps and kills viruses. One study found that the tissues, made by Kleenex, reduced the spread of colds and respiratory infections by 10 percent.

Bare your arm. The best way to avoid the flu is to get a flu shot. Studies show that it's effective in 70 to 90 percent of healthy people under age 65, as long as the vaccine and the circulating virus are a close match. Among those over age 65 who don't reside in nursing homes, the flu shot is 30 to 70 percent effective in preventing

Don't take aspirin for a cold! Research has shown that using aspirin to treat cold symptoms increases the amount of virus shed in nasal secretions, possibly making you more of a hazard to others. Plus, aspirin—as well as acetamino-phen (Tylenol)—can suppress certain immune responses and increase nasal stuffiness.

hospitalization for the flu or pneumonia. It's 50 to 60 percent effective for nursing-home residents over age 65. If the vaccine is in short supply, ask for FluMist nasal spray vaccine. It received FDA approval in 2003 and is recommended for healthy people ages 5 to 49.

Heal Yourself

If despite your best efforts you end up with a cold or the flu, it's time to hunker down, manage your symptoms, and get on the road to recovery as quickly as possible. The flu, in particular, should prompt a trip to the doctor. Prescription antiviral drugs, such as oseltamivir (Tamiflu) and zanamivir (Relenza), can ease your misery and shorten symptoms. The catch is, you must take them within 48 hours of the onset of symptoms.

Eat right. Though a cold or the flu can sap your appetite, it's important to maintain optimal nutrition while you're sick. Otherwise, your body won't be able to fend off the invading germs. A study at Stanford University found that virus-fighting helper T cells depend on the nutrients in foods to do their jobs properly.

Sip some soup. "Chicken soup is the ideal remedy for the common cold," Dr. McAllister says. "Its healing powers have been proven in the laboratory." In one study conducted at Nebraska Medical Center in Omaha, researchers found that chicken soup contains a number of medically beneficial substances. Its mild anti-inflammatory effect soothes many of the miseries that accompany upper respiratory tract infections. "In the laboratory, chicken soup has been shown to stop the migration of white blood cells to the site of infection," she notes. "This action helps reduce the production of mucus and the degree of congestion experienced by cold sufferers."

Consider adding some garlic to your chicken soup recipe. Garlic contains potent compounds that attack viruses. Mash or mince it finely to release allicin, garlic's active component, before tossing it into your soup pot.

Try a berry good remedy. Elderberry extract fights the flu. A study conducted in Norway showed that people who took the herb recovered from the flu 4 days faster than people who didn't. In addition, their symptoms were less severe, and they didn't experience any side effects. At the first sign of symptoms, take either 1 tablespoon of elderberry syrup or 1 lozenge four times a day.

Send out for seafood. You probably don't feel like cooking or even going out, so have someone bring you oysters, clams, lobster, or crab. All of these shellfish are rich in the mineral selenium. In a British study, getting enough selenium increased immune cell production of proteins called cytokines, which can help clear the flu virus from your body.

Relax. Even if you're not a stress-prone person, just having a cold or the flu taxes your body. Any relaxing activity can help reduce your stress level and enhance your immune function. (For suggestions, see pages 92 and 254.) In fact, if you're able to relax, you may not get as sick. A Carnegie Mellon study revealed that the most stressed-out people have the worst flu symptoms.

TEST YOURSELF

Is It a Cold or the Flu?

Ask yourself the following questions.

1. Did your symptoms come on suddenly, like getting hit by a Mack truck (A), or did they sneak up over time (B)?
2. Do you have a fever of 102°F or higher (A) or no fever (B)?
3. Are you exhausted (A), or can you push through your symptoms? (B)
4. Do you have a headache (A) or not (B)?
5. Do your muscles ache (A) or not (B)?
6. How's your stomach? Do you have nausea, vomiting, or diarrhea (A) or no digestive symptoms (B)?

More As than Bs suggests that you probably are down with the flu. More Bs than As suggests that it's more likely a cold.

Still not sure? Your doctor can confirm a flu diagnosis in 10 minutes by swabbing the back of your throat or nose and testing the specimen.

On the Horizon

"We may not find a cure for the common cold in our lifetimes," Dr. Marcus says. "But we may be in a position that we won't feel its effects so badly.

"The interactions between our mental health and our immune function will continue to be a fascinating area of exploration," he adds. "Another area of exploration will be the impact of nutrition and specific nutrients on immunity. A third area will involve determining how different portions of the immune system communicate with each other through a variety of chemical transmitters and mediators. The better we're able to understand the interaction between sections of the immune system, the better we'll be able to influence and improve this interaction."

Crohn's Disease

A life with Crohn's disease is not a spontaneous one. Needing to always know the location of the nearest bathroom and perhaps even packing toilet paper and a change of clothes "just in case" can make going out seem like more trouble than it's worth. Yet this is the reality for the more than 500,000 Americans with Crohn's disease, a chronic condition that's characterized by inflammation in the digestive tract. It can affect any part of the digestive tract, but it most commonly strikes the lower section of the small intestine, causing diarrhea and abdominal pain, often in the lower right abdomen. Rectal bleeding, joint pain, skin problems, fever, and weight loss also may occur. The symptoms can be mild or severe, waxing and waning without warning.

The Immunity Link

The exact cause of Crohn's disease remains a mystery. Some experts, though, believe that it stems from a problem in the body's immune response. "The immune system has T-helper cells and T-suppressor cells," explains Mark Fleisher, MD, director of the Infusion Therapy and Immune Mediated Inflammatory Disorder Clinics at the Borland-Groover Clinic in Jacksonville, Florida. "In AIDS patients, for example, the T-suppressor cells are overactive, so the immune system is underactive. In conditions such as Crohn's disease, however, it's the opposite. The T-helper cells are overactive, which means that the immune system is overactive. It goes into overdrive making cytokines, which are inflammatory mediators. It's as though a firework shoots into the air, releasing a plume of cytokines.

"For some people, this manifests as digestive problems such as Crohn's disease," he continues. "For others, it manifests as skin problems such as psoriasis or as joint problems such as rheumatoid arthritis. Basically, all of these people have the same illness; it just has been given different names."

Other experts suspect that a protein produced by the immune system, called antitumor necrosis factor, may cause the inflammation of Crohn's. Yet another theory is that the disease may be triggered by a fundamental flaw in the body's immune response: The immune system mistakes foods and other substances as foreign invaders and attacks them. During this process, white blood cells accumulate in the lining of the intestines, producing chronic inflammation and eventually leading to the ulcerations associated with Crohn's.

Protect Yourself

Crohn's disease seems to have a genetic link. People of Jewish heritage are at higher-than-average risk for Crohn's, while African Americans are at lower-than-average risk. Of course, you can't choose your parents or ethnicity. However, you can do at least one thing to reduce your own risk: If you smoke, quit. Smoking increases your chances of developing Crohn's.

Heal Yourself

If you have Crohn's disease, you should be under a doctor's care. The following measures are meant to complement conventional therapies. Be sure to discuss them with your doctor before adding them to your treatment regimen.

Supplement. Research from the United Kingdom suggests that taking a combination of fish oil and antioxidants may help control Crohn's symptoms. In one small study, researchers observed that symptoms declined by almost half among people with Crohn's who were given 2.7 grams of fish oil and a mixture of antioxidants each day. The researchers theorize that the omega-3 fatty acids in fish oil prevent white blood cells from attacking the intestinal lining, while the antioxidants repair previously damaged areas. If you'd like to try this remedy, take a multivitamin—which will contain plenty of antioxidant vitamins C and E—and a fish-oil capsule with an enteric coating. This will ensure that the capsule dissolves in your small intestine, where it's needed most. (The volunteers in the study took more than 2 grams of fish oil a day.)

Eat right. No specific dietary guidelines seem to improve or worsen the symptoms of Crohn's. That said, maintaining a healthy diet is important for people with the disease to avoid malnutrition and weight loss. It may help to keep a food diary to see if any particular foods worsen diarrhea. Then you can avoid those foods in the future.

Know that it's not your fault. For a long time, conventional wisdom held that Crohn's disease was associated with having a certain personality type or being "overly emotional." Researchers now know that this is not the case. "Patients and families need to remember that Crohn's disease is a blameless illness," Dr. Fleisher says. It isn't your fault, and "just calming down"—as some well-meaning people may suggest—won't help. As Dr. Fleisher observes, "There are plenty of surfers in Laguna Beach with Crohn's, and they're pretty mellow folks.

"Stress, such as having a hard time at work, has not been shown to cause a flare-up of Crohn's disease," he says. "However, having a flare-up is likely to cause stress and problems at home or at work."

Push to get better. "It's a sad truth that many people with chronic conditions such as Crohn's disease have very low expectations," Dr. Fleisher says. "Many of them have had their illnesses for decades and have seen five or six doctors. My job is to raise their expectations. 'Don't settle for this level of discomfort,' I tell them. 'Push me to help you get better.'

"One patient of mine with Crohn's disease had to use an ostomy bag for 25 years," he recalls. "After 6 months of maximizing her treatment, including inflix-imab (Remicade) therapy, she used toilet paper for the first time in almost 3 decades. That's the best present I've ever given anyone."

Food Poisoning

The stories never fail to make headlines: "*E. coli* sickens 39 in New York and New Jersey," "500 stricken by hepatitis A from a Pennsylvania Mexican restaurant." Outbreaks of food-borne illness definitely should be taken seriously. But the fact is, you're more likely to contract food poisoning at home than at a restaurant. (After all, the local health inspector probably hasn't knocked on your door asking to see your kitchen.) When researchers at Tennessee State University in Nashville checked the refrigerators in 210 homes, they found moldy, spoiled, or outdated foods inside almost one-quarter of them.

Commonly referred to as the stomach flu or a 24-hour bug, food poisoning typically strikes within hours or days of eating an offending food. Typically, the culprit is any one of a number of bacteria—such as *Escherichia coli, Campylobacter, Listeria,* or *Salmonella*—although viruses, parasites, and chemicals also can cause trouble.

According to the Centers for Disease Control and Prevention, there are more than 250 types of food-borne illnesses. In the United States, the incidence of food poisoning is on the rise. Our food chain is longer today than it was in the past, which means our food supply passes through numerous hands before it reaches our tables. Consider that up to 80 percent of supermarket chickens are contaminated with *Salmonella* or *Campylobacter* during the production process.

Symptoms of food poisoning can be mild or severe, depending on the status of your immune function and the amount of contamination. Nausea, vomiting, diarrhea, fever, and body aches are most common, but certain food-borne illnesses can produce long-term health effects, such as arthritic conditions, heart complications, kidney failure, and central nervous system disorders.

Each year, 76 million Americans—one in five of us—fall sick with food-borne illnesses, and 5,000 die. Among the most vulnerable to infection are pregnant women and their fetuses; young children, whose immune systems aren't fully developed; the elderly, whose immune systems have weakened with age; and those with compromised immune systems, as in cases of cancer and AIDS. Alcoholism and depleted stomach acid (due to surgery or regular use of antacids) also can raise risk.

The Immunity Link

All food contains bacteria. Normally these bacteria are present only in small amounts, so the body's natural defense system is able to destroy them. If conditions are right, however, the bacteria can rapidly multiply within the food to dangerous levels. Once inside the body, the microorganisms continue to multiply in the digestive tract, causing an infection.

In addition, bacteria growing on a food sometimes produce a toxin that causes illness when eaten.

Protect Yourself

Though it's impossible to completely eliminate disease-causing bacteria from food, you can minimize your exposure to them—and therefore lower your risk of food-borne illness. Here's how.

Practice safe cooking. The following tips can help ensure the safety of your family's food supply, from the moment you buy it until the moment you eat it.

■ Keep track of when you purchase and open each item in your refrigerator, freezer, and pantry. You might want to write the date right on the packaging with a marker.

■ Pay attention to the recommended storage times on food labels. (See "Safe to Eat or Time to Pitch?" on page 329.)

■ Wash your hands before handling food, as well as after using the bathroom, sneezing, or touching your face or hair.

■ Consider all animal products and their juices to be contaminated. Be especially clean and careful when handling them.

■ Disinfect your kitchen sink once a week with ½ cup of bleach or a cleaner labeled as a disinfectant, paying close attention to the faucet and handles. The sink and faucets are hotbeds of germs because of their moist conditions and their contact with hands and uncooked foods.

■ Cool food properly. Set your refrigerator at 40°F or below. (A recent study found that 59 percent of fridges run warmer than that.) Check the temperature with a refrigerator thermometer, which you can buy in supermarkets for less than $12.

■ Freeze food at the correct temperature—0°F.

■ If possible, don't rewrap packaged meat before freezing it. Rewrapping requires more handling and increases the risk of contamination. If you must rewrap, work in a clean area with clean hands and use freezer containers, foil, or moisture-proof freezer wrap.

■ Thaw frozen foods in the refrigerator or microwave, never on the counter. Bacteria can start multiplying on the food's outer layer long before the inner layer thaws.

■ Keep raw foods away from cooked foods.

■ Thoroughly wash produce to remove bacteria. Fully immerse in water and rinse, or use a vegetable wash product.

■ Don't wash meat, fish, and poultry before cooking, despite what you learned in home ec. Doing so allows bacteria to spread all over the kitchen.

■ Use separate utensils and cutting boards for foods that need to be cooked (such as raw meats, poultry, seafood, and eggs) and those that may not be cooked (produce and sandwiches). You could buy cutting boards of different colors, or simply label them with a permanent marker.

■ Wash utensils and cutting boards either by hand (with soap and hot water) or in the dishwasher after each use.

■ Monitor the cooking temperature of foods so that it's hot enough to destroy bacteria. (See "Hot Stuff" on page 330.) Cook food to the proper temperature and without interruption.

■ Cook stuffing separately from poultry. The turkey or chicken cavity is the perfect environment for bacterial growth.

■ Make leftover marinade safe for basting by boiling it for 5 minutes to kill any bacteria the uncooked meat may have left behind.

■ Wash your hands immediately after handling raw meat or poultry.

■ Wipe down countertops and sinks with a disinfecting spray or hot soapy water, using disposable cloths or paper towels.

Safe to Eat or Time to Pitch?

It's not likely to surprise anyone that food left out on the counter isn't safe to eat for long. But while refrigeration slows bacterial growth, it doesn't stop the process. Even freezing doesn't kill bacteria. It just puts them to sleep for a while.

Yet most people overestimate how long their foods are safe to eat. Researchers at Utah State University in Logan discovered that 31 percent of people ate leftovers that were more than a week old, which is several days past the danger zone.

Here are guidelines for the storage limits of some common foods.

FOOD	KEEP IT FOR
In the Refrigerator	
Cheese, hard, opened	3–4 weeks
Cheese, hard, unopened	6 months
Cheese, soft	1 week
Condiments	6 months
Leftovers	3–4 days
Lunchmeat, opened	3–5 days
Lunchmeat, unopened	2 weeks
In the Freezer	
Fruit	12 months
Ground meat, raw	3–4 months
Ice cream	2–4 months
Meat, cooked	3–4 months
Meat (steaks and roasts), raw	12 months
Pork, raw	12 months
Poultry, raw	12 months
Vegetables	12 months
In the Pantry	
Baking powder	3 months
Baking soda	12 months
Canned goods, unopened	2–5 years
Herbs	6 months
Oils, opened	1–3 months
Oils, unopened	6 months
Pasta	12 months
Rice	12 months
Spices, ground	6 months
Spices, whole	2 years
Sugar	12 months

■ Throw out your kitchen sponge. It's party central for bacteria. Use paper towels instead.

■ Never eat raw shellfish. They can harbor bacteria or viruses.

■ Don't eat undercooked eggs. Even sampling uncooked cake batter or cookie dough is risky. (Cookie dough ice cream is okay because it uses pasteurized eggs.)

■ Don't eat foods from bulging cans. The swelling could be a sign of bacterial contamination.

■ Hold foods at the proper temperature—for example, keep them hot (or cold) while they're being transported or set out for a buffet.

Wash up. Wash your hands before eating—especially in scenarios such as stopping for gas and buying food inside the minimart, where your hands come into contact with tons of germs. This is when an alcohol-based hand sanitizer can come in handy. When researchers from Children's Hospital Boston tracked 292 families over 5 months, they found that the families who used hand sanitizers developed 59 percent fewer gastrointestinal infections than those who didn't. If it just isn't possible to scrub up or sanitize, then try to keep your fingers away from your eyes, nose, and mouth.

Go organic. Research has shown that conventionally raised chickens are more likely to carry bacteria than organically raised chickens. Scientists at Johns Hopkins University in Baltimore tested four brands of chicken for drug-resistant *Campylo-*

Hot Stuff

To kill bacteria, it's critical to heat foods to certain temperatures. Common indicators such as pink meat or clear juices are no guarantees. Use an instant-read food thermometer to be sure. Measure at the thickest part of the meat toward the end of the cooking time.

FOOD	HEAT IT TO
Chicken breasts	170°F
Fish	140°F
Ground meat	160°F
Lamb	145–170°F (depending on thickness)
Pork	160°F
Roast beef	145–160°F (depending on thickness)
Whole poultry	180°F

bacter, a cause of food poisoning. They found bugs in a whopping 96 percent of Tyson and 43 percent of Perdue chickens but only 13 percent of organic Bell & Evans and 5 percent of organic Eberly chickens.

Pick a dry plate. At a salad bar or buffet, don't take a wet plate. Plates stacked before they're dry may be a breeding ground for bacteria.

Beware the buffet. Who knows how long that food has been sitting there and how warm or cold it's been kept?

Be like Sally. Like Meg Ryan's character in *When Harry Met Sally . . . ,* don't be afraid to make your preferences clear when ordering in a restaurant. Ask for meat to be cooked well done, never rare or medium. Send back any food that you think is undercooked, such as chicken that is pink near the bone.

Order the red. Drinking wine with your meal actually may ward off food poisoning. Scientists at Oregon State University in Corvallis discovered that wine kills three common food-borne bugs: *E. coli, Listeria,* and *Salmonella.* In laboratory studies, the ethanol, organic acids and low pH of wine appear to scramble the genetic material of bacteria. Although all wines help, red offers the most protection.

Wash up after touching animals. It's possible to contract *E. coli* and other germs at petting farms. So pack away any food when in the animal area; keep your hands away from your eyes, nose, and mouth; scrub your hands and fingernails with soap and water after touching the animals; and change your clothes and shoes as soon as you get home.

Heal Yourself

If you contract food poisoning, you surely will feel it. The nausea, vomiting, diarrhea, fever, and body aches can be quite debilitating. Try the following strategies to help speed your recovery.

Drink up. Drinking fluids is critical for preventing dehydration and flushing out the bug that caused your food poisoning in the first place. "At the first sign of diarrhea, you should start chugging fluids," advises Rallie McAllister, MD, MPH, a board-certified family physician and author of *Healthy Lunchbox: The Working Mom's Guide to Keeping You and Your Kids Trim.* "Water and clear broth are okay, but sports drinks may be even better because they replace minerals that are lost in stool. Usually they're loaded with sugar, an ingredient that can cause diarrhea on its own, so it may be a good idea to dilute them with equal parts water."

While you're sick, avoid beverages that contain alcohol and caffeine. Both work as diuretics and can rob your body of additional fluids.

Eat chocolate! Yes, you read that right. Chocolate may help ease diarrhea.

According to one study, catechin—a flavonoid in cocoa—blocks CFTR, the gene that regulates fluid loss in your small intestine and causes diarrhea. Try one or two snack-size bars of dark chocolate. White and milk chocolate don't contain as many flavonoids, and too much cocoa can cause constipation.

Sprinkle on some cinnamon. It's a home remedy for diarrhea. Try adding it to food or stirring it into tea.

Be a BRAT. "When you have diarrhea, drinking definitely is more important than eating," Dr. McAllister says. "But if you're starving, it's okay to eat as long as you stick to foods that are easy on your innards." Most doctors recommend the BRAT diet—bananas, rice, applesauce, and toast. These foods are easy to digest, she explains, so they won't add insult to your intestinal injury.

Take a break. "When you have diarrhea, it's a good idea to get plenty of rest," Dr. McAllister says. "You'll need to save your strength for the 100-yard dash to the bathroom."

On the Horizon

Stay tuned for these possible breakthroughs in preventing and treating food-borne illnesses.

Using fish mucus. Trout secrete mucus that battles bacteria. Researchers in Britain are studying the mucus to see which bugs it can beat. So far, it has stopped both *E. coli* and *Salmonella*, with more tests to come.

Destroying germs by shock waves. Scientists in Mexico are developing a system that uses shock waves to kill germs in food. So far it's most successful against *Listeria* bacteria, which can infect poultry and deli meats.

Posting health department grades. Since 1997, Los Angeles restaurants have been required to post their grades where customers can see them. Since then, food poisonings have fallen by 13 percent. Perhaps other cities will follow suit.

HIV/AIDS

In the United States, the first reported case of AIDS occurred in 1981—though in fact, the disease probably arrived on our shores several years earlier. Since then, AIDS—shorthand for "acquired immunodeficiency syndrome"—has become a major pandemic. As of the end of 2003, HIV/AIDS affected an estimated 38 million people worldwide.

In the United States, as many as 950,000 people may be infected with HIV (human immunodeficiency virus, which causes AIDS), though one-quarter of them may not realize it. Here's why: A few weeks after infection, up to 70 percent of people experience fever, headache, fatigue, and enlarged lymph nodes. But because these symptoms usually linger for only a short time, perhaps a week to a month, they're often mistaken for the flu. Ironically, it's during this time that people are especially contagious because the virus is present in large quantities in genital fluids. Then the immune system fights back, and the person is symptom free, at least for a while.

The duration of this "honeymoon period" varies from one person to the next. Some people develop more severe symptoms within a few months; others may remain symptom free for more than 10 years. All the while, the virus is quietly doing its dirty work, infecting and killing CD4+ T cells and replicating rapidly. (CD4+ T cells, also known as T-helper cells, are white blood cells that orchestrate the body's immune response by signaling other immune cells to perform their special functions.)

As time goes on, the immune system starts to lose its battle with the virus. This is when complications set in. Among the late-onset symptoms are persistently swollen glands, low energy, weight loss, frequent fevers and night sweats, persistent or frequent yeast infections, persistent skin rashes or flaky skin, pelvic inflammatory disease, and short-term memory loss. It's at this point that a person is said to have full-blown AIDS.

AIDS is the most advanced stage of HIV infection. By definition, a person has AIDS when he or she has fewer than 200 CD4+ T cells per cubic millimeter of blood. A healthy adult has more than 1,000.

The Immunity Link

A person contracts HIV from contact with an infected person's blood, semen, or breast milk. The virus progressively destroys the body's ability to fight infections and certain cancers. Even though the aggressive immune response handily wipes out most viral infections, some of the HIV manages to escape. This is largely because of how quickly the virus mutates. HIV also can hide out for long periods within the chromosomes of an infected immune cell, effectively shielded from surveillance by the immune system.

As the body's immune defenses falter, a person with AIDS falls prey to unusual, often life-threatening infections that generally do not make healthy people sick. People with AIDS are particularly prone to certain cancers—especially those caused by viruses (such as Kaposi's sarcoma and cervical cancer) and those that affect the immune system (known as lymphomas). These cancers tend to be more aggressive and more difficult to treat in the presence of AIDS.

Protect Yourself

Not much in life is black-and-white, but the things to do to prevent HIV infection are pretty clear-cut. Just as you can't be "a little bit" pregnant, you can't have "a little bit" of HIV.

Avoid unprotected sex. Of new HIV infections, approximately 70 percent are spread through unprotected sex with an infected partner. The virus can enter the body through the lining of the vagina, vulva, penis, rectum, or mouth. "Right now the only preventive measure for HIV/AIDS is to use condoms and avoid unprotected sex," says Alan L. Landay, PhD, professor and chairman of the department of immunology/microbiology at Rush University Medical Center in Chicago.

Don't share drug paraphernalia. The remaining 30 percent of new HIV infections are associated with the injection of recreational drugs. Don't engage in these risky behaviors, either. Needles and syringes can be contaminated with very small quantities of blood from someone infected with the virus.

Fortunately, it's rare for HIV to pass from a patient to a health care worker, or vice versa, through accidental sticks with contaminated needles or other medical instruments.

Heal Yourself

When AIDS first surfaced in the United States, we had no medications to combat immune deficiency and no treatments for the opportunistic diseases that resulted. Medical science has made great strides since then, developing drugs to fight both the HIV infection and its associated infections and cancers. "When you have HIV/AIDS, taking the medications that you have been prescribed is the most important thing that you can do," Dr. Landay says. The following measures also are beneficial.

Maintain your weight. The Multicenter AIDS Cohort Study—conducted in Baltimore, Pittsburgh, Chicago, and Los Angeles—found that HIV-infected men who maintain their weight prior to an AIDS diagnosis live longer than men who lose a lot of weight. But eating right may not be so easy for someone with AIDS. It may help to work with a nutritionist to come up with a healthy, sustainable eating plan.

Protect unborn children. Approximately one-quarter to one-third of women infected with HIV transmit the virus to their babies during birth. However, if the mother takes certain drugs during pregnancy and delivers her baby by Caesarean section, the chances of the baby getting infected drop to just 1 percent. According to the National Institutes of Health, HIV infection in newborns in the United States has been almost eradicated because of these practices.

Don't breastfeed. New moms with HIV can pass the virus to their babies in their breast milk.

On the Horizon

A small number of people infected with HIV 10 or more years ago have yet to develop AIDS symptoms. These people are known as long-term nonprogressors. Scientists are trying to figure out how they stay healthy for so long. For example, do their immune systems have particular characteristics? Here are other frontiers that AIDS researchers are exploring.

Less toxic therapies. "The most realistic hope for the future with AIDS is the same as our most realistic hope for cancer—to take it from a fatal disease to a chronic disease," says John Rothman, PhD, vice president of clinical development at Advaxis, a biotechnology company. "Eventually, it will become something that you can live with. It won't go away, but it won't kill you, either."

New drug treatments. Researchers are working overtime trying to develop new, better drugs for AIDS. "We're just in the early stages, but one immune modulator that's being studied as a possible treatment for AIDS is a cytokine called interleukin-2," Dr. Landay says. "We also are looking at agents that block immune activation or inflammation, which may help reduce the ability of the virus to replicate because it requires an activated immune system.

"Another avenue of exploration involves drugs that have been used for autoimmune conditions or organ transplants as treatments for AIDS," he continues. "That's a faster route than developing an entirely new drug."

Microbicides. "Researchers are developing microbicides, products that women will apply vaginally before having sex to help prevent infection," Dr. Landay says. "These are currently in clinical trials." A new antiviral gel called PRO 2000 is one example. Researchers from Mount Sinai School of Medicine in New York City reported that a single vaginal dose reduced both HIV and herpes simplex virus infectivity (their capacity to produce infection) by at least a thousandfold. The product still requires much testing, but if all goes well, it could be widely available within a few years.

HIV vaccine. The first clinical trial of an experimental HIV vaccine began in 1987. Today, several vaccines are in preclinical development or clinical trials. Scientists hope that understanding the body's natural method of controlling infection may lead to ideas for vaccines that both protect against HIV infection and prevent the virus from spreading.

Lupus

Lupus is a mysterious condition. Ask anyone about it, and if they've heard of it at all, they probably don't know much about it—despite the fact that more than 16,000 Americans develop lupus each year. The condition is believed to affect between 500,000 and 1.5 million people in the United States.

The symptoms of lupus creep up slowly, over time. Its hallmark is a butterfly rash across the nose and cheeks. In fact, the name *lupus* comes from the Latin for "wolf"—a reference to the red facial rash, which can resemble a wolf's snout. Other symptoms include rashes on sun-exposed skin, sores in the mouth or nose, painful or swollen joints, hair loss, fatigue, painful breathing, purple or pale fingers or toes, headaches, and abdominal pain.

The Immunity Link

Lupus is what's known as an autoimmune disease, in which the immune system's recognition apparatus breaks down. The body begins to manufacture T cells and antibodies (called autoantibodies) directed against its own cells and organs. People with lupus have antibodies to many of their own cells and cell components, which may be why the condition causes such diverse symptoms affecting so many body parts.

"Lupus is an inflammatory autoimmune condition," says David Grotto, RD, LDN, president and founder of Nutrition Housecall and a spokesperson for the American Dietetic Association. "Some forms of it are mild and do not seem to impact quality of life at all, but other forms can be severely debilitating."

No one knows what causes autoimmune conditions like lupus, but it's likely that a few things are at work.

- First, elements in the environment—such as viruses, certain drugs, and sunlight—may damage or alter healthy cells.

- Second, because most autoimmune diseases afflict more women than men—particularly during their childbearing years—hormones such as estrogen may play a role in determining who gets an autoimmune disease and how it progresses. Lupus, in particular, strikes women 10 to 15 times more often than men. Symptoms often increase before menstrual periods and during pregnancy.

- Third, ethnicity may be a factor. Lupus is two to three times more common in African Americans, Hispanics, Asians, and Native Americans than in Caucasians. Curiously, though, only 10 percent of people with lupus have a parent or sibling who has or may develop lupus.

Protect Yourself

Scientists aren't sure what triggers lupus in a susceptible person. In some people, exposure to the sun causes a sudden rash, followed by other symptoms. In others, an infection—even a cold—doesn't get better, and then complications arise. In still others, drug therapy for another illness, especially antibiotics in the sulfa and penicillin groups, can lead to symptoms. Extreme stress can be a factor, as can pregnancy or childbirth.

Because of all the uncertainty surrounding lupus, effective preventive measures are few and far between. One that may help: Stink up the place. "It might be beneficial to increase your intake of what I call stinky vegetables, such as broccoli and cauliflower," Grotto says. "According to one study involving laboratory mice, indole-3-carbinol, a substance found in these vegetables, may prevent or delay lupus."

Heal Yourself

Just as the causes of lupus remain elusive, so does a cure. That said, your doctor can offer medications to help manage symptoms. These self-care measures may provide relief as well.

Shun the sun. For people with lupus who are sensitive to the sun, limiting exposure may reduce flare-ups. When you do head outdoors, slather on lots of sunscreen to help prevent rashes.

Try fish oil. Irish researchers found that fish oil may help treat lupus symptoms. For the study, 27 women with lupus took a 3-gram fish-oil supplement every day for half a year. Another 13 women took a look-alike placebo. Nearly half of the women who took fish oil experienced relief from facial rashes, fatigue, and joint pain. In the placebo group, 69 percent got worse or stayed the same.

"Increase your intake of omega-3 fatty acids, and go easy on omega-6 fatty acids, which are thought of as being more proinflammatory," Grotto says. "Omega-3s are found in fish and flaxseed, while omega-6s are in animal fats as well as corn, sunflower, and safflower oils. The new mid- or high-oleic versions of sunflower and safflower oils are okay." If you prefer supplements to eating fish or flaxseed, Grotto recommends taking at least 2 to 3 grams of omega-3 fatty acids per day.

Follow a balanced diet. The dietary guidelines recommended for the general population are especially important for people with lupus. Because both antibodies and other immune cells may be adversely affected by nutritional deficiencies or imbalances, not eating a healthful diet may have profound effects on immune function. "Consider limiting your protein intake, especially from dairy foods, and adopting a more plant-based vegetarian diet," Grotto says. "Scant research suggests a possible link between the dairy protein casein and autoimmune conditions such as lupus."

Multiple Sclerosis

Life with multiple sclerosis (MS) can seem like a roller-coaster ride. About 85 percent of patients have a form of the disease called relapsing-remitting MS: flare-ups characterized by worsening neurological function, followed by periods of remission. The flare-ups tend to strike without warning, causing tremendous physical, mental, and emotional distress.

In the United States, a new case of MS is diagnosed every hour. About 400,000 people have been diagnosed so far, though an unknown number may have the disease and not know it. The initial onset usually occurs between ages 20 and 40. It can be quite sudden, with symptoms such as blurred or double vision, fatigue, tingling, dizziness, lack of coordination, tremors, and diminished concentration. The mix and severity of symptoms depends on where in the brain or along the spine MS strikes. It is a progressive disease, which means it gets worse over time.

The Immunity Link

"Multiple sclerosis is considered to be an inflammatory autoimmune disease of the central nervous system," says David Grotto, RD, LDN, president and founder of Nutrition Housecall and a spokesperson for the American Dietetic Association. "It is diagnosed via MRI detection of sclerotic lesions throughout the central nervous system and brain."

Normally, nerve fibers are coated with a protective sheath called myelin. In MS, immune cells turn on and attack myelin, destroying nerves and building up scar tissue in the brain and spinal cord. Without myelin, electrical signals become scrambled. The brain can't send or receive messages, so the patient gradually loses muscle control throughout the body. MS can affect speech, vision, movement, memory, concentration, and even swallowing.

While the exact cause of MS isn't known, much is understood about its effects on the immune system. In general, people with MS have a larger number of immune cells than a healthy person. This suggests that the immune response might contribute to the disease in some way.

Protect Yourself

Since it's not clear what triggers MS, how to prevent it also remains something of a mystery. Still, research points to a few self-care measures that may help reduce your risk for the disease.

D-fend against MS. Flash back to middle school geography: If you draw a line around the earth at 45° latitude, you'll find the greatest incidence of MS above that line. It's too late to relocate, however. Studies show that it's where you lived as a child that influences your risk.

One theory about the connection between "location, location, location" and MS is that vitamin D deficiency may be a factor in the disease. Indeed, much research has focused on the relationship between vitamin D and MS. "Vitamin D deficiency is becoming more common in this country," Grotto notes. "We have an indoor society, for several reasons. One is the increased risk of skin cancer from sun exposure. Along with the rise in vitamin D deficiency, we have seen an uptick in the number of MS cases."

So how much vitamin D do you need? The current Daily Value is 400 IU, with a safe upper limit of 2,000 IU. "But some research is calling that upper limit into question," Grotto says. "Many experts think that 2,000 IU should be the starting point and that the Daily Value is just skimming the surface of how much vitamin D we should be getting."

Manufacturers have been fortifying dairy products with vitamin D for years. But other fortified foods may be available soon, Grotto says, and amounts of D are increasing. "Years ago, you'd see only about 400 IU of vitamin D per serving," Grotto notes. "But it's becoming more common to see 1,000 IU per serving." Some companies take an even more aggressive approach, putting 2,000 IU of vitamin D into each serving of their products.

Be healthier with B$_{12}$. Vitamin B$_{12}$ deficiency also is quite prevalent in MS patients. "B$_{12}$ is important to the development of the myelin sheath," Grotto says.

"When Japanese researchers gave very aggressive doses of B$_{12}$—60 milligrams per day—to people with MS, they saw improvement in sensory nerve potential." The Daily Value for B$_{12}$ is 6 micrograms, but taking up to 500 micrograms per day may be safe, Grotto says. Talk with your doctor to be sure.

Multiply your odds with a multi. "Another theory about MS is that the immune dysfunction associated with the disease is caused by oxidative stress," Grotto says. "So taking a multivitamin containing antioxidants such as vitamins C and E is a good idea.

"Eating a healthy diet rich in whole grains and fresh fruits and vegetables is optimal," Grotto adds. Good food sources of vitamin E are whole grains and vegetable oils, while you can get vitamin C from citrus fruits, sweet peppers, strawberries, and kiwifruit.

Heal Yourself

If you've been diagnosed with MS, you most likely are under a doctor's care. Treatment usually involves medications that can help modify the progression of the disease. Here are a few additional things that you might want to try, with your doctor's blessing.

Learn what aggravates your symptoms. Perhaps you feel worse when you become overly tired; adjust your daily routine accordingly. It may help to keep a journal to track your activities and identify patterns in your symptoms.

Change your oil. "The fats that you eat may be especially important when you have MS," Grotto says. "The myelin sheath and nervous system tissue depend heavily on fatty acid metabolism, so it's advisable to get more omega-3 fatty acids in your diet. These fats come primarily from fish, but if you're fish-challenged, you might take a supplement instead. Aim for at least 2 to 3 grams of omega-3 fatty acids each day."

Keep symptoms at bay with GLA. "There has been some research showing a deficiency of gamma-linolenic acid [GLA] in MS patients," Grotto says. "In fact, a meta-analysis that examined very high-dose GLA supplementation—20 grams per day—in 181 MS patients found that it reduced the severity of disability and shortened the duration of relapses." Typically, you can't get enough GLA through food, so you need to take supplements. Grotto recommends black currant oil, primrose oil, or borage oil. "Most people with MS probably should take between 1 and 2 grams of GLA each day," he says.

Go low—fat, that is. Roy L. Swank, MD, PhD, was an early pioneer in the study of dietary interventions for MS patients. Dr. Swank advocated limiting total fat intake to 20 grams per day or less—very low in fat by American standards, for sure. "But in his research, Dr. Swank demonstrated that 95 percent of his patients who were on the diet after being diagnosed with MS but before developing clinical impairment [manifesting major symptoms] did not have signs of disease progression for 35 years," Grotto says. "That's impressive. Many other practitioners have since shown less dramatic benefits with higher amounts of fat."

Get moving. Exercise such as tai chi can be helpful to manage symptoms, maintain muscle tone, and increase relaxation. According to the Multiple Sclerosis International Federation, any exercise that you enjoy and are able to do comfortably will be beneficial.

On the Horizon

Researchers are working on blood tests to diagnose MS much earlier in its onset. Studies suggest that early intervention can dramatically slow the disease's progression.

Pneumonia

Sir William Osler, often called the father of modern medicine, referred to pneumonia as the old man's friend because it offered a reasonably quick and painless trip to the afterlife. Ironically, Osler himself died from the disease.

The advent of antibiotics and supportive therapies has rendered pneumonia much more treatable than it once was. Still, it claims more than 60,000 lives a year in the United States alone. Together with influenza, it's the seventh leading cause of death in this country. It also sends about 1.2 million people to the hospital each year, making it the third most frequent cause of hospitalizations (after childbirth and heart disease).

Pneumonia is an inflammation of the lung. Most cases result from viral infections, though sometimes bacteria, fungi, or parasites are to blame. Among pneumonia's symptoms are chest pain, fever, shaking, chills, shortness of breath, and rapid breathing and heartbeat. With treatment, bacterial pneumonia usually clears up within 1 to 2 weeks. Viral pneumonia can last longer.

The Immunity Link

Unbeknownst to you, you frequently come into contact with the viruses and bacteria that cause pneumonia. You don't know it because your immune system keeps these bugs from entering your lungs and causing a problem. But sometimes, for reasons that aren't entirely clear, the bugs manage to evade your body's defenses. Once deep inside your lungs, the invading microorganisms are attacked by white blood cells (leukocytes). The accumulating pathogens, white blood cells, and immune proteins cause the air sacs of your lungs to become inflamed and filled with fluid. This leads to the breathing difficulties that characterize many types of pneumonia.

Pneumonia usually occurs when a person's immune system is weakened, most often by a simple viral infection of the upper respiratory tract or by influenza. Symptoms can set in after 2 or 3 days of a cold or sore throat. Such illnesses don't cause pneumonia directly, but they do alter the mucus blanket of the lungs, thus encouraging bacterial growth.

Pneumonia can be particularly serious for people with impaired immune function, such as those with HIV/AIDS or chronic illnesses such as cardiovascular disease, emphysema, or diabetes.

Protect Yourself

The general guidelines for staying healthy—eating a diet rich in fruits, vegetables, and whole grains; engaging in moderate exercise; and getting enough sleep—can help strengthen your immune system so that it's better able to intercept and destroy pneumonia-causing germs. You also can reduce your chances of getting sick by heeding this advice.

Fend off pneumonia with flaxseed. Alpha-linolenic acid (ALA), an omega-3 fatty acid in flaxseed, can help prevent pneumonia. When a research team from Harvard University compared the diets of 38,378 men with their disease rates over 10 years, the researchers found that a 1-gram increase in daily intake of ALA reduced a man's chances of developing pneumonia by 31 percent. The researchers think that ALA lowers the risk of infection by reducing inflammation and regulating blood sugar.

You can buy flaxseed in the health-food section of your grocery store. Grind it in a clean coffee grinder and eat 2 teaspoons each day. You can stir it into smoothies or applesauce, roll it on a banana, sprinkle it on cooked grain or cereal, or serve it on a salad or steamed vegetables.

Another source of ALA is canola oil. Get your extra gram by eating vegetables or chicken sautéed in 1 tablespoon of the oil.

Practice good hygiene. The viruses and bacteria that cause pneumonia can be spread by sneezing, sharing drinking glasses and eating utensils, or touching the used tissues of an infected person. It isn't uncommon for people, especially children, to carry the bacteria in their throats without getting sick.

Your hands, in particular, are in almost constant contact with the germs that cause pneumonia. These germs enter your body when you touch your eyes, rub your nose, or put food into your mouth. Washing your hands thoroughly and often can help reduce your risk.

An alcohol-based sanitizer can be handy if you don't have easy access to water at any given moment; in fact, it may be even more effective than water in destroying viruses and bacteria. Also, hand sanitizers contain ingredients that moisturize your skin. This is good because healthy skin without cracks or scrapes is your most effective barrier against foreign microorganisms. You might think of your skin as your immune system's first line of defense. Its protectiveness is enhanced by secretions that contain chemicals toxic to bacteria.

Curb your vices. Both smoking and heavy drinking are risk factors for pneumonia. Smoking damages your lungs' natural defenses against respiratory infections. Millions of microscopic hairs called cilia cover the surface of the cells lining your bronchial tubes. Normally, the hairs beat in a wavelike fashion to clear your airways of normal secretions. But irritants such as tobacco smoke paralyze them, allowing secretions to accumulate. If these secretions contain bacteria, they can set the stage for pneumonia.

People who drink excessively are at risk for a certain type of pneumonia called aspiration pneumonia. Alcohol inhibits the gag reflex, which normally keeps foreign materials, such as food and liquids, from entering the lungs and causing infection. Alcohol also interferes with the activity of infection-fighting white blood cells.

Get out and mingle. Spending more time with others can help strengthen your immune system to fight off pneumonia, among other infections. One study found that the more social interactions people have, the less likely they are to get colds, possibly because of declines in levels of stress hormones that can suppress immune function.

Get vaccinated. Because pneumonia can be a complication of the flu, it makes sense to get an annual flu shot, especially if you have a chronic condition such as asthma. "Everyone with asthma should receive the flu shot prior to the start of flu season," advises Michele Columbo, MD, a specialist in allergy and immunology in private practice in Bryn Mawr, Pennsylvania. "The occurrence of flu in an asthmatic patient poses an increased risk of pneumonia."

One study, conducted at the Research Institute at the Hospital for Sick Children in Toronto, found that people hospitalized for pneumonia are about one-third less likely to die if they are up-to-date on their flu vaccines.

People over age 65 should consider getting a pneumonia vaccine. However, as Dr. Columbo notes, this vaccine protects against only one common type of pneumonia. It does not prevent other types of bacterial or viral pneumonia.

Heal Yourself

Most cases of viral pneumonia clear on their own—which is a good thing, since medical science has yet to identify an effective treatment. Bacterial pneumonia generally responds to antibiotics, provided the infection is caught early on. The bacteria are becoming more resistant to drugs, which will make treating pneumonia more difficult over time.

Regardless of the type of pneumonia that fells you, these tips can help ease your symptoms and speed your recovery.

Drink plenty of liquids. This will not only prevent dehydration but help loosen mucus in your lungs. Drinking enough water keeps your immune cells plump and healthy, just as it does all your body's cells.

Cough. You may be tempted to take cough medicine, but resist. Coughing can actually help clear your lungs. Instead, use a warm heating pad to alleviate chest pain.

On the Horizon

Ongoing research may lead to new advances in preventing and treating pneumonia. Here's a snapshot of what's in development.

New drug interventions. Physicians and researchers are very concerned about certain types of bacterial pneumonia becoming resistant to standard drug therapy. One-third of cases of streptococcal pneumonia, the most frequently identified cause of pneumonia, already are resistant to many antibiotics. As bacteria develop resistance to more classes of existing antibiotics, pharmaceutical companies are racing to create new ones.

New diagnostic tool. The Cyranose 320—an electronic nose device originally developed for industrial quality control—sparked the interest of medical researchers, who have long known that smell can assist in disease diagnosis. Researchers at the University of Pennsylvania in Philadelphia tested the Cyranose 320 to see if it could

Immunity Alert

Antibiotics, which are necessary to treat bacterial pneumonia, double a woman's risk of vaginal infections. Take acidophilus or eat yogurt with active cultures to protect against vaginal infections while taking antibiotics.

diagnose pneumonia. They found a good correlation between the device and the actual clinical pneumonia score, which is the traditional way to identify pneumonia. Smiths Detection, the manufacturer of the Cyranose 320, has not pursued FDA approval to use the device for disease detection. Perhaps in the future, this technology will help doctors diagnose pneumonia more quickly and accurately.

Psoriasis

The life of a normal skin cell is rather slow-paced. The new cell forms deep beneath the skin, matures, and journeys to the surface, where it dies and sloughs off the body—all in 28 to 30 days. By comparison, a psoriatic skin cell is an overachiever. It takes only 3 to 4 days to mature and move to the skin's surface. In the most common type of psoriasis, called plaque psoriasis, psoriatic cells don't slough off but instead pile up to form thick, scaly, silvery-white plaques.

Psoriasis plaques tend to occur on the scalp, elbows, torso, and knees. Once in a while they appear in places that are more difficult to hide: on the face, nails, and palms of the hands, as well as on the soles of the feet and the genitals. Often the plaques appear symmetrically, or similarly on both sides of the body.

The classic symptom of psoriasis is itchy skin, sometimes severe enough to disrupt sleep—if not a person's entire daily routine. The skin can crack and bleed, too. Perhaps that's what inspired the old television ad catchphrase "the heartbreak of psoriasis." That certainly can ring true for the 7.5 million Americans who have this chronic skin condition.

The Immunity Link

The exact cause of psoriasis remains a mystery, though genetics may play a role. Someone whose parent has psoriasis has a 20 percent chance of developing the condition herself. It seems to be most common in Caucasians—especially people of Scandinavian descent—and less so among people of Asian, African American, or Hispanic descent. Native Americans rarely develop the condition.

Most researchers agree that in psoriasis, something prompts the immune system to shift into overdrive. The immune system consists of T-helper cells and T-suppressor cells, explains Mark Fleisher, MD, director of the Infusion Therapy and the Immune Mediated Inflammatory Disorder Clinics at the Borland-Groover Clinic in Jacksonville, Florida. In conditions such as psoriasis, there's an overexpression of the T-helper cells, prompting the immune system to accelerate production of inflammatory mediators called cytokines.

The outcome of this process can vary from one person to the next. Some people develop psoriasis; others have Crohn's disease or rheumatoid arthritis. Still others show signs of all three conditions. "The incidence of psoriasis is much higher in people with Crohn's disease than in the general population," Dr. Fleisher notes. "And people with psoriasis or Crohn's are more prone to rheumatoid arthritis. These people accumulate dermatologists, gastroenterologists, and rheumatologists, all of whom are doing the same thing—tinkering with the immune system."

Protect Yourself

Researchers believe that psoriasis requires both a genetic predisposition and then a "trigger" to actually cause the disease. With that in mind, we offer the following strategies to help prevent flare-ups if you already have psoriasis—and to reduce your risk of the disease if you don't.

Relax. According to the National Psoriasis Foundation, one of the known triggers of psoriasis is stress. It can cause a first-time flare-up, as well as a recurrence. Stress hormones compromise your health by binding to immune cells, which short-circuits the cells' ability to fight off illness. Less stress helps keep your immune system working as it should.

So take steps to keep your stress level in check. A meditation or yoga class might help you recognize the stressors in your life and teach you how to manage them. One study found that skin healed faster in people with psoriasis who listened to meditation-based relaxation tapes while using light therapy than those who didn't listen to the tapes.

Be safe. Another factor in triggering psoriasis—whether for the first time or a recurrence—is trauma or injury to the skin. It can be as innocuous as a bruise, burn, cut, or scrape. Shaving, sunburn, tattoos, vaccines, and acupuncture cause flare-ups, too. This is known as the Koebner phenomenon, named after a 19th-century doctor who discovered that a patient with psoriasis had developed new skin lesions in areas where his horse had bitten him.

People with psoriasis often notice new lesions within 10 to 14 days after skin sustains damage. According to research, this happens to about 50 percent of people with psoriasis. The good news is, it's possible to prevent a full-blown flare-up by treating the trauma or injury as quickly as possible.

Stay well. Catching a cold can have an especially unpleasant side effect for people with psoriasis. "Twenty percent of psoriasis flare-ups occur after upper respiratory infections," Dr. Fleisher says. In many cases, treating the infection alleviates psoriasis symptoms and sometimes clears up the skin completely. (See page 317 for ideas on how to enhance your body's natural defenses against these virulent viruses.)

Although it hasn't been proven, some people with psoriasis suspect that allergies can bring on a flare-up. (If you have allergies, see page 293 for ways to keep them under control.)

Follow a healthy lifestyle. The stock advice for a healthy lifestyle—eat right, sleep well, drink plenty of water—is especially important to avoid psoriasis flare-ups. "Certain lifestyles are not beneficial for chronic illnesses such as psoriasis," Dr. Fleisher says. "If you have poor dietary habits, you're not getting enough rest, or you're dehydrated, you're going to have trouble managing your condition."

Check your medicine cabinet. Some medications for other conditions can aggravate psoriasis. Among the potential offenders are antimalarials, propranolol (Inderal, for high blood pressure), indomethacin (for arthritis), lithium (for bipolar disorder and other psychiatric disorders), and quinidine (for heart conditions). If you're taking any of these medications, talk with your doctor. Perhaps your dosage can be adjusted or your medication changed.

Keep a food diary. Although unproven, dietary changes have helped some people with psoriasis minimize flare-ups. It may be helpful to keep a record of the foods you eat and the symptoms you experience to see if you notice any correlations between the two.

Moisturize. The weather can dry out skin and leave it more susceptible to a flare-up. Winter tends to be the most challenging season. Numerous studies have shown that cold, dry air is a trigger for many people, while hot, sunny climates help clear the skin. If moving to Florida isn't an option, do your best to keep your skin from drying out. Stock up on emollients and moisturizers and apply them at least twice a day, especially in winter and after bathing.

Curb your vices. Some studies suggest a link between smoking and several types of psoriasis. Smoking also may be a factor in the severity of flare-ups. Some smokers see improvement in their symptoms once they quit. Interestingly, nicotine patches actually can aggravate psoriasis because they're applied to the skin, so talk with your doctor about other options.

As with smoking, excessive drinking appears to not only trigger psoriasis but also influence the severity of flare-ups. It can undermine the effectiveness of certain treatments, too.

Heal Yourself

"There is no 'best' way to treat psoriasis," says Rallie McAllister, MD, MPH, a board-certified family physician and author of *Healthy Lunchbox: The Working Mom's Guide to Keeping You and Your Kids Trim*. "People respond favorably to different treatments, making psoriasis therapy highly individualized. Often the best course of treatment is discovered only by trial and error."

There are three main avenues of psoriasis treatment: topical preparations, medicines delivered by pills and shots, and phototherapy. According to Dr. McAllister, most creams and lotions contain steroids, though some older remedies contain crude coal or wood tar. Both work well to alleviate redness and swelling.

Your best bet is to work with your doctor to develop a regimen that's tailored to your particular symptoms. You might want to discuss the following self-care options, too.

Catch some rays. "If creams, lotions, and medications don't work, phototherapy is the next line of treatment," Dr. McAllister says. "Sunbathing in the great outdoors is the easiest method. It reduces the frequency of flare-ups in 80 percent of people with psoriasis." Bear in mind that short, multiple exposures to sunlight are recommended. You don't want to end up with a sunburn, which could trigger a flare-up. "Fair-skinned folks may benefit from just a few minutes of sunshine, while those with darker skin may be able to tolerate longer periods," she says. "It's a good idea to wear sunscreen on areas of the body unaffected by psoriasis to prevent sun damage."

Soothe your skin. Applying moisturizer regularly can help prevent itchy, painful, dry skin and reduce scaling and inflammation. Try using a lotion (which seals in your skin's own moisture) during the day and after bathing and a thicker cream or ointment at night. One technique is to coat each plaque with a thick layer of over-the-counter emollient cream and then cover it with plastic wrap, which you leave on overnight. In the morning, wash away the scales in the shower. Another option is to soak your skin in warm water and bath oil for 10 to 15 minutes. Then gently rub your skin with a towel to remove scales.

Avoid scratching. This is a tall order, we know. Psoriasis itches. In fact, the word *psoriasis* comes from the Greek *psora*, meaning "itch." But while scratching may make you feel better momentarily, it could leave you feeling worse in the long run. Itching can injure your skin, allowing bacteria to enter and cause an infection. If you scratch enough, your skin may bleed, which can worsen your flare-up. To relieve itchy skin, apply moisturizer, press a towel against the itchy spot, soak in a warm oatmeal bath, or apply a cold pack.

Maintain a positive attitude. Research has shown that stress, anxiety, loneliness, and low self-esteem are common among people with psoriasis. One study found that thoughts of suicide are three times more common among those with psoriasis than in the general population. "If you have a chronic condition such as psoriasis, you have to keep a good attitude," Dr. Fleisher advises. "It will raise your endorphin levels, which in turn will make you feel better."

Be a good student. "Read about psoriasis," Dr. Fleisher urges. "The more you know about your condition, the more you can actively participate in your care. I understand that medicine is not your field of expertise. But actually, it is your field when you're talking about *your* body.

"As you read and learn about your condition, you feel better—not so helpless," he adds. "I tell my patients to read what I read by searching the medical journals at www.pubmed.gov. I give them homework!"

On the Horizon

"In the past 15 years, we have seen remarkable changes and major advances in treating psoriasis," says Steven R. Feldman, MD, PhD, professor of pathology and dermatology at Wake Forest University School of Medicine in Winston-Salem, North Carolina. "But none of these advances has been even a baby step toward taking out psoriasis at its source." However, he continues, "our ability to control the disease has improved dramatically, and I think that it will continue to improve." Among the more fascinating and promising developments to date:

Genetics advances. "Genetics experts are studying people with psoriasis to determine what genes they have that people without psoriasis don't have," Dr. Feldman says. "I think that within the next 10 to 20 years, we'll come to understand the genes that cause psoriasis. Then we'll be able to find a treatment that will affect those genes specifically."

Honey-based treatments. "Scientists believe that psoriasis sufferers may benefit from the application of a mixture of honey, beeswax, and olive oil," Dr. McAllister says. "In a study of people suffering from psoriasis and other inflammatory skin conditions, 60 percent showed significant improvement when treated with this mixture."

Rheumatoid Arthritis

Curl your fingers to grip a pen, turn your wrist to unlock a door, bend your knees to tie your shoelaces—you make thousands of small movements like these every day. Who knows, perhaps it's millions. When they don't cause pain, you don't give them more than a second's thought. But for the 2.1 million Americans with rheumatoid arthritis (RA), even small movements can be excruciating. RA, one of more than 100 different types of arthritis, is a chronic disease, which means that it's unlikely to go away.

According to the Arthritis Foundation, RA progresses through three stages. First, the lining of the joints (called the synovium) becomes inflamed. The affected joints may be red, swollen, stiff, and painful and feel warm to the touch—all signs of inflammation. Next, the cells begin to rapidly divide and grow, causing the synovium to thicken. Finally, the inflamed cells release enzymes that may digest bone and cartilage. When this occurs, the joint loses its shape and alignment, leading to more pain as well as loss of movement.

Though RA can originate in any joint, it most commonly starts in the smaller joints of the fingers, hands, and wrists. Usually it progresses symmetrically, meaning that it affects the same joint on both sides of the body at once. RA also can cause fatigue, weakness, muscle aches, and even flulike symptoms.

The Immunity Link

RA is an autoimmune disease, which means it occurs when the immune system turns on the body—in this case, attacking the joints. This prompts white blood cells to flood the synovial fluid inside the joints, causing RA's characteristic symptoms.

As with other autoimmune diseases, researchers have yet to pinpoint the cause of RA. It's much more common in women than in men; in fact, women account for 70 percent of the population with RA. Interestingly, the likelihood of onset seems to increase in the year after a woman gives birth, though the condition often goes into remission during pregnancy. While men are less likely to develop RA, their symptoms tend to be more severe.

People with a specific genetic marker called HLA-DR4 may be at increased risk for RA. This marker, found in white blood cells, plays a role in helping the body distinguish between its own cells and foreign invaders.

Some experts believe that some sort of infection may trigger the onset of RA. The theory is that a germ to which almost everyone is exposed may prompt an abnormal immune response in those who have a predisposition to RA.

Protect Yourself

You may have been born with certain risk factors for RA, including having a family history of the condition and being female. Even so, you may be able to reduce your risk. Here's how.

Get some orange aid. Researchers in the United Kingdom found that people with the highest intakes of beta-cryptoxanthin (a compound found in fruits and vegetables that makes them yellow or orange) were half as likely to develop inflammatory polyarthritis, a precursor to RA, as those with lower intakes. According to the research team, the antioxidants in citrus fruits help protect joints. Drinking one 8-ounce glass of freshly squeezed orange juice or eating 1 tablespoon of cooked pumpkin, a handful of carrots, or ¼ cup of cooked red bell peppers each day supplies enough beta-cryptoxanthin to reduce your risk.

Drive by burger joints. Cutting back on red meat, such as hamburgers, may offer some protection against RA if you're prone to the disease. When researchers in Great Britain tracked a group of 264 volunteers, they found that the people who ate 2 or more ounces of red meat a day had almost twice the risk of RA as those who ate less than 1 ounce a day. Why is this so? One possibility is that red meat contains a lot of collagen, which may activate the antibodies thought to trigger RA in those who are susceptible to it.

Heal Yourself

If you've been diagnosed with RA, you likely are following a treatment regimen to help alleviate symptoms and reduce flare-ups. Consider the following self-care measures as adjuncts to any therapies that your doctor has prescribed.

Get a move on. Moderate physical activity can reduce fatigue, strengthen muscles and bones, increase flexibility and stamina, and provide a sense of general well-being. It also helps to manage stress and depression and improve sleep. All of these benefits are very important for anyone with RA. "People with rheumatoid arthritis need to exercise," says Mark Fleisher, MD, director of the Infusion Therapy and Immune Mediated Inflammatory Disorder Clinics at the Borland-Groover Clinic in Jacksonville, Florida. But not during a flare-up—wait until your symptoms subside. Then get moving as soon as you feel well enough to do so. "You don't have to enter the ESPN strongman competition," Dr. Fleisher says. "Just do something to be active."

Besides the physical and mental benefits, exercise offers a welcome opportunity to socialize. People with chronic conditions such as RA can easily become isolated from the rest of the world. Make a point to get out and interact with others.

Fight fire with fire. In the past decade, more than 1,300 scientific studies have confirmed the benefits of capsaicin—the compound that puts the heat in hot peppers—for the treatment of arthritis pain. "Capsaicin inhibits the action of substance P, the chemical messenger responsible for transmitting pain signals from nerves in the skin to the brain," explains Rallie McAllister, MD, MPH, a board-certified family physician and author of *Healthy Lunchbox: The Working Mom's Guide to Keeping You and Your Kids Trim*. "When capsaicin-containing creams are applied to painful joints, nerve cells are stimulated to release their entire supply of substance P. Once depleted of the substance, nerve fibers are incapable of relaying pain messages to the brain for several hours."

Capsaicin creams, such as Capzasin-P and Zostrix, are available at drugstores and some supermarkets. Follow the label directions, but the general recommendation is to apply a thin film to the affected area three or four times daily, gently rubbing the cream into the skin until it's completely absorbed.

Eliminate food triggers. For a small number of people with RA, certain foods could trigger or worsen symptoms. It might be helpful to keep a food diary for a few weeks, making note of what you eat and how you feel. Pay attention to any correlation between certain foods and your symptom patterns. A diet high in saturated fats or vegetable oils, for example, may increase the inflammatory response, contributing to joint and tissue inflammation.

Stress less. Because stress can trigger a flare-up of RA, it's important to have an arsenal of relaxation techniques at the ready. (See page 255 for suggestions.) Besides, research suggests that people with RA who have optimistic outlooks and feel in control of their conditions tend to fare better over the long term than people who don't.

Let yourself go. Guided imagery appears to help alleviate RA pain. In one study, conducted at Albert Einstein College of Medicine in New Hyde Park, New York, researchers enlisted 13 children with RA. Through eight sessions, the children learned guided-imagery techniques in combination with progressive muscle relaxation and meditation breathing. Their pain declined substantially over the course of the study, and it remained in check at their 6- and 12-month follow-ups.

You can do guided imagery on your own or with a trained practitioner. During a session, you hear and internalize therapeutic suggestions to help bring about relaxation and relief. To locate a practitioner in your area or to purchase tapes, visit www. academyforguidedimagery.com.

Sleep tight. Two-thirds of people with RA report that they don't get enough sleep. Part of the problem may stem from their medications. Research suggests that certain drugs commonly prescribed for RA inhibit slow-wave sleep. That's cause for concern, since your immune system can't perform at its best if you're sleep-deprived.

One study found that taking the herb valerian (*Valeriana officinalis*) allowed people with RA to get some much-needed slow-wave sleep. This, in turn, helped ease their pain and tension. As with any herb, you should talk with your doctor before adding valerian to your RA treatment regimen. The usual dose is 1 teaspoon of valerian root tincture or two 500-milligram valerian root tablets 30 minutes before bedtime. Side effects may include headache and stomach upset.

Be kneaded. Massage therapy can ease the pain and stiffness of RA. According to various studies, it works by improving immune function and sleep, reducing stress hormones and depression, easing muscle pain and spasms, and increasing production of endorphins, the body's natural painkillers. If you decide to try massage, it's important to find a massage therapist who has experience in treating people with arthritis. While a rubdown may provide short-term relaxation and relief, if it's too rough, it could actually aggravate arthritis pain and other symptoms.

Try acupuncture or acupressure. Like massage, these ancient therapeutic disciplines may release pain-relieving endorphins. They also may have anti-inflammatory properties. To find a certified practitioner in your area, visit the Web site for the National Certification Commission for Acupuncture and Oriental Medicine at www. nccaom.org.

Do your homework. "I think that people who confront their illnesses and are proactive about developing partnerships with their doctors tend to do better," Dr. Fleisher says. "I tell my patients, 'Don't go by my opinion alone. Check into it, and let's discuss the benefits, risks, and options.'

"When you're learning about your condition, you need to read double-blinded, placebo-controlled studies," he adds. "This means researchers took a group of people—let's say 1,000—and gave 500 of them a drug and the other 500 a placebo—a pill that looks just like the drug. [This way neither the patients nor the scientists know who got the drug and who got the placebo.] What many people don't realize is that placebos evoke a positive response 25 to 65 percent of the time. But what studies using placebos tell us is the absolute reduction of risk. For instance, if the drug worked 80 percent of the time, and the placebo worked 65 percent of the time, the therapeutic gain from taking the drug is 15 percent."

Say a prayer. Public opinion polls show that prayer is one of the most commonly used complementary therapies for arthritis. While no studies to date have found a specific connection between prayer and RA symptoms, research shows that the mind can have a powerful effect on health. So prayer certainly won't hurt.

On the Horizon

An article published in the *British Medical Journal* identified the following areas of RA research as ripe for breakthroughs.

Genetics advances. Using gene characteristics, researchers hope to identify people at risk for aggressive RA earlier—and treat them sooner.

Improved drugs. Pharmaceutical companies are pursuing several avenues of drug therapy for RA. These include more selective nonsteroidal anti-inflammatory drugs, redesigned COX-2 inhibitors, new drugs to induce immune cells in joints to self-destruct or at least stop accumulating, and new drugs to keep harmful blood vessels from forming in joints.

Shingles

Like a driver's test or the SATs, chickenpox may have been one of the least pleasant rites of passage of our youth. It's over and done with, and we have no desire to repeat it.

Unfortunately, varicella zoster—the virus that causes chickenpox—may have other ideas. Sometimes it resurfaces in adulthood. When it does, it's referred to by another name—shingles, or herpes zoster.

One-quarter of Americans get shingles, usually after age 40. Often the first sign is burning or tingling pain or an itch in one particular location. After several days to a week, a rash of fluid-filled blisters appears on one side of the body.

For most people, shingles rashes heal within a few weeks. Sometimes, though, the pain can linger for weeks, months, or even years. This condition, called postherpetic neuralgia, can be agonizingly painful. "The older you are and the more shingles blisters you have, the more likely you are to get postherpetic neuralgia," says M. Susan Burke, MD, FACP, clinical assistant professor of medicine at Thomas Jefferson University in Philadelphia and director of the Internal Medicine Clinical Care Center at Lankenau Hospital in Wynnewood, Pennsylvania.

The Immunity Link

Once you've had chickenpox, the virus lies dormant in some of your nerve roots, Dr. Burke explains. Initially, your immune system is able to keep the virus in check. But as you get older and your immune function declines, the virus can come out of hibernation, causing shingles. "Sometimes younger people get shingles, but it doesn't necessarily indicate a problem with their immune systems," Dr. Burke says. "Perhaps they didn't have an especially dramatic case of chickenpox in the first place. Or they had chickenpox as babies, and so they didn't build strong immunity to the virus, as they might have if they'd been older when they got sick."

Shingles also can occur in people with compromised immune systems, such as those who have HIV/AIDS or are taking immune-suppressing medications.

Protect Yourself

Anyone who has had chickenpox is at risk for shingles. That includes most of us! Though there's no fail-safe way to keep the virus at bay, these strategies can help.

Ask your doctor about vaccination. Dr. Burke advises her adult patients to get a shingles vaccine once they reach age 60. "With the vaccine, your body is more likely to keep the virus in check," she explains. "If you do develop shingles, it's less likely to progress to postherpetic neuralgia."

If you've never had chickenpox, you're a candidate for the vaccine. But there is a catch: Even though you probably won't get chickenpox, you still might develop shingles later on. "Both the chickenpox vaccine and the shingles vaccine are live attenuated vaccines, which means that they contain a small dose of the virus," Dr. Burke explains. "So with the chickenpox vaccine, you still are at risk for shingles."

Try tai chi. One study found that tai chi offered protection against shingles in older adults. The 18 seniors who participated in a tai chi program showed a nearly 50 percent increase in immune cell levels after only 1 week, compared with the seniors who didn't practice tai chi.

If you'd like to try tai chi, it's best to start out by working with a qualified tai chi instructor, who can teach proper body position and movement. Once you're comfortable with the moves, you can continue on your own by choosing from among the many available tai chi videos and DVDs.

Heal Yourself

"If you break out with shingles, head to your doctor as quickly as possible for a prescription for an antiviral medication," Dr. Burke advises. "Studies have shown that if you begin taking the medication within 3 days, you have the best results." For additional relief, try these tips.

Soothe the itch. To ease the pain and itch of shingles, Dr. Burke suggests applying cool compresses to your skin or taking an oatmeal bath. Other options include calamine lotion and a prescription burn treatment called Silvadene cream. "Sometimes it's soothing, and it has a mild antibacterial effect to cut down on the chance of developing a bacterial infection on top of the shingles rash," she says.

Ease the pain. Unlike chickenpox, shingles can hurt far more than it itches. "If you develop postherpetic neuralgia, your doctor may prescribe a few different types of medication to deal with the pain," Dr. Burke says. "These include any medicine that is usually reserved for nerve pain, such as anticonvulsants and certain antidepressants. Opiate medications also may help."

Among over-the-counter remedies, you might try acetaminophen or a nonsteroidal anti-inflammatory medication such as ibuprofen. "Or apply capsaicin cream, also called Zostrix, three or four times a day," Dr. Burke says. "But don't start using the cream until your rash is completely healed. It can make your skin burn even on a good day."

Type 1 Diabetes

When most people hear the word *diabetes,* they tend to think of type 2, the most common among the 20.8 million Americans with diabetes. It results from insulin resistance, a condition in which the body can't properly use insulin, the hormone that "unlocks" the body's cells and allows glucose (blood sugar) to enter and fuel them.

Of the total population with diabetes, about 5 to 10 percent have type 1. In this version, the body is unable to produce its own insulin because the beta cells in the pancreas—the only cells in the body that can make insulin—have been destroyed.

Until recently, type 1 diabetes was thought to affect primarily children and young adults (hence its alternative name, juvenile diabetes). But now more adults are being diagnosed with type 1. "You can see forms of it develop in people up to age 90," says Claresa Levetan, MD, clinical professor at the Lankenau Institute for Medical Research at Lankenau Hospital in Wynnewood, Pennsylvania.

Among the symptoms of type 1 diabetes are increased thirst and urination, weight loss despite increased appetite, nausea, vomiting, abdominal pain, fatigue, and absence of menstruation. Left untreated, type 1 diabetes can lead to serious complications such as heart disease, blindness, and nerve and kidney damage.

The Immunity Link

Unlike type 2 diabetes, which is a metabolic disorder, type 1 has a very strong link to the immune system. Specifically, the immune system is responsible for destroying the insulin-producing beta cells. In other words, type 1 diabetes is an autoimmune disease. "An autoimmune disease occurs when the immune system makes a mistake and starts attacking the body's own cells and tissues," explains Alberto Pugliese, MD, research associate professor of medicine, microbiology, and immunology and head of the immunogenetics program at the Diabetes Research Institute at the University of Miami Miller School of Medicine. "Some people have multiple autoimmune diseases, while others have one disease that affects multiple organs.

"Type 1 diabetes is a classic example of an organ-specific autoimmune disease," he adds. "It affects only one organ—the pancreas. And even within that organ, it targets just the beta cells."

But what causes the immune system to run amok? According to Dr. Levetan, it's a combination of genetic predisposition and an environmental trigger. "If you have a genetic predisposition to type 1 diabetes, it means that there is a mistake in your immune mechanism," she explains. "So let's say that you get an illness such as the mumps. Your body will make antibodies to fight the mumps. After you've gotten over the illness, the antibodies will begin attacking the beta cells in the pancreas because of that mistake in the immune mechanism. Once you've lost 90 percent of your beta cells, you no longer have the ability to process glucose."

Protect Yourself

Doctors have come to view type 2 diabetes as a lifestyle disease, meaning that certain lifestyle choices—especially diet and exercise—can influence risk for better or worse. Not so with type 1 diabetes. "We know that a person must have the genetic predisposition in addition to the environmental trigger, but we don't know what the trigger might be," Dr. Levetan says. "We've seen some associations with babies who were fed cow's milk in their first year and with people who have low levels of vitamin D. But for now, we can't do much to prevent type 1 diabetes."

One strategy that you may want to try: Battle vitamin D deficiency, which appears to contribute to autoimmune disorders such as type 1 diabetes. It's on the rise in the United States, at least partly due to our indoor, sunlight-deprived society. "In a study of more than 10,000 children, researchers found that those who took a recommended dose of vitamin D during infancy were far less likely to develop type 1 diabetes than those who did not," says Rallie McAllister, MD, MPH, a board-certified family physician and author of *Healthy Lunchbox: The Working Mom's Guide to Keeping You and Your Kids Trim*. "Although some foods are fortified with vitamin D, the amounts are relatively low. It's probably best to take a supplement."

But how much to take is the subject of great debate. "According to the Institute of Medicine, kids under age 19 and adults under age 50 should get 200 IU of vitamin

D a day, adults ages 51 to 70 should get 400 IU a day, and adults older than age 71 should get 600 IU a day," Dr. McAllister says. "Among nutrition experts, these recommended daily intakes are widely believed to be inadequate. Many experts recommend a daily intake of 1,000 IU for adults [over age 19]."

Heal Yourself

People with type 1 diabetes need insulin to survive (which is why you may hear it described as insulin-dependent diabetes). It's different from type 2 diabetes, in which the body makes insulin but the hormone isn't working as it should. If you have type 1, you should definitely work closely with your doctor to develop and fine-tune your treatment plan. The following measures may help balance your blood sugar and prevent diabetes complications down the road.

Check and recheck. "It's critical for people with type 1 diabetes to monitor their blood sugar levels throughout the day," Dr. Levetan says. "Keep a journal of what foods you eat and how your blood sugar levels change to understand how your body responds to different foods. That way, you can tailor the insulin that you take to mimic what your own pancreas would do. Every 10 minutes, the pancreas releases a burst of insulin; within 1 minute of eating, it makes the perfect amount of insulin. You want to do as much as you can to follow that pattern."

Be healthy. "The best things to complement the treatments that your doctor prescribes are the same things that anyone should do to maintain good health," says Luigi Meneghini, MD, associate professor of clinical medicine and director of the Eleanor and Joseph Kosow Diabetes Treatment Center at the Diabetes Research Institute at the University of Miami Miller School of Medicine. "Eat reasonably, exercise regularly, and maintain an ideal body weight."

Move it. Historically, studies have shown that people with type 1 diabetes live longer if they exercise regularly. More recently, the Finnish Diabetic Nephropathy Study found that women with type 1 diabetes who did not exercise had worse blood sugar control than women who did. But you need to be smart about how you exercise— and definitely talk to your doctor before you start a fitness routine. "People with type 1 diabetes need to be mindful of how exercise affects their blood sugar levels," Dr. Meneghini says. "The combination of exercise and high insulin levels tends to lower blood sugar much more than either exercise with basal insulin levels or no exercise. For example, let's say that you're planning to eat a meal containing 60 grams of carbohydrates, and your blood sugar level is 200. You calculate that you need to take eight units of insulin. If you're planning to exercise within a couple of hours of taking the insulin, you may need to reduce your dose.

"We give patients with type 1 diabetes some guidelines about how exercise affects blood sugar levels and some suggestions about how to alter their insulin dosing. But since everyone responds differently to exercise, the rest is trial and error," he adds. "For instance, one patient of mine—a high school basketball player—noticed that his blood sugar level would go low during practice, but it would go high during a game. The higher adrenaline levels during his games were pushing up his blood sugar level."

Chill out. People with type 1 diabetes need to learn how stress affects their blood sugar. "During times of stress—both psychological and physiological, such as illness—your body releases stress hormones, which raise blood sugar levels," Dr. Meneghini explains. "So when you're under stress, there's a good chance that your blood sugar levels will rise. For some people, it can be as much as 200 to 300 mg/dl [milligrams per deciliter of blood]. It depends how sensitive you are to stress.

"Also, during times of stress, your body may not respond to insulin as it usually does," he adds. "So you need to check your blood sugar level more often, take insulin more frequently, and increase your dose if necessary. When the stress goes away, go back to what you were doing before."

On the Horizon

"I hope that we will have a cure for type 1 diabetes in our lifetime," Dr. Pugliese says. "For sure, we will have treatments and other measures that will have an even greater impact on the condition than the ones we already have." Here's just a sampling.

Better diagnostic measures. Researchers know that when immune cells attack beta cells, they're responding to specific molecules that beta cells make. "We call these target molecules," Dr. Pugliese says. "In many patients, one of the target molecules actually is insulin itself. This explains in part why beta cells are the only cells killed off. It's as though insulin is waving a flag and saying, 'Come shoot me.'

"Now that we know what some of these target molecules are, we know what the immune system goes after," he adds. "So we are learning how to identify people who are developing type 1 diabetes, before they even have symptoms, by measuring certain markers in their blood. These markers are the antibodies that are directed against the same target molecules that the lymphocytes go after. Sometimes these antibodies are present years before symptoms develop, when insulin production appears to be normal."

Improved treatments. As researchers are able to determine at an earlier stage who will develop type 1 diabetes, their next step is to find ways to disrupt and perhaps even halt the disease process. "One possibility is to put a person on immune-suppressive drugs," says Dr. Pugliese, who has participated in a number of clinical trials. "The problem with this treatment is that it may work for a time, but then the disease comes back. Also, the drugs suppress all of the immune cells, not just the small number causing trouble. The drugs can have a lot of unpleasant side effects, so they could not be taken indefinitely." Current trials are exploring the use of immunosuppressive drugs for a limited time and with an emphasis on immune regulation rather than immune suppression.

Another possibility is to treat people with one or more target molecules to help regulate the immune system and specifically control the "bad" immune cells that kill off beta cells. "In one double-blind, randomized study, the Diabetes Prevention Trial, we found a significant effect in people who had developed antibodies to insulin," Dr. Pugliese notes. "We're going to expand this study in the near future."

Ultimately, Dr. Pugliese says, the best approach may be a combined one. "We may treat people with one or more target molecules—insulin, for example—and also with immune-suppressing drugs for short periods. The goal is to get rid of the immune cells that destroy beta cells with drug therapy, while regulating the immune system with administration of the target molecules. Perhaps once the immune system stops destroying beta cells, we'll see regeneration or the formation of new beta cells."

Islet transplants. Islets are clusters of cells in the pancreas that consist of several types of cells, including the beta cells that produce insulin. In a recent study conducted by the National Institutes of Health, 60 percent of people with type 1 diabetes who underwent islet transplants didn't need daily insulin shots a year later. The downside is that transplant patients need to take powerful immune-suppressing drugs for life, which come with a host of nasty side effects. Also, islet transplants begin to lose functioning after a year. Further research may help troubleshoot and refine this experimental procedure.

Ulcers

At one time, ulcers were a dubious badge of honor, "awarded" to hardworking business types in high-stress positions. Only fairly recently has medical research determined that most ulcers result not from stress but from bacteria called *Helicobacter pylori* that nestle into the stomach wall and wreak havoc.

As their name suggests, ulcers are sores in the lining of the digestive tract, usually in the stomach or possibly in the upper part of the intestines. They make their presence known with symptoms that include stomach pain that disrupts sleep, a heavy feeling in the stomach, a sense of fullness or bloating, vomiting, unexplained weight loss, and a burning discomfort under the notch of the sternum.

The Immunity Link

As much as half of the world's population is infected with *H. pylori*—but up to 90 percent of people who have it don't know it. As it turns out, the bacteria are very tricky. They can co-opt the body's immune system for their own hostile purpose.

Once *H. pylori* get into your stomach, the infection causes mild inflammation. The cells that line the stomach produce a specific kind of sugar molecule, called sLex, on their surface to direct immune cells to the infection site. But the tenacious bacteria use an adhesion protein to latch on to the sugar molecules. In this way, they're able to alter certain immune factors, which allows them to evade detection and cause persistent inflammation—but never an ulcer.

So why do some people get ulcers? Experts suspect that these people have an abnormality in their immune response that allows the bacteria to burrow into the stomach lining and weaken the protective layer of mucus. As stomach acid eats into the lining, an ulcer occurs.

Protect Yourself

Worried about getting an ulcer? These tips may reduce your risk.

C some relief. It might seem odd that something as acidic as oranges could help prevent ulcers. But because of their high vitamin C content, they may do just that. When researchers measured the blood levels of vitamin C in more than 6,000 people, they discovered that the people with the most C were the least likely to have *H. pylori*. One 8-ounce glass of orange juice provides a day's supply of vitamin C.

Lay off the meds. Infection with *H. pylori* isn't the only cause of ulcers, though it is the most common one. Long-term use of certain medications also can increase risk. If you're taking a nonsteroidal anti-inflammatory drug such as aspirin, ibuprofen, naproxen, or ketoprofen or using an arthritis drug, you may want to talk with your doctor about other treatment options.

Curb your vices. Both smoking and excessive alcohol consumption can damage the lining of your digestive tract, paving the way for an ulcer to form.

Heal Yourself

Though you may be inclined to just tough out ulcer symptoms, it's important to get proper treatment. An ulcer can perforate, which requires surgery. Also, ulcers are a risk factor for gastric cancer. In fact, *H. pylori* may be responsible for up to 55 percent of gastric cancer cases.

If *H. pylori* is the culprit behind your ulcer, your doctor likely will prescribe antibiotics to clear the infection. You may want to ask your doctor about these home remedies, too.

Drink grapefruit juice. No kidding! When scientists in Poland gave a concentrated grapefruit-seed extract to laboratory rats with ulcers, the rats' acidic stomach secretions slowed by 50 percent, and their ulcers healed. The researchers suspect that the high level of antioxidants in grapefruit enhanced bloodflow to the rats' stomachs and kept the ulcer sites clear of harmful microbes.

Take a tip from the bog. Another type of juice, cranberry juice, may help heal ulcers. In one study, drinking a tall glass of cranberry juice every day for 3 months significantly suppressed *H. pylori* bacteria.

Blast ulcers away. Capsaicin, the compound that gives hot peppers their heat, may help treat stomach ulcers. "While most people with stomach irritation are warned to avoid spicy foods, research suggests that capsaicin actually may be beneficial," says Rallie McAllister, MD, MPH, a board-certified family physician and author of *Healthy Lunchbox: The Working Mom's Guide to Keeping You and Your Kids Trim.* "It stimulates bloodflow to the stomach, nourishing the lining and speeding repairs. It also stimulates peristalsis, the muscular contractions of the intestines that propel food through the digestive tract. Several studies have shown a lower incidence of stomach ulcers among pepper-eating populations."

Calm down. It's true that stress won't necessarily cause an ulcer. However, it can aggravate one you already have. (See page 255 for on-the-spot stress reduction techniques.)

Watch what you eat. Avoid foods that can aggravate ulcer pain, such as caffeinated coffee and tea, chocolate, black pepper, mustard seed, and nutmeg. Eating small but frequent meals can help as well.

On the Horizon

Researchers are working to develop a vaccine that would prevent ulcers. Because *H. pylori* uses a specific kind of adhesion protein to latch on to sugar molecules, this attachment mechanism is the most likely target for the vaccine.

TEST YOURSELF

Is It an Ulcer or Just a Stomachache?

Have something to eat. If you feel better initially but worse 1 to 2 hours later, it could be an ulcer in your duodenum, the first section of your small intestine. When you have an ulcer, eating food buffers it and quickly relieves the pain, unlike with a stomach bug, when eating often makes you feel worse.

Index

Antibiotics *(cont.)*
  vaginal infections and, <u>347</u>
  viral diseases not treatable by, <u>8</u>
Antibodies
  autoantibodies, 17
  B cells' production of, 14
  with lupus, 337
  positive emotions increasing, 109–10
  received by babies from mother, 12
  smoking lowering levels of, 20
Antidepressants, 259
Antigens, 12–14, <u>12</u>, <u>16</u>
Antimalarials, 351
Antioxidants. *See also specific kinds*
  conditions benefited by
    asthma, 305
    chronic inflammation, <u>6</u>
    Crohn's disease, 324
    multiple sclerosis, 342
    smoking, 252–53
  decline of levels with age, 34
  free radicals combated by, 34
  immune function preserved by, 34–35
  sources of
    chocolate, 62, <u>226</u>
    coffee, 59, 313
    EpiCor, 279
    flaxseed, 183
    fruits and vegetables, <u>6</u>, 46
    tea, 58, 313
Antiviral drugs, 320
Antiviral tissues, 319
Apoptosis (programmed cell death), 14
Apples
  overview, 46–47
  recipes, 167, 218, 231
Apricots, 185
Arachidonic acid, 54
Aricept (donepezil), 301
Aromatherapy, 78, 99, <u>184</u>, <u>202</u>
Aromatic diffusers, 286
Arthritis. *See* Rheumatoid arthritis
Ashwagandha, 287
Asian pears, 221
Asthma
  allergies with, 303
  colds vs., <u>307</u>
  costs of caring for, 303
  future breakthroughs, 307
  healing, 305–7
  immunity link to, 303–4
  omega-3 fatty acids for, 52
  prevalence of, 303
  protection from, 304–5
  qigong for treating, 73
  vitamin D for improving, 125
Atherosclerosis, 81. *See also* Cardiovascular
    disease

Attitude. *See* Mood
Autoantibodies, 17
Autoimmune diseases
  aging and increase in, 275
  overview, 17–18
  smoking linked to, 20, 250
  stress as risk factor for, 255
  tai chi beneficial for, 73
  tryptophan for treating, <u>52</u>
  vitamin D for improving, 122
Avian or bird flu (H5N1), 3, <u>4</u>
Avocado, 166, 225, 227

B

Bach flower essences, 267–68
Bacteria, beneficial, 7, 13. *See also* Probiotics
Bacteria, harmful
  adaptive immunity to, 12–14
  antibiotic resistant, 7, <u>8</u>
  antigens for, 12–13, <u>12</u>
  beta-glucan as protection against, <u>39</u>
  catching from children, 279
  from contaminated food, 11
  EpiCor for, 279
  food poisoning culprits, 326
  glutathione as protection against, 50
  immune response to, <u>12</u>
  innate immunity to, 12, 13
  malnutrition aggravating infection, 34
  as pathogens, 12
  perspiration as protection against, 69
  pets and infection risks, <u>21</u>
  vitamin A as protection against, 36
BactoShield, 138
B cells
  described, 14, 238
  exercise for activating, 63, 72
  obesity impairing function of, 238
  soy for increasing, 55
  stimulated by helper T cells, 14
  stress and reduced levels of, 20
  suppressor T cells and, 14
B-complex vitamins. *See also specific vitamins*
  depression reduced by, 261
  in grains, 38
  stress counteracted by, 98
  supplements, <u>37</u>
Beans and legumes. *See also* Soybeans and soy
    foods
  baked, 209
  canned, 167, 225, 227
  dried, 190
  isoflavones in, 54–55
  recipes, 166, 171, 178, 206, 225
  refried, 227
  salads as chips replacement, 225
Bean soups, 163
Bedclothes, 90

Beef
   choices recommended, 51
   healthier alternatives, 223
   recipes, 164, 171, 198, 221
   rheumatoid arthritis risk and, 355
Bell peppers
   roasted red peppers, 167
   Sunflower and Three-Pepper Salad, 198
Bench pushups, 216
Benzethonium chloride, 138, 139
Berries. *See also specific kinds*
   for Alzheimer's protection, 299
   recipes, 157, 160, 166, 197
   reduced-fat sour cream with, 207
   as vitamin C source, 276
Beta-amyloid proteins, 299, 300
Beta-carotene, 43, 211, 305, 312. *See also*
      Vitamin A
Beta-cryptoxanthin, 355
Beta-endorphins, 131
Beta-glucan, <u>39</u>, 44, 66–67, 256
Beverages. *See* Fluids
Biceps curl, 177
Bifidobacterium breve, 247
Bifidobacterium lactis, 49, 247
Biofeedback asthma treatment, 307
Bioflavonoids, 5
Biological weapons, 3
Bird or avian flu (H5N1), 3, <u>4</u>
Blackberries, 198
Black mold, 286–87
Bladder cancer, 19, 250
Blood pressure, high
   lowering, 44, 61, 73, 116
   medications and target heart rate, 70
   worsened by alcohol, 61
Blood sugar, 82, 84, 364, 365
Blueberries
   for Alzheimer's protection, 299
   health benefits of, 240
   immune system enhanced by, 198
   pancakes and muffins, 192, 205
   recipes, 166, 197
   reduced-fat sour cream with, 207
Body mass index (BMI), 238
Bowing shoulder stretch, 176
Brain, 97–98, 143, 298, 300
BRAT diet, 332
Breakfast. *See also* Menus
   Better Breakfast Sandwich, 164
   Cheddar Scrambled Eggs, 218
   Cinnamon French Toast, 222
   exercise and, 79
   Ginger Peach Smoothie, 204
   Lox and Cream Cheese on Bagel, 208
   meat choices recommended, 165
   Mixed Berry Yogurt Parfait, 197
   Mushroom and Cheddar Omelet, 187

Sausage and Egg Burrito, 202
   Super Blueberry Smoothie, 166
Breast cancer
   exercise reducing risk of, 67
   massage benefits for, 105
   smoking as risk factor for, 19
   soybeans for preventing, 55–56
   vitamin D for preventing, 122, 125, 126
Breastfeeding, <u>53</u>, 293, 304, 335
Breathing
   deep, enhanced by laughter, 116–17
   in meditation practice, 103, 256–57
   regulating during exercise, 77
   sleep apnea, 266
   for stress reduction, 98–99
Broccoli, 42–43, 299, 338
Bronchitis, 19, 278
Brushing teeth, 153–54
Butterbur for allergies, 293

C

Cabbage
   coleslaw, 171–72, 202
   sauerkraut, 207
Caffeine
   diuretic effect of, 56–57
   sleep disruption by, 59, 86, 90, 267
   ulcers aggravated by, 369
Calcium, 48, 248
Calorie restriction. *See also* Dieting;
      Weight loss
   cutting menu plan for weight loss, 150
   exercise with, 65
   immune system enhanced by, 35, 319
   immune system impaired by, 245–46
   life span extension from, 35
   not restricting protein, 248
Calories
   burned by muscle tissue, 151
   chores for burning, <u>224</u>
   with Immune Essentials Plan menus, 150
   lawn mowing for burning, <u>208</u>
   margarine for reducing, 158
   sugar-free spreads for reducing, 171
Campylobacter, <u>21</u>, 326, 330–31
Canadian bacon, 164, 165
Cancer. *See also specific kinds*
   checking with doctor about symptoms, 309
   early warning signs, 308–9
   exercise during treatment of, 67
   immunity link to, 309–10
   malnutrition risk from, 23
   prevalence of, 308
   protective factors
      broccoli and tomatoes, 42–43
      exercise, 67
      lycopene, 40, 41
      omega-3 fatty acids, 53

Cold-fX ginseng product, 318
Colds
    allergies vs., <u>296</u>
    antibiotics not suitable for, <u>8</u>
    asthma vs., <u>307</u>
    echinacea for, <u>228</u>
    feeding, <u>62</u>
    flu vs., <u>321</u>
    future breakthroughs, 322
    healing, 281, 320–21
    immunity link to, 316–17
    optimism and risk for, 112
    protection from, 52, 58, 65–66, 317–20
    psoriasis flare-ups with, 351
    as sign of poor immunity, 19
    smoking as risk factor for, 19
    washing hands to avoid, 135–36
Coleslaw, 171–72, 202
Colon cancer prevention, 40, 122, 126, 314
Colorectal cancer prevention, 53, 60
Congestive heart failure, 61
Constipation, preventing, 38
Contract for exercise, 78
Cooking. *See also* Kitchen safety
    avoiding food poisoning, 141–42, 327–31
    with garlic, 44
    meat and poultry, 51
    with mushrooms, 45
    reheating leftovers, 142
    temperatures for, 141–42, <u>330</u>
    tomatoes, 42
    vegetables, 40–41
Cordyceps (*Cordyceps sinensis*), 45
Core exercises, 156, 177, 197, 217
Corn, 206, 293
Corpse Pose, <u>166</u>
Cortisol. *See also* Stress
    aging and levels of, 97
    chronically elevated, 93, 254–55, 257
    circadian rhythm and, 271
    exercise increasing levels of, 71
    insufficient, 93
    massage for reducing, 104
    overview, 92
    Seriphos for lowering levels, 267, 273
    sleep and, 265
Cosmetics, natural, <u>212</u>
Coughing, with pneumonia, 347
Coumaric acid, 41
Couscous, 158, 219
Crabmeat, 200. *See also* Shellfish
Crackers, 243
Cranberries, 160, 368
C-reactive protein, 81, 110
Crohn's disease, 52, 323–25
Crouch step exercise, 157
Croutons, whole grain, 169
Curl-up exercise, 156

Cynical distrust, 111
Cyranose 320, 347–48
Cystein, 50
Cytokines
    allergic response and, 292
    defined, 21
    fasting vs. eating and, <u>62</u>
    inflammation regulated by, 21
    selenium increasing production of, 36
    sleep deprivation and, 22, 82–83
Cytomegalovirus (CMV), 275

D

Daidzein, 54–55
Dairy products. *See also specific kinds*
    cancer risk and, 311
    fat content of, 48
    food group, 48–51
    in Immune Essentials Plan, 49
    lactose intolerance, 48
    probiotics, 49–51
    safe storage times, 142, <u>329</u>
    tips for using, 48
    as vitamin D sources, <u>131</u>
DanActive yogurt, 49, 247, 280
Danimals yogurt, 247
Dates (fruit)
    nutritional benefits, 232
    recipes, 202, 231
Dates on food products, <u>141</u>
Dehydration, 56–57, 241. *See also* Fluids
Dehydroepiandrosterone (DHEA), 260
Dendritic cell vaccines for cancer, <u>16</u>
Depression
    aging and risk for, 275
    cold and flu risk with, 319
    coping with, 259–63
    immune system impaired by, 259
    major vs. mild, 258
    omega-3 fatty acids for, 52
    pregnancy and postpartum, 104–5
    sleep deprivation and, <u>87</u>
    worsened by alcohol, 61
Dessert, fruits for, 46
DHA (docosahexaenoic acid). *See* Omega-3
        fatty acids
Diabetes
    Alzheimer's possibly related to, 300
    chronic inflammation linked to, 21
    coffee for protection against, 59
    exercise possibly helpful for, 22
    future breakthroughs, 365
    healing from type 1, 364–65
    immunity link to type 1, 362–63
    pneumonia with, 345
    protection from type 1, 363–64
    qigong for treating, 73
    red wine for preventing, 59

household toxins, avoiding, 134, 144, 146, <u>212</u>, 215, <u>233</u>, 287
  in Immune Essentials Plan, 153–54, 175, 195, 214–15
  immune-friendly, indoors, 285–88
  indoor air pollution, <u>145</u>, <u>233</u>, 284–85, 305
  as key to maximum immunity, 7
  pollution's effect on immune system, 143
  primary sources of contaminants, 133–34
  surfaces, contaminated, 133, 134, <u>135</u>
  washing hands for safety, 135–39, <u>135</u>
EPA (eicosapentaenoic acid). *See* Omega-3 fatty acids
EpiCor, 281
Epigallocatechin gallate, 191
Epigallocatechin-3-gallate (EGCG), 313
Epinephrine, 63, 71, 92. *See also* Stress
Escherichia coli, 60, 139–40, 326, 331, 332
Esophageal cancer, 19, 250
Ethnicity
  Crohn's disease risk and, 324
  lupus risk and, 338
  psoriasis risk and, 349
Exercise. *See also* Aerobic exercise; Resistance training; Workouts
  aches and pains, reducing, <u>75</u>
  asthma and timing of, 306
  benefits of
    with aging, 67–69
    Alzheimer's protection, 299
    cancer prevention, 67, 310–11
    cold and flu protection, 318–19
    immune system enhanced, 5, 63–64, 67
    infection reduced, 65–66
    quitting smoking aided, 67
    rheumatoid arthritis eased, 356
    stress counteracted, 98
    type 1 diabetes eased, 364–65
    weight loss, 64–65, 242, 246
  breath regulation during, 77
  calorie restriction with, 65
  checking with doctor before starting program, 75
  chores for, <u>224</u>
  close to bedtime, avoiding, 90, 267
  daily amount of, 63, 64, 70, 77
  excessive, poor immunity from, 23, 63, 70–71, 318–19
  getting started, 74–77
  heart rate during, 69–70
  home gym for, <u>161</u>
  hydration important with, 57
  lack, as risk factor for poor immunity, 22
  laughter as, 117
  moderate, defined, 69–70
  mowing your lawn, <u>208</u>
  MS eased by, 343
  nonregimented workouts, 79

  for older persons, 68–69, 278
  outdoors, avoiding skin damage, 76
  qigong, <u>73</u>
  skipping when ill, 77, <u>78</u>
  staying motivated, 77–80
  tai chi, <u>73</u>, 156–57, 256, 360
  tips for, 76
  warming up before, 77, 154–55, 176, 196, 215–16
  yoga, <u>166</u>, 242, 262
Expiration dates on food products, <u>141</u>

F

"Fantasy" to-do list, 214
Fat, body. *See* Obesity; Overweight; Weight loss
Fatigue, as sign of poor immunity, 19
Fats, dietary. *See also* Omega-3 fatty acids
  cancer link to saturated, 311
  for carotenoid absorption, 42
  chronic inflammation reduced by, <u>6</u>
  immune function and, 23, 52
  limiting with MS, 342–43
  mushrooms aiding metabolism of, 44
  saturated, avoiding, 311
  sources of
    avocado, 225
    dairy products, 48, 160
    ice cream, 172
    margarine, 158, 305
    nut butters, 160
    salad dressings, 200
    trans fats, avoiding, 240–41, 305
Feed a cold, starve a fever, <u>62</u>
Fevers, starving, <u>62</u>
Fexofenadine (Allegra), 294
Fiber, 38, 40, 240
Fight-or-flight response, 20, 93. *See also* Stress
Figs, 190
Filters for air and water, <u>145</u>, <u>233</u>, 287
Fish. *See also* Shellfish
  for Alzheimer's protection, 298–99
  arachidonic acid in, 54
  for cancer prevention, 314
  lox, about, 209
  mercury in, <u>53</u>
  for older persons, 277
  omega-3 fatty acids in, 52–54, <u>53</u>, 239, 248, 260, 277
  recipes, 158, 169, 187, 198, 208, 218, 225
  recommended kinds, 54
  temperatures for cooking, 141–42, <u>330</u>
  as vitamin D sources, <u>131</u>
Fish oil, benefits for. *See also* Omega-3 fatty acids
  Alzheimer's disease, 299
  asthma, 306
  Crohn's disease, 324

immunity link to, 316–17
obesity and increased risk for, 23–24
omega-3 fatty acids for preventing, 52
omega-6 fatty acids contributing to, 53
optimism and risk for, 112
pandemics, 4
pneumonia risk with, 345
positive mood for preventing, 109–10
protection from, 317–20
as sign of poor immunity, 19
Spanish flu, 3
tea for preventing, 58
vaccine effectiveness and age, 319–20
vaccine effectiveness and social network,
    113–14
vaccines aided by exercise, 67
vaccines blunted by sleep deprivation, 83
vaccines for asthmatic patients, 307
vitamin D as protection against, 7
washing hands to avoid, 135–36
Injury, psoriasis risk and, 350–51
Innate or passive immunity, 12–13. *See also*
    Antibodies
Inole-3-carbinol, 42
Insomnia. *See* Sleep deprivation
Insulin, Alzheimer's disease and, 300
Interferon
    described, 5
    gamma, 52, 118
    raising levels of, 5, 37, 52, 58, 118
Interleukin
    interleukin-2, 81, 335
    interleukin-6, 22, 110, 259
    sleep deprivation disturbing balance of,
        82–83
    vitamin E for raising levels of, 37
Internet resources. *See* Web sites
Intestinal bacteria, 13, 49. *See also* Probiotics
Intimacy, immune system enhanced by, 115–16
Ion generators, 145
IQ quiz, immunity, 26–30
Islet transplants, 366
Isoflavones, 54–55

J

Jicama, 211
Journal (Immune Essentials Plan), 152, 210
Junk food, 23, 243

K

Kaposi's sarcoma, 334
Kashi crackers, 243
Kefir. *See also* Dairy products
    in Immune Essentials Plan, 150
    overview, 167
    as probiotics source, 49, 50–51
    smoothies, 166, 204
    yogurt vs., 50, 167

Keys, duplicating to avoid stress, 100
Kidney cancer, 53, 250
Killer T cells. *See also* T cells
    chronically elevated cortisol and, 93
    described, 14
    sleep deprivation reducing, 81
Kitchen safety. *See also* Food poisoning
    cleanup after handling meat, 141
    disinfecting sponges and scrubbers, 140
    E. coli contamination issues, 139–40
    germ-proofing, 175
    interpreting expiration dates, 141
    reheating leftovers, 142
    safe storage times, 142, 329
    temperatures for cooking, 141–42, 330
    washing fruits and vegetables, 141
Kleenex antiviral tissues, 319
Knee pull (stretch), 154
Koebner phenomenon, 350
Krill oil, 240

L

Lactobacillus acidophilus, 49
Lactobacillus bulgaricus, 49
Lactobacillus casei, 49, 247
Lactobacillus reuteri, 49–50, 247
Lactobacillus rhamnosus GG, 247
Lactose intolerance, 48
Laughter. *See* Humor
Lawn, mowing, 208
Lead, affect on glial cells, 143
Leeks, 44
Legumes. *See* Beans and legumes
Lettuce wraps, 220, 221
Leukemia, 310
Licorice for asthma relief, 306
Life span extension, 35. *See also* Aging
Lifeway Kefir, 51
Lighting, indoor, 286
Lignans, 299
Lingzhi. *See* Reishi mushrooms
Listeria, 60, 326, 331, 332
Lithium, psoriasis aggravated by, 351
Liver cancer, vaccine for, 16
Liver disease, 61
Live vaccines, 15
Lower body exercises, 156–57, 178, 197, 217
Lox, 208, 209
L-theanine, 267
Lunch. *See also* Menus
    Apple Turkey Pocket, 218
    Cheese and Avocado Quesadilla, 227
    Chicken Spinach Strawberry Salad, 157
    Citrus Salad with Shrimp, 211
    Crabmeat Melt, 200
    Crunchy Coleslaw, 202
    Crunchy Tuna Salad Pocket, 187
    Easy Three Bean Salad, 225

Minerals. *See also specific kinds*
  aiding immune response, 36, 37–38
  in grains, 38
  multivitamin supplements, 150
Mineral water, 248
Mitochondria, 60
MLD (manual lymph drainage), 17
Modified Triangle Pose, 215–16
Mold, black, 286–87
Monocytes, 123
Montelukast sodium (Singulair), 294
Mood. *See also* Depression; Humor
  aromatherapy for brightening, 184
  attitude for stress reduction, 99
  diary for tracking, 153
  diary review, 175
  dieting and, 159
  "fantasy" to-do list for improving, 214
  flower essences for balancing, 267–68
  in Immune Essentials Plan, 153, 175, 195,
    214
  intimacy and immunity, 115–16
  as key to maximum immunity, 7
  negative, immune system harmed by, 110–11
  optimistic, range of effects from, 111–12
  personality types and, 111–12
  positive, for cold and flu protection, 319
  positive, immune system enhanced by,
    109–10
  positive, sleep aided by, 268–69
  psoriasis and, 353
  psychological conditioning and immune
    function, 108
  psychoneuroimmunology findings, 108–9
  scheduling happy activities, 195, 214
  sex for improving, 189
  social interaction, 113–15
  sunlight for improving, 285–86
Morning sickness, 18
Mouth cancer, 40
Mowing your lawn, 208
MRSA (methicillin-resistant *Staphylococcus
    aureus*), 21
MS2 bacteriophage, 138, 139
Mucous membranes, 37, 67
Multiple sclerosis (MS)
  future breakthroughs, 343
  healing, 342–43
  immunity link to, 340–41
  prevalence of, 340
  protection from, 341–42
  relapsing-remitting form, 340
  smoking linked to, 20
  symptoms, 340
  tai chi beneficial for, 73
  tryptophan for treating, 52
  vitamin D for improving, 122, 125
Multivitamin supplements, 150, 342

Mumps, vaccine for, 15
Mushrooms
  cooking with, 45
  immune system enhanced by, 44–45, 188
  Mushroom and Cheddar Omelet, 187
  reishi, 39, 44–45, 306
Myeloma, 310

N

N-acetylcysteine (NAC), 253
Napping, 182
Natural killer (NK) cells
  described, 13
  factors aiding
    AHCC, 278, 283
    beta-glucan, 67
    drumming, 173
    EpiCor, 279
    exercise, 22, 63, 72
    humor, 118, 119
    lycopene, 41
    mushrooms, 44
    vitamin D, 123
    vitamin supplements, 35
  factors harmful for
    depression, 259
    sleep deprivation, 22, 81, 265
    smoking, 20
    stress, 20
    yo-yo dieting, 24, 64–65, 245
Needles, not sharing, 334
Negative ions, 284–85
Negative thinking, ill effects of, 110–11
Neuropeptides, 108–9
Neutrophils, 22, 67, 123
Niacin, 44. *See also* B-complex vitamins
Non-Hodgkin's lymphoma, 125
Nonsteroidal anti-inflammatory drugs, 361,
    368
Nursing. *See* Breastfeeding
Nut butters, 160
Nutrition. *See also* Cooking
  balanced diet, 33
  for conditions (*see also* Eating; Menus)
    cold and flu recovery, 320
    Crohn's disease, 324–25
    lupus, 339
    swing-shift schedule, 272
  dairy products food group, 48–51
  decline in America, 238–39
  fruits food group, 45–47
  grains food group, 38–40
  as key to maximum immunity, 5
  people at risk for malnutrition, 23
  proteins food group, 51–56
  as risk factor for poor immunity, 23–24, 24,
    34–35
  vegetables food group, 40–45

Pizza, 191–92
Plagues, pandemics vs., 4
Plank lift, 217
Pneumonia, 19, 34, 278, 344–48
Polio vaccine, 15
Pollutants. *See* Environment
Polyphenol oxidase, 296
Polyphenols, 46–47, 75, 313
Polyporus umbellatus (Zhu ling), 44
Polyunsaturated fat, 23
Pomegranate, 185, 205, 222
Pork
    baked beans, 209
    as beef alternative, 223
    choices recommended, 51
    recipes, 220, 221, 231
    tenderloin, 162
Portions. *See* Servings
Portobello mushrooms, 188
Positive ions, 284–85
Positive mood. *See* Mood
Positive self-talk, 261–62
Postherpetic neuralgia, 359, 361
Potassium, 41
Potatoes, 206, 229
Poultry
    chicken recipes, 157, 169, 192, 200, 209,
        221, 227
    choices recommended, 51
    cooking, 51
    safe storage time, 142, 329
    temperatures for cooking, 141–42, 330
    turkey recipes, 160, 185, 218, 223,
        229–30
Prayer, 103–4, 358
Prebiotics, 280
Pregnancy
    with AIDS, protecting the unborn, 335
    allergic response during, 292
    avoiding mercury in fish during, 53
    depression reduced by massage, 104–5
    quitting smoking, 305
    risks from cat droppings, 21
Premature infants, 304–5
Preparedness, for stress reduction, 101
Prevacare, 139
Prima-Kare, 138
Probiotics
    aging and need for, 49, 50
    bacteria strains in, 49, 247, 280
    daily amount of, 50
    hospital-borne infections and, 50
    in Immune Essentials Plan, 150
    immune response improved by, 247
    in kefir, 50–51, 167
    for those around children, 280
    with weight-loss programs, 247
    in yogurt, 49–50, 247

Procyanidins, 226
Produce. *See* Fruits; Vegetables
Programmed cell death (apoptosis), 14
Progressive muscle relaxation
    HIV benefited by, 102–3
    immune response improved by, 7
    for sleep improvement, 91
    for stress reduction, 99, 187
Prophylactic vaccines for cancer, 16
Propranolol (Inderal), 351
Prostaglandins, 317
Prostate cancer, 42–43, 122, 125, 126
Protein. *See also specific kinds*
    in dairy products, 48
    dried beans as, 190
    essential for immune system health, 51
    food group, 51–56
    in Immune Essentials Plan, 51
    immune function during exercise and,
        75
    meat choices recommended, 51
    need when dieting, 248
    omega-3 fatty acid sources, 52–54
    ounce portions of, 51
Protozoan diseases, 39
Pseudoephedrine hydrochloride (Sudafed
        24 Hour), 294
Psoriasis, 349–53
Psychoneuroimmunology, 108–9
Pumpkin, 355
PureWorks products, 139
Pushups, 152, 156, 216
Pyridoxine. *See* Vitamin B$_6$

Q

Qigong, 73
Quercetin, 44, 46
Quinidine, 351

R

Radiation therapy, 44
Radon, 146, 215
Rashes, 19
Raspberries, 197, 198
Reconditioning therapy, 91
Rectal cancer, 314
Refried beans, 225
Reishi mushrooms, 39, 44–45, 306
Relaxation
    for cold and flu recovery, 321
    immune response improved by, 7
    progressive muscle relaxation, 7, 91, 99,
        102–3, 187
    for psoriasis protection, 350
    before sleep, theanine for, 267
Relenza (zanamivir), 320
Remicade (infliximab), 325
Renal cell carcinoma, 53

Repetitions or reps in resistance training, 151
Reptiles, infection risks from, <u>21</u>
Resistance training. *See also* Exercise; Workouts
  abdominal crunch, 177
  aerobic exercise vs., 72
  aerobic exercise with, 74
  avoiding overstraining, 152
  biceps curl, 177
  choosing right weight for, 152
  core exercises, 156, 177, 197, 217
  curl-up exercise, 156
  diamond crunch, 197
  dumbbells for, 151, 152, <u>161</u>
  elbow-to-knee situp, 217
  growth hormone and, 74
  immune system enhanced by, 72, 74
  lower body exercises, 156–57, 178, 197, 217
  lunge exercise, 197
  modified pushups, 156
  overview, 151–52
  plank lift, 217
  squat exercise, 178
  tai chi–inspired moves, 156–57
  terminology, 151
  T-raises, 217
  triceps extension, 197
  upper body exercises, 156, 177, 197, 217
  for weight loss, 74
Respiratory infections
  catching from children, 279
  smoking as risk factor for, 19
  vitamin D as protection for, 123
  washing hands to avoid, 135–36
Respiratory syncytial virus (RSV), 304–5
Resveratrol, 59–60, 240, 298
Reverse osmosis filters, <u>145</u>
Rheumatoid arthritis (RA)
  autoantibody contributing to, 17
  chronic inflammation linked to, 21
  future breakthroughs, 358
  healing, 355–58
  immunity link to, 354–55
  omega-3 fatty acids for, 52
  protection from, 355
  qigong for treating, 73
  smoking linked to, 20
  stress as risk factor for, 255
  symptoms, 354
  tumor necrosis factor-alpha and, 42
  vitamin D for improving, 122
Rice, 198, 209
Rigid personality type, 112
Ringworm, <u>21</u>
Rooster pose, 157
Rosacea, 283
RSV (respiratory syncytial virus), 304–5

S

Sage, for Alzheimer's disease, 301
St. John's wort, 261
Salads
  Apple Walnut Salad, 167
  bean, replacing chips with, 225
  Chicken Spinach Strawberry Salad, 157
  Citrus Salad with Shrimp, 211
  Crunchy Coleslaw, 202
  Crunchy Tuna Salad Pocket, 187
  Easy Three Bean Salad, 225
  Fruit and Spinach Salad, 205
  Greek Salad with Chicken, 200
  Italian Bean Salad, 178
  Mixed Greens and Fruit Salad, 185
  reduced-fat dressings for, 200
  Salmon Caesar Salad, 225
  Sensible Chef's Salad, 229–30
  Smoked Salmon Caesar Salad, 169
  Southwest Salad, 189
  Strawberry Almond Spinach Salad, 222
  Sunflower and Three-Pepper Salad, 198
  Tossed Vegetable Salad, 162
Saliva, defenses against pathogens, 13
Salivary immunoglobulin A (sIgA), 7
S-allylcysteine, 44
Salmon
  lox, about, 209
  omega-3 fatty acids in, 169
  recipes, 158, 169, 208, 225
  smoked, purchasing, 169
Salmonella
  food poisoning by, 326
  pets and infection risks, <u>21</u>
  in pet treats, <u>21</u>, <u>136</u>
  red wine inhibiting, 60, 331
  trout mucus for battling, 332
Salt-free seasonings, 162
Sandwiches
  Apple Turkey Pocket, 218
  Better Breakfast Sandwich, 164
  Crabmeat Melt, 200
  Crunchy Tuna Salad Pocket, 187
  Grilled Cheese Sandwich, 205
  Ham and Swiss on Rye, 209
  Ham Sandwich, 171, 224
  increasing nutritional value of, 165
  Roast Beef Sandwich, 164, 198
  Super Sloppy Joes, 223
  Turkey and Cranberry Sandwich, 160
  Turkey Veggie Wrap, 185
  Veggie Cheeseburger, 180
Sauerkraut, 207
Savasana yoga posture, <u>166</u>
Scharffen Berger Bittersweet chocolate, <u>170</u>
Scratching with psoriasis, 352–53
Scrubbers, disinfecting, <u>140</u>
Seated shoulder/wrist stretch, 176

Lose up to 11 inches of body fat in 32 days!

INTRODUCING
Flat Belly Diet!

Finally, the editors of *Prevention* have developed a science-based diet that directly targets harmful belly fat! Lose up to 15 pounds while you slash your risk of heart disease, stroke, and type 2 diabetes. Here's just a sampling of what you'll get by signing up for the *Flat Belly Diet* online.

- **Easy-to-Use Food Logs and Meal Plans**
- **Access to Expert Help**
- **Daily Video Inspiration and Tips**
- **Community Support**

SIGN UP TODAY FOR YOUR 10-DAY RISK-FREE TRIAL AT:

flatbellydiet.com/max